Substance Abuse Education in Nursing

Volume I

Curriculum Modules

Substance Abuse Education in Nursing

Volume I

Curriculum Modules

Madeleine A. Naegle, Editor

National League for Nursing Press • New York
Pub. No. 15-2407

Copyright © 1991
National League for Nursing
350 Hudson Street, New York, NY 10014

ISBN 0-88737-523-5

This book was set in Caledonia by Publications Development Company. The editor and designer was Allan Graubard. Northeastern Press was the printer and binder. The cover was designed by Lillian Welsh.

Printed in the United States of America.

CONTENTS

CONTRIBUTORS

Janet S. D'Arcangelo, MA, RN, C, is Clinical Instructor of Community Health at New York University, and is a practicing psychotherapist and community health educator in Darien, Connecticut.

Elizabeth A. Duthie, MA, RN, is Assistant Clinical Professor, New York University, and Assistant Director of Nursing for Interdepartmental Coordination and Special Projects, New York University Medical Center, Tish Hospital.

Patricia I. Hogan, PhD, Assistant Professor of Health Promotion, Northern Michigan University.

Jeremy Leeds, PhD, is Assistant Professor, School of Education, Health, Nursing and Arts Professions, New York University.

Phyllis Lisanti, PhD, RN, is Clinical Assistant Professor and Undergraduate Program Director, Division of Nursing, New York University.

Kem Louie, PhD, RN, CS, is Associate Professor, Division of Nursing, Lehman College, City University of New York.

Madeline A. Naegle, PhD, RN, FAAN, is Associate Professor and Principal Investigator, Faculty Development Program in Alcohol and Other Drug Abuse Education, Division of Nursing, New York University.

James P. Santomier, PhD, is Associate Professor and Director of the Program in Physical Education and Sport, New York University.

Rothlyn P. Zahourek, MS, RN, CS, is Clinical Assistant Professor, School of Nursing, University of Massachusetts.

ACKNOWLEDGMENTS

The development of a model curriculum in substance abuse education for nursing was supported by the NIDA-NIAAA contract number 88-008. The award and successful completion of this contract was greatly facilitated by the guidance of contract officers Frances Cotter, MPH, and Dorynne Czechowicz, MD, and project officers Claire Callahan, MSW, and Donna English, RN, MPH. We thank them for their consistent support of substance abuse education in nursing and their efforts to make the curriculum project a reality.

Throughout the development and implementation of Project SAEN, the project coordinator, Janet D'Arcangelo, RN, MA, C, has demonstrated exceptional commitment and effort to this task in a variety of ways. From the completion of administrative details to the authorship, careful refinement of modules and study guides, Ms. D'Arcangelo has performed every assignment professionally and in a manner supportive of working committee members, authors and the project director. As assistant editor of this publication, she has demonstrated a broad knowledge of nursing and substance abuse education for professionals.

Members of the working committee of Project SAEN, Margret Wolf, EdD, RN, Gean Mathwig, PhD, RN, Cassie Greeley, MA, RN, Eileen Wolkstein, PhD, Joanne Griffin, PhD, RN, Beth Duthie, BSN, MA, RN, and Vivian Clarke, EdD, were the architects of the curriculum as well as authors of several modules. Their careful assessment of curricular issues and their recommendations for module development was comprehensive and visionary. The support of the Division of Nursing, New York University, in particular, its head, Diane O'Neill McGivern, PhD, RN, FAAN, was essential to the implementation of the modules in the standing curriculum and the acceptance of the content in the core curriculum.

The expertise of several consultants enriched the contents and scope of the modules. It is because of their suggestions and guidance that the project reflects not only the thinking of the members of the Project SAEN but current educational trends in substance abuse education today. They were Rothlyn Zahourek, MS, RN, CS, Sandra Jaffe-Johnson, EdD, RN, Marc Galanter, MD, John Morgan, MD, and Richard Frances, MD.

The modules were authored by faculty members at the School of Education, Health, Nursing and Arts Professions in the Division of Nursing and other departments, New York University, and nurses specializing in treatment of clients with drug and alcohol problems. Special thanks are extended to the authors who generously shared their thinking and clinical expertise.

Ms. Bonnie Johnson, Ms. Maureen Doyle, and Ms. Linda Patterson rotated as Research Assistants to the project, and were unable to remain with the project due to curricular demands of the doctoral programs in which they were enrolled. Research assistants were responsible for identifying resources and establishing a data base of over 500 entries.

Central to the final form and high quality of these final products has been the assistance of the New York University SEHNAP Office of Research and Development.

Acknowledgments

Mr. Charles Sprague, Director, and his staff have contributed many hours to the organization of content, formatting and final production of the learning modules. Special thanks are extended to him and to Leslie Anndeherz for her skillful reproduction of many graphics as well as key modules.

These volumes are dedicated to advancing the knowledge of health professionals, especially nurses, about alcohol and other drug abuse, and to the many health professionals recovering from the personal experience of the addictions and their devastating consequences.

Eleanor J. Sullivan, PhD, RN, FAAN
Dean, School of Nursing, University of Kansas

PREFACE

New York University Division of Nursing, under the leadership of Dr. Madeline A. Naegle and with the support of a curriculum development grant from the National Institute on Alcohol Abuse and Alcoholism (NIAAA) and the National Institute on Drug Abuse (NIDA), has prepared an extensive and well-developed set of materials appropriate for use in nursing and other health care professional programs. The curriculum has been designed in modules for three levels of instruction: beginning baccalaureate (Volume I); advanced baccalaureate (Volume II); and master's degree level (Volume III). The materials include a content outline for each topic and an instructor's guide presenting learner objectives, audiovisual resources, overhead and handout masters, recommended teaching strategies, test questions and answers, and a faculty and student reading list.

A comprehensive substance abuse education curriculum for both baccalaureate and master's nursing and other health care professional education is provided. Baccalaureate level modules specifically include physiological consequences, pharmacology, psychological manifestations, specific nursing care, care of special populations, and attitudes regarding drug and alcohol use. Master's level modules cover nursing intervention in client populations, advanced practice in addictions nursing, alcohol and drug research, and management of impaired practice. Alternative course placement in the nursing curriculum are presented with each module. Thus, the materials may be used in any program's specific curricular arrangement.

The extent of alcohol and drug abuse problems in the population, and the absence of a concerted effort to provide education content on the topic to health professions' students in the past, increases the importance of providing relevant and extensive information to nursing students. NIAAA has estimated that at least 30 percent of acute care patients have a health problem directly or indirectly related to alcohol or drug use or abuse. While recipients of nursing care are frequently suffering from alcohol or drug related problems, most nurse (and other health care providers) ignore both symptomatology and intervention with these problems. The primary reason for ignoring an obvious health problem is the health professionals' lack of educational preparation regarding addictions. If medical and nursing schools have included alcohol or drug content, it usually has been concerned with the pharmacology of alcohol and drugs or pathology caused by substance use. Recent initiatives by NIAAA and NIDA have targeted nursing and medical schools to support and improve alcohol and drug abuse education.

The strengths of this project include its breadth and depth. The scope of this work is extensive, exhaustive, and comprehensive. It is scientifically sound, including essential and current findings, and integrating the body of knowledge into useful materials. These materials provide an invaluable resource to the nursing and other health care professional educator and curriculum planner in offering current and complete information about alcohol and drug abuse relevant to nursing and other health care practice.

Eleanor J. Sullivan, PhD, RN, FAAN
Dean, School of Nursing,
University of Kansas

Foreword

This volume on substance abuse education in nursing represents an important step in the development of sophisticated health care for addicted people in the United States. The nursing profession is, at the very least, the body of health professionals who work most closely and intimately with our hospitalized ill. More broadly, however, it is the profession that organizes care, provides bedside treatment, and serves as the primary health provider for millions of Americans. Because of this, the establishment of effective treatment options in addiction for nursing is a *sine qua non* for such care nationwide.

The issues dealt with here represent a particularly important perspective on the role that nurses play in the addiction treatment system. "Dysfunctional Patterns in Families with Drug and Alcohol Problems," for example, lays out the basic issues in which the social context of addiction is played out outside the health care system. It suggest the systemic changes that will be necessary to stabilize abstinence. A section on "Special Populations" deals with the increasing importance of subgroups within the addiction patient population whose special needs must be attended to. Women, minorities, and the psychiatrically ill have unique needs which cannot be merged into a homogeneous body of care. Finally, the "Fetal Effects of Maternal Alcohol and Drug Use" is an area of grave concern within the medical context, and one that must be addressed in pre-natal care, as well as in the public health context.

In order to understand the importance of these nursing initiatives, it is useful to look at some of the background of the development of medical care in this field.

The magnitude of the alcohol and drug abuse problem today is well-documented, with the cost to the public calculated at over $125 billion per year in health care and lost work. In general medical facilities alone, on average 20 percent of patients present with such problems, many of which go undiagnosed. Only when the sequelae of addiction, such as cirrhosis, trauma, and infection present, may such patients receive proper medical attention. Nonetheless, the patients' primary addictive problems go untreated. Furthermore, the rate of substance abuse among general psychiatric patients with non-addictive disorders has been found to be 25 to 60 percent, depending on the region and clinical setting. Despite this, medical education has been seriously lacking in the addictions until recently. For example, training in this area was not formally required of psychiatrists until 1985, and is not required in other medical specialties.

Clearly we need to assure greater medical sophistication in substance abuse. Where, however, do we stand in developing the needed teaching faculty and specialists in the field? In 1972, the federal government initiated a program of three-year grants for Career Teachers in Alcoholism and Drug Abuse, but in 1981, after only one grantee had been funded in each of 55 of the 124 eligible schools, the program was terminated. Subsequently, modest grants have addressed nursing and curriculum development, but have failed to provide meaningful support for training positions. Recent federal faculty development awards have provided partial support for training faculty, but none for residents or fellows.

Foreword

Given this perspective on the evolution of nursing and medical care in the field, it is clear that the development of this nursing curriculum package represents an important stage in our growing sophistication of care for addictive illness. Further evolution in this regard will provide an important assurance for effective treatment of addicted patients across the country.

Marc Galanter, MD
Professor of Psychiatry
Director of the Division of Alcoholism and
  Drug Abuse
New York University School of Medicine

MODULE I.1
ATTITUDES AND VALUES
ABOUT DRUG AND ALCOHOL USE

Rothlyn P. Zahourek, MS, RN, CS

Madeline A. Naegle, PhD, RN, FAAN
Project Director
Janet S. D'Arcangelo, MA, RN, C
Project Coordinator

Project SAEN
SUBSTANCE ABUSE
EDUCATION IN NURSING

CONTENT OUTLINE

I.   Contemporary Societal Patterns and Drug Use
    A. Historical Influences
    B. Alcohol as a Drug
    C. Caffeine and Nicotine
    D. Pharmacologic Trends in Society
    E. Patterns of Use by Special Populations
    F. Patterns of Use in Social Settings
    G. Patterns of Use and Lifestyles

II. Motives for Drug Use
    A. Drugs of Abuse (in Addition to Alcohol)
    B. Group and Societal Patterns
    C. Factors Contributing to Drug Use
    D. Choices About Drug Use

III. Biased Attitudes About Drug-Abusing Populations
    A. Addiction as a Moral Failing
    B. The Disease Model and Social Definitions of Drug
       Abuse
    C. Effects of Bias on Access to Health Care
    D. Attitudes Which Influence the Nurse-Client
       Relationship

IV. Drug Use by Health Professional Students and
     Practitioners
    A. Reported Patterns of Use
    B. Determining Risk Factors for Health Care
       Workers
    C. Legal Implications
    D. Ethical Implications
    E. Attitudes of Caregivers
    F. Treatment for Chemical Dependence

CONTENTS

I. CONTEMPORARY SOCIETAL PATTERNS AND DRUG USE

A. Historical Influences

1. Alcoholic beverages have been made since the beginning of time. Beer and wine are the end result from a natural process resulting from fermentation. Distillation was used much later.

2. Ancients had gods of wine: Egyptians, Osiris; Romans, Bacchus; Greeks, Dionysus; Biblical references and uses of wine in sacrifices and rituals are commonplace.

3. Ritual to convivial use: Includes the use of alcohol as part of meals, a staple in many early cultures' diets; it became a part of Roman orgies and was used to reward the Hebrews after battle.

4. By the Middle Ages alcohol permeated many events: Births, marriages, deaths, treaty signings, crowning of kings and queens. Monasteries were the inns and taverns. Alcohol was also used medicinally as an antiseptic, for salves, anesthesia, and tonics.

5. Alcohol was important in the settling of the New World. It was purported that the settlers on the Mayflower landed at Plymouth because they had spent their victuals, especially their "bere."

6. Prohibition (1920–1933) attempted to limit or eliminate alcohol use:

   a. In 1919, Congress passed the 19th amendment, making it illegal to manufacture and sell alcohol; it was based on the Volstead Act which had 16 cumbersome provisions, all controlling alcohol manufacture and consumption.

   b. Prohibition grew out of the temperance movement, which started as a humanitarian movement. Temperance was grounded in the belief that human problems could be solved through laws; originally the movement only condemned drunkenness and drinking distilled spirits.

   c. Prohibition was a method to control drinking with legislation which shaped much of our economic and social life, and did nothing to control drunkenness or alcoholism.

B. Alcohol as a Drug

1. Alcohol is classified as a central nervous system (CNS) depressant.

2. Alcohol is soluble in water and distributed throughout the body by diffusion.

3. Alcohol is addicting and, when consumed over time and in increasing quantities, can produce withdrawal symptoms if its use is abruptly stopped.

4. Alcohol behaves as an aberrant nutrient; it serves as a substitute for body repairing nutrients.

4

C. Caffeine and Nicotine

1. These substances are commonly used and legal in our society.

2. Increased awareness of negative effects of nicotine on the body and the addictive nature of smoking are more evident.

   a. A 1989 report by Johnston, O'Malley, and Bachman on drinking and smoking high school seniors found: 18% of all seniors smoked one or more cigarettes a day in the last 30 days and 10.6% smoked a half pack or more.

3. Increased awareness of negative effects of caffeine; use continues to be widespread.

D. Pharmacologic Patterns in Society

1. In 1988, the NIDA National Household Survey on Drug Abuse reported that 37% of U.S. household population ages 12 and older had used illicit drugs one or more time in their lives; 85% had used alcohol and 75% had used cigarettes.

2. The same survey (NIDA, 1988) stated that, in the month before the survey, 7% of the population had used illicit drugs, 53% had used alcohol, and 29% had used cigarettes. The alcohol use rate is higher than that of cigarette smoking.

3. Our society is anti-discomfort and is impatient for relief.

4. Advertising and cultural norms support the avoidance of discomfort as a desirable goal.

5. Advertising links many drugs of common use (alcohol, caffeine, nicotine) with success, power, sexuality, romance, and being socially and personally adept.

E. Patterns of Use by Special Populations

1. *Drug of choice remains alcohol in all groups.*

2. *Adolescents:* A high percentage have been drunk by their senior year and some have already become regular drinkers. A sizeable number of high school students have also smoked marijuana and have experimented with other hallucinogens; cocaine use has decreased in the adolescent population except in poverty-bound inner city areas, where "crack" continues to be problematic.

3. *Women:* New research indicates that women are more sensitive to effects of ETOH and have more difficulty metabolizing alcohol. While the number of alcoholic men still exceeds women, the number of women identified as alcoholics has increased. Whether this is due to decreased stigma and more female role models obtaining treatment, or due to more women actually suffering from alcoholism, is unclear. A NIDA (1988) population prevalence study of white men and women indicates that women born recently are at the same risk for alcoholism as were men in their fathers' generation. Age of onset is earlier in more recently born individuals.

4. *The elderly:* It is now more common to find elderly persons addicted to prescribed medications. They often share medications with each other; family

physicians prescribe minor tranquilizers and addicting sleeping medications to help relieve problematic symptoms related to losses and numerous life changes.

5. *The socially and economically disadvantaged:* Alcohol and drug use continue to be problems for this population. Chemical dependency is often the result of social pressures to use drugs, the need to use drugs to relieve tension, a pervasive sense of powerlessness, and the need to find even temporary pleasure. Drug dealing is seen as a way out of an impoverished life. Physiological and genetic influences are important as well: Children of addicted persons and alcoholic mothers and fathers are at high risk.

F. Patterns of Use in Social Settings

1. Alcohol use is linked with celebrations, transitions (graduation), funerals, and general social occasions.

2. Social caffeine use is common; e.g., you invite someone to meet you for a cup of coffee. The need for a coffee pick-up is common.

G. Patterns of Use and Lifestyles

1. Daily wine drinking with meals.

2. Daily drinking; e.g., the ritual cocktail before dinner.

3. Alcohol (wine) use for religious purposes; e.g., the Jewish Seder.

4. Cultures that prohibit alcohol use for any purpose; e.g., Jehovah's Witnesses, Muslims, other religious or cultural groups.

5. Groups that promote or encourage use: Marijuana use in a college fraternity—how is that different or is it different from regular alcohol use in another cultural group?

II. MOTIVES FOR DRUG USE

A. Drugs of Abuse (in Addition to Alcohol)

1. *Stimulants:* Amphetamines (uppers, speed); cocaine (coke, crack, snow, rock).

2. *Hallucinogens:* Lysergic acid diethylamide (LSD, acid); phencyclidine (PCP, angel dust); mescaline, MDA, DMT, STP, psilocybin, shrooms, designer drugs, ecstasy.

3. *Cannabis:* Marijuana (grass, pot, weed); hashish (hash).

4. *Depressants:* Barbiturates (barbs, goof balls); tranquilizers (Valium, Xanax, Librium); methaqualone (quaaludes, soapers, ludes, quads).

5. *Narcotics:* Heroine (H, scag, junk, smack); morphine (M, dreamer); codeine, opium.

6. *Deliriants:* Aerosol products, lighter fluid, paint thinner, amyl nitrite (poppers), white out.

7. *Alcohol:* Booze, hootch, white lightning, liquid courage. Mood elevator and CNS depressant.

8. *Designer drugs:* Fentanyl analogues (China white); synthetic heroin; analgesics. Mood elevators.

B. Group and Societal Patterns

1. Use depends on what is in fashion, affordable, and accessible; e.g., in the late 1970s it was chic to "coke."

2. Drinking in many circles is still considered the social norm; however, abstinence or drinking less is now being met with more social acceptance.

3. Some influences have helped alcohol consumption to be more moderate in the last few years:

   a. MADD (Mothers Against Drunk Driving) and SADD (Students Against Drunk Driving).

   b. Designated driver programs.

   c. Legal suits testing the liability of hosts who let guests leave and drive cars while drunk.

   d. More and better information on the dangers and health effects of drugs and alcohol.

   e. Famous people publicly declaring their illness and recovery: Jason Robards, Liza Minelli, Kitty Dukakis, Betty Ford.

C. Factors Contributing to Drug Use

1. Young adults and adolescents often experiment:

   a. Peer pressure: Wanting to do what your friends do; wanting to appear sophisticated and "cool."

   b. Adult examples: See adults in one's life smoking cigarettes and drinking alcohol; parental drinking correlates closely with adolescent consumption.

   c. Curiosity: Interest in novel experiences.

   d. Rebellion: Deviation from parental values.

   e. Boredom.

   f. To escape painful emotions or dissociate one's self from reality.

2. Factors influencing drug use later in life:

   a. To relieve unpleasant feelings: Boredom, anger, anxiety, depression, and/ or physical or mental pain.

   b. To increase energy, creativity, self-esteem.

   c. To feel more capable of solving problems, relating to others.

   d. To get high, euphoric.

3. Social factors contributing to drug use:

   a. Poverty.

   b. Peer pressure.

   c. Social norms.

D. Choices about Drug Use

1. Influence of personality types:

   a. Some theorists believe that the drug chosen for abuse is related to one's individual psychology, biology, and heredity. Those choosing depressant drugs, for example, tend to be more anxious while those choosing stimulants tend to be more depressed.

   b. Edward Khantzian (1980), a psychiatrist at Cambridge Hospital in Massachusetts, theorizes that specific personality types go with specific types of drug use:

      (1) Opiate users tend to be aggressive and violent.

      (2) Alcohol is disinhibiting and is preferred by people who have difficulty expressing feelings.

      (3) Stimulants are used as energizers and appeal to people who are feeling high or low. When low the stimulant provides a pick-up; when on the high side the stimulant makes it easier to maintain the high.

   c. The "Just Say NO" campaign has been aimed at elementary, junior, and senior high school children. The message is that people can say "no" to experimentation.

III. BIASED ATTITUDES ABOUT DRUG-ABUSING POPULATIONS

A. Addiction as a Moral Failing

1. Until recent times, addictions and alcoholism were seen as moral failings, including a lack of values, as being purely psychological phenomena and definitely under the individual's control.

2. In the 1800s, the Temperance Society started with efforts to control heavy drinking; when this failed the emphasis was on controlling alcohol. The abstinence focus produced a conflict between the "wets" and the "drys." An alcoholic was seen as morally evil, a disgrace, as having a self-inflicted condition, sub-human, and having no will power or character.

B. The Disease Model and Social Definitions of Drug Abuse

Early attempts in this country to define alcoholism as a disease:

1. In 1804, Dr. Thomas Trotter wrote the first scientific formulation of "drunkenness" on record in "An Essay, Medical, Philosophical and Chemical, on Drunkenness and Its Effects on the Human Body" (excerpted in Marconi, 1959). He stated, "In medical language, I consider drunkenness, strictly speaking, to be a

disease, produced by a remote cause, and giving birth to actions and movements in the living body that disorder the functions of health."

2. The 1930s impact on changes:

   a. Richard Peabody (1936) coined the term "alcoholic" to replace the term "drunkard."

   b. At Yale, Yandell Henderson, Howard Haggard, Leon Greenberg, and later E. M. Jellinek founded the *Quarterly Journal of Studies on Alcohol* (1949).

   c. Formation of Alcoholics Anonymous by Bill Wilson and Dr. Bob Smith.

3. Later institutions which influenced the exploration of alcoholism as a disease:

   a. Yale Center of Alcohol Studies, founded in the early 1930s.

   b. Yale Summer School for Alcohol Studies (now at Rutgers University).

   c. National Council on Alcoholism, founded in 1944.

   d. National Institute of Alcohol Abuse and Alcoholism, founded in 1971.

4. Conceptualization of drug addiction as a disease has been influenced by the alcoholism field but drug addiction has had less benefit from genetic and biological research. Drug addiction is still looked at more as a learned, behavioral, psychological, socioeconomic, and cultural phenomenon.

   a. Concept of the "addictive personality": A term that has not been useful but which guided psychiatrists in the 1950s. The addictive personality was the orally dependent, manipulative, lying person. What is generally believed now is that people who become addicted often do so as a result of unhappy childhoods, marriages and as a reaction to losses. The alcoholism or drug abuse often causes chaos in the person's life, as it requires lying and manipulation to maintain the dependency behaviors.

   b. Coinage of the term and definition of "chemical dependency": Progressive, problematic use of a mind-altering substance that affects, on a more or less consistent basis, the individual's mental health, physical health, and/or his or her interpersonal, family, social, or financial life. This definition applies to substances ranging from caffeine and alcohol to heroin. The definition is also being used to explain other problematic behaviors; e.g., gambling, compulsive shopping, compulsive sexual activity, and dependency on destructive relationships, as well as exercise.

   c. Robert Millman et al. (1981) are now describing two basic models for addiction:

      (1) *Psychological model:* Compulsive behavior due to psychological difficulties; the behavior of the substance is soothing and masks pain. Edward Khantzian (1985) has studied the psychological aspects of narcotic addictions specifically and explains drug addiction as a form of self-medication and not as part of pleasure seeking or self destructive behavior. Khantzian believes that choice of drug is not random.

      (2) *Chemical dependency model:* Addicts are the same as everyone in society until they drink or use a drug. They quickly become dependent and then suffer physical and mental changes.

9

C. Effects of Bias on Access to Health Care

1. Treatment centers will not exist in a society that does not see chemical dependency as a disease. In the extreme, chemical dependence at different times in history has been managed in the criminal justice system or asylums for the severely mentally ill.

2. People with chemical dependency will use treatment more often if their particular cultural or social groups believe chemical dependency is a treatable problem or illness.

D. Attitudes Which Influence the Nurse-Client Relationship

1. Many research studies describe nurses' attitudes toward alcoholic patients as moralistic, pessimistic, stereotypical, and authoritarian. Older nurses with less education have a more negative attitude toward the substance abuser.

2. Alcoholics are frequently labeled as "difficult" by caregivers; and drug addicts are usually seen as even more difficult, suffering from untreatable personality disorders and having strong connections with the underworld of crime.

3. Nurses' past experience: Many nurses, as with other health care workers, have come from dysfunctional and often alcoholic families. As a result, their attitudes and subsequent care of patients will reflect that experience. This is often seen in nurses becoming angry with chemically dependent patients and subsequently avoiding them.

4. Many nurses have seen patients admitted numerous times for medical/surgical complications of drinking or taking drugs. Nurses seldom have contact with recovering people. As a result, nurses begin to view chemical dependency as a hopeless, untreatable problem.

5. If nurses view chemical dependency as a moral problem or due to a weak character, it will be harder for them to interact with clients non-judgmentally and therapeutically.

6. In a 1988 study, Cannon and Brown found that nurses' attitudes toward substance abusers reflected a belief in the disease concept for both alcoholism and drug addiction; i.e., that the diseases are treatable but not curable, and that even with several relapses the patient could still be helped. Scores on measures of the nurses' attitudes had a wide range and, when further analyzed, indicated many individuals believed that substance abuse was both a disease and a moral blemish.

IV. DRUG USE BY HEALTH PROFESSIONAL STUDENTS AND PRACTITIONERS

A. Reported Patterns of Use

1. Physicians, nurses, and pharmacists are most likely reported to their state regulatory boards for diverting drugs.

2. American Nurses' Association (1984) estimates that 6–8% of nurses have a substance abuse problem.

3. New York State Board for Nursing (1986) estimates are only for those cases reported and estimates will be low, since only the most severe cases are reported. The 1985 statistics indicate that 67% of cases reported (1,520 cases for the year) were for chemical dependency.

4. Recent studies (Sullivan, 1989) support earlier findings that nurses in recovery tend to be exceptional students in the top third of their class who have earned, or were earning, degrees beyond their basic training; they were often viewed as exceptional by their colleagues.

B. Determining Risk Factors for Health Care Workers

1. Role strain and stress of work may result in greater consumption, although a direct relationship between stress and addictive behavior has not been demonstrated.

2. High demands and few options for coping; health care workers are taught to suppress feelings and control one's self.

3. Demands to work long hours; physical and emotional exhaustion.

4. Awareness of drug's effectiveness to change feelings.

5. Accessibility of drugs and casual attitude toward their use, dangers and potential for addiction.

6. The grandiose belief that "it will never happen to me."

C. Legal Implications

1. It is illegal to take certain classes of nonprescription drugs.

2. Practicing while impaired from drugs and/or alcohol is prohibited, according to professional state regulatory boards, as well as standards of practice and codes of ethics.

3. Risks to patients and subsequent malpractice suits for impaired practice.

D. Ethical Implications

1. Health care workers and professionals have an obligation to their clients, and to society at large, to practice as safely and effectively as they are able.

2. Health care consumers, as opposed to others, are often dependent on the provider.

E. Attitudes of Caregivers

1. Many are judgmental of colleagues who become chemically dependent.

2. Many are frightened and shy about confronting a coworker about decrease in performance, particularly when it is related to substance abuse.

3. Attitudes of colleagues: Cannon and Brown (1988) studied nurses in Oregon; found generally an optimistic attitude and a willingness to confront a colleague. Bissell and Haberman (1984) found that 75% of impaired nurses were never confronted by colleagues. They also found that many coworkers would approve the alcoholically impaired nurse's return to work and would accept their colleague back as a coworker. These figures were lower with the drug-abusing nurse. More also would report the drug-abusing nurse to the regulatory board than they would report an alcoholic nurse.

F. Treatment for Chemical Dependence

1. Nurses and health care workers have special needs for treatment: Difficulty in accepting their illness; a tendency to intellectualize; extreme guilt and shame; fear of rejection by colleagues; legal problems if charges have been filed or if they have been reported to regulatory boards.

2. Programs providing peer intervention and peer assistance often have support from state and district nurses' associations.

3. Employee assistance programs are operated in health care facilities.

4. Specialized inpatient treatment facilities are now available to treat the health professional.

5. There are specialized Alcoholics Anonymous (A.A.) and Narcotics Anonymous (N.A.) meetings for health care professionals.

6. Reentry to the workplace is an important issue for the health care worker. Special back-to-work contracts are often implemented to aid that process including: not handling medications and/or addicting substances; regular attendance at outpatient treatment and A.A. or N.A. meetings; urine screens for drugs/alcohol, etc.

7. Many state regulatory boards and professional associations have developed guidelines and programs to aid in intervention and to help monitor treatment and recovery.

MODULE I.1
ATTITUDES AND VALUES
ABOUT DRUG AND ALCOHOL USE

INSTRUCTOR'S GUIDE

Rothlyn P. Zahourek, MS, RN, CS

Madeline A. Naegle, PhD, RN, FAAN
Project Director
Janet S. D'Arcangelo, MA, RN, C
Project Coordinator

Project SAEN
SUBSTANCE ABUSE
EDUCATION IN NURSING

CONTENTS

MODULE DESCRIPTION

This module assists the student in understanding the various meanings of drug use and attitudes about it in Western society. The use of drugs medicinally, in rituals, and in social settings will be reviewed in relation to attitudes about drugs and drug users. The development of personal and professional attitudes will be explored in relation to drug use by health professionals and the implications for delivery of nursing care.

TIME FRAME

2 hours

PLACEMENT

Elective: Health Education, Introduction for Health Professional Courses

LEARNER OBJECTIVES

Upon successful completion of this module, the learner will:

1. Describe attitudes about drug use in contemporary Western society.

2. Identify personal patterns of licit and illicit drug use.

3. List common societal values associated with drugs and their various uses.

4. Describe the effects of provider bias about drug use on client-health provider relationships.

5. Identify attitudes commonly held by health professionals toward alcoholics and individuals with drug dependencies.

6. Describe drug-using patterns reported by nursing students, nurses, and other health professionals.

RECOMMENDED READINGS

FACULTY READINGS

Baum, C. D., Kennedy, M. F., Forbes, T., & Jones, J. (1984). Drug use in the United States. *Journal of the American Medical Association, 251*(10), 293–297.

Clark, M. D., Kachoyeanos, M., & Twadell, A. S. (1986). Educating the educators on alcoholism. *Nursing Success Today, 3*(12), 21–22.

Schoenborg, C. A. (1988). National health interview survey: 1985 statistics on smoking and alcohol use. In *Vital and Health Statistics, Series 10, No. 163* (DHHS Publication No. PHS 88-1591). Washington, DC: U.S. Government Printing Office.

Sullivan, E. J., & Hale, R. E. (1987). Nurses' beliefs about the etiology and treatment of alcohol abuse: A national study. *Journal of Studies on Alcohol, 48,* 456–460.

STUDENT READINGS

Barber, J. G., & Grichting, W. L. (1987). Assessment of drug attitudes among university students using the short form of Drug Attitudes Scale. *International Journal of Addictions, 22*(10), 1033–1039.

Cornish, R. D., & Miller, M. V. (1976). Attitudes of registered nurses toward the alcoholic. *Journal of Psychiatric Nursing and Mental Health Services, 14*(2), 19–22.

Nurco, D. N., Shaffer, J. W., Hanlon, T. E., Kinlock, T. W., Duszynski, K. R., & Stephenson, P. (1987). Attitudes toward narcotic addiction. *Journal of Nervous and Mental Disease, 175*(11), 653–660.

Peele, S. (1982). Love, sex, drugs and other magical solutions to life. *Journal of Psychoactive Drugs, 14*(1–2), 125–131.

Swanson, A., & Hurley, P. (1983). Family systems: Values and value conflicts. *Journal of Psychosocial Nursing and Mental Health Services, 21*(7), 25–30.

RECOMMENDED AUDIOVISUAL AND OTHER RESOURCES

AUDIOVISUAL RESOURCES

1. Cause the Effect/Affect the Cause

This film deals with the influence of hospital personnel's attitudes on a patient's willingness to cooperate. It demonstrates that when negative attitudes on the part of the hospital staff are perceived by the patient, the patient-staff relationship may be put in jeopardy. Useful as a staff development tool; a classic. 23 minutes. Available from the New York State Council on Alcoholism, Film Library, 155 Washington Avenue, Albany, New York 12210. Telephone: (518) 432-8281 or 1-800-252-2557.

2. Staff Attitudes Toward Alcoholism

Demonstrates how negative attitudes of hospital staff not directly involved with alcohol treatment affect the quality of care given to patients in alcohol treatment programs. Released in 1983. 30 minutes. Available from National Audiovisual Center, National Archives and Records Administration, Customer Services Section PY, 8700 Edgeworth Drive, Capitol Heights, Maryland 20743-3701. VHS # A10908/PO, purchase ($110).

GROUP ACTIVITY

1. Activity Sampler for College Prevention Programs

Includes lectures, workshop outlines, guidelines for resident assistants, etc. 1985. Publication No. MS314. Available from NIAAA, National Clearinghouse for Alcohol Information, P.O. Box 2345, Rockville, Maryland 20852. Telephone: (301) 468-2600 or 1-800-729-6686.

OVERHEAD MASTERS

MODULE I.1 ATTITUDES AND VALUES ABOUT DRUG AND ALCOHOL USE

1. Myths about Alcoholics
2. Myths about Drugs of Abuse
3. List of Drugs of Abuse
4. Sources of Negative/Positive Attitudes in Health Care
5. Effects of Nurses' Attitudes on Care
6. Characteristics of Health Care Professionals Who Are Chemically Dependent
7. Risk Factors for Health Care Professionals
8. Factors Contributing to Impairment of the Health Care Worker
9. Factors Contributing to Rehabilitation of the Impaired Professional

Myths About Alcoholics

VERY FEW WOMEN BECOME *Alcoholic!*

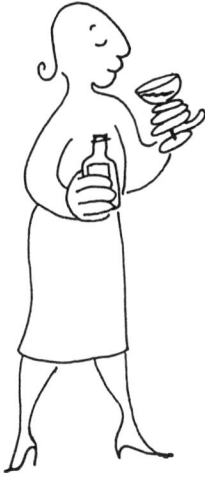

MOST *Alcoholics* ARE SKID-ROW BUMS!

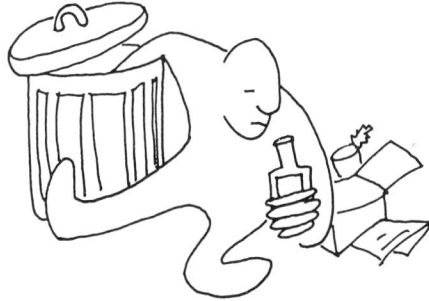

Alcoholics DRINK *Every Day!*

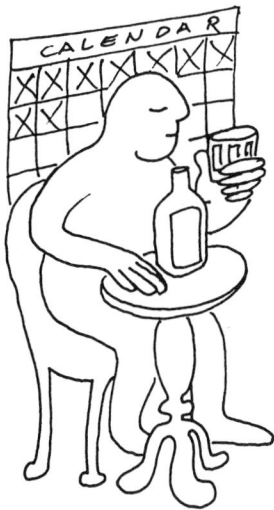

Alcohol IS A STIMULANT!

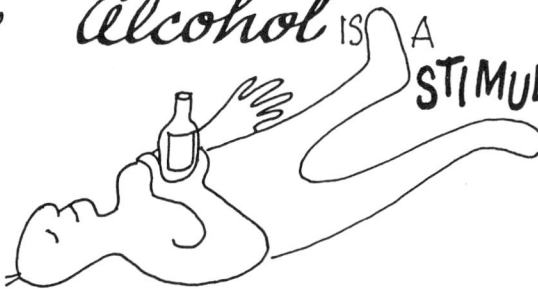

A MYTH IS A HALF-TRUTH interpreted as a WHOLE TRUTH

MYTHS ABOUT DRUGS OF ABUSE

MYTHS ABOUT THEM . . .

- Narcotic users are sociopaths who frequently commit murder, rape, and other crimes of violence while under influence of dope.

- Narcotic parties are characterized by highly stimulating sexual activities.

- Drug dependents are easily distinguished from other people by their appearance and behavior.

- Professional pushers hang around schools and street corners waiting to introduce innocent victims to narcotics.

- Marijuana use inevitably leads to a dependence upon heroin.

- Users can control casual use of narcotics without becoming dependent.

TRUTHS ABOUT THEM . . .

- Narcotic users, alone or in groups, prefer a quiet, secluded place where they can enjoy their contentment in peace and quiet.

- Narcotics reduce sexual drives.

- It is often difficult for police and medical experts to identify a user without specific medical tests or interview.

- Individuals are generally introduced to the use of narcotics through their friends.

- Marijuana does not produce physical dependence; it can lead to emotional dependence which can be equally habit-forming. Most heroin dependents started with marijuana or pills.

- No one can predict at what point one can or will lose control. The occasional joy popper is highly vulnerable to getting hooked.

LIST OF DRUGS OF ABUSE

1. *Stimulants:* Amphetamines (uppers, speed); cocaine (coke, crack, snow, rock). Stimulation; mood elevator.

2. *Hallucinogens:* Lysergic acid diethylamide (LSD, acid); phencyclidine (PCP, angel dust); mescaline, MDA, DMT, STP, psilocybin, shrooms, designer drugs. Altered perceptions.

3. *Cannabis:* Marijuana (grass, pot, weed); hashish (hash). Altered perceptions; relaxant and depressant.

4. *Depressants:* Barbiturates (barbs, goof balls); tranquilizers (Valium, Xanax, Librium); methaqualone (quaaludes, soapers, ludes, quads). Muscle relaxant; depressant.

5. *Narcotics:* Heroine (H, scag, junk, smack); morphine (M, dreamer); codeine, opium. Pain killer, mood elevator; depressant.

6. *Deliriants:* Aerosol products, lighter fluid, paint thinner, amyl nitrite (poppers), correction fluid. Altered perceptions; hallucinogenic.

7. *Alcohol:* Booze, hootch, white lightning, liquid courage. Mood elevator and CNS depressant.

8. *Designer drugs:* Fentanyl analogues (China white); synthetic heroin. Pain killers; mood elevators.

SOURCES OF NEGATIVE/POSITIVE ATTITUDES IN HEALTH CARE

1. Past experience: Family, friends, work.
2. Cultural attitudes: Alcohol, drugs, intoxication, addiction.
3. One's own habits.

EFFECT OF NURSES' ATTITUDES ON CARE

1. Avoidance of involvement with patients.

2. Appreciation of disease concept: Increased ability to assess, intervene, and plan for additional treatment.

3. Nurse's positive attitudes enable patient to cope with stigma, shame, as well as avoidance and denial.

4. Nurse's positive attitudes enhance a positive attitude toward recovery and counter hopelessness.

CHARACTERISTICS OF HEALTH CARE PROFESSIONALS WHO ARE CHEMICALLY DEPENDENT

1. Nurses and pharmacists, compared to the other groups, most often abused narcotics in addition to alcohol.

2. Nurses were least likely to be cross-addicted to many different classes of drug.

3. Pharmacists were most likely to abuse stimulants and sedatives.

4. Alcohol is the drug most often abused by all health care professionals.

5. No significant difference among the groups regarding cocaine use.

RISK FACTORS FOR HEALTH CARE PROFESSIONALS

1. Role strain and stress of work itself.

2. High demands and few options for coping; taught to suppress feelings and control one's self.

3. Demands to work long hours; physical/emotional exhaustion.

4. Awareness of the effectiveness of drugs on changing feelings.

5. Accessibility of drugs and casual attitude toward their use, dangers, and potential for addiction.

6. The grandiose belief that "it will never happen to me."

FACTORS CONTRIBUTING TO IMPAIRMENT OF THE HEALTH CARE WORKER

1. Genetic predisposition and environmental exposure.

2. Stress and poor coping skills.

3. Lack of education regarding chemical dependence.

4. Absence of effective prevention and control strategies.

5. Drug availability in a permissive professional and social environment.

6. Denial.

FACTORS CONTRIBUTING TO REHABILITATION OF THE IMPAIRED PROFESSIONAL

1. Involvement of professional associations.
2. Clear standards of practice and codes of ethics.
3. Peer assistance programs.
4. Hospital-based employee assistance programs.
5. Treatment programs for the health professional.
6. Reentry programs.

HANDOUT MASTERS

MODULE I.1 ATTITUDES AND VALUES ABOUT DRUG AND ALCOHOL USE

1. List of Drugs of Abuse
2. Sources of Negative/Positive Attitudes in Health Care
3. Effects of Attitudes on Care
4. Characteristics of Health Care Professionals Who Are Chemically Dependent
5. Risk Factors for Health Care Professionals
6. Factors Contributing to Impairment of the Health Care Worker
7. Factors Contributing to Rehabilitation of the Impaired Professional

Module I.1—Handout #1

LIST OF DRUGS OF ABUSE

1. *Stimulants:* Amphetamines (uppers, speed); cocaine (coke, crack, snow, rock). Stimulation; mood elevator.

2. *Hallucinogens:* Lysergic acid diethylamide (LSD, acid); phencyclidine (PCP, angel dust); mescaline; MDA; DMT; STP; psilocybin, shrooms; designer drugs. Altered perceptions.

3. *Cannabis:* Marijuana (grass, pot, weed); hashish (hash). Altered perceptions; relaxant and depressant.

4. *Depressants:* Barbiturates (barbs, goof balls); tranquilizers (Valium, Xanax, Librium); methaqualone (quaaludes, soapers, ludes, quads). Muscle relaxant; depressant.

5. *Narcotics:* Heroine (H, scag, junk, smack); morphine (M, dreamer); codeine, opium. Pain killer, mood elevator; depressant.

6. *Deliriants:* Aerosol products, lighter fluid, paint thinner, amyl nitrite (poppers), correction fluid. Altered perceptions; hallucinogenic.

7. *Alcohol:* Booze, hootch, white lightning, liquid courage. Mood elevator and CNS depressant.

8. *Designer drugs:* Fentanyl analogues (China white); synthetic heroin. Pain killers; mood elevators.

Module I.1—Handout #2

SOURCES OF NEGATIVE/POSITIVE ATTITUDES IN HEALTH CARE

1. Past experience: Family, friends, work.
2. Cultural attitudes: Alcohol, drugs, intoxication, addiction.
3. One's own habits.

Module I.1—Handout #3

EFFECTS OF ATTITUDES ON CARE

1. Avoidance of involvement with patients.

2. Appreciation of disease concept: Increased ability to assess, intervene, and plan for additional treatment.

3. Nurse's positive attitudes enable patient to cope with stigma, shame, as well as avoidance and denial.

4. Nurse's positive attitudes enhance a positive attitude toward recovery and counter hopelessness.

Module I.1—Handout #4

CHARACTERISTICS OF HEALTH CARE PROFESSIONALS
WHO ARE CHEMICALLY DEPENDENT

1. Nurses and pharmacists, compared to the other groups, most often abuse narcotics in addition to alcohol.

2. Nurses are least likely to be cross-addicted to many different classes of drug.

3. Pharmacists are most likely to abuse stimulants and sedatives.

4. Alcohol is the drug most often abused by all health care professionals.

5. No significant difference among the groups regarding cocaine use.

RISK FACTORS FOR HEALTH CARE PROFESSIONALS

1. Role strain and stress of work itself.

2. High demands and few options for coping; taught to suppress feelings and control one's self.

3. Demands to work long hours; physical/emotional exhaustion.

4. Awareness of the effectiveness of drugs on changing feelings.

5. Accessibility of drugs and casual attitude toward their use, dangers, and potential for addiction.

6. The grandiose belief that "it will never happen to me."

Module I.1—Handout #6

FACTORS CONTRIBUTING TO
IMPAIRMENT OF THE HEALTH CARE WORKER

1. Genetic predisposition and environmental exposure.
2. Stress and poor coping skills.
3. Lack of education regarding chemical dependence.
4. Absence of effective prevention and control strategies.
5. Drug availability in a permissive professional and social environment.
6. Denial.

FACTORS CONTRIBUTING TO
REHABILITATION OF THE IMPAIRED PROFESSIONAL

1. Involvement of professional associations.
2. Clear standards of practice and codes of ethics.
3. Peer assistance programs.
4. Hospital-based employee assistance programs.
5. Treatment programs for the health professional.
6. Reentry programs.

RECOMMENDED TEACHING STRATEGIES AND SAMPLE ASSIGNMENTS

RECOMMENDED TEACHING STRATEGIES

- Lecture
- Audiovisual materials
- Community self-help meetings (such as Alateen, Al-Anon)
- Small group discussion
- Role-playing
- Clinical placement in residential and ambulatory settings

CASE VIGNETTE

Annie Lennon

Annie Lennon is a 20-year-old nursing major who is starting her first nursing course that involves a clinical laboratory experience. Annie comes from a very strongly religious family and is an only child. Although they were quite strict, Annie felt very close to her parents and has been experiencing a recurrence of her initial homesickness and loneliness while away from home at college. She has found it comforting to indulge in high calorie snacks while studying and feels embarrassed that she has gained 25 pounds since graduating from high school. She feels frightened that she will not meet her parents' expectations for her to be an excellent nurse, as her grades are declining. She blames herself for the fact that she has few friends and feels very unsure that nursing is her preferred career. Annie is quite distressed that the first client she was assigned to is a "drunk." Although neither of her parents drink, her father is currently undergoing chemotherapy for lung cancer that followed many years of heavy smoking. She approaches her instructor to say she is leaving nursing.

SAMPLE ASSIGNMENT

Role-Play Teaching Format

1. Explore Annie's attitude about caring for alcoholic clients.

2. Identify the relationship between Annie's personal experience and her current attitude.

3. Intervene with Annie to relieve her distress; e.g., by:

   a. Providing an opportunity to verbalize her feelings.

   b. Assisting her to see alternative coping mechanisms.

   c. Encouraging her to use campus socialization resources.

WARM UP EXERCISE

Imagery Exercise to Elicit Stereotypes

Have the participants close their eyes, and visit in their imagination a pleasant place. It could be a place where they had a wonderful vacation or a place they are most comfortable in now. It could be a beach or a vacation cabin or even their favorite chair in their own living room. As they are relaxing, they should fully enjoy where they are. Now they should realize that an alcoholic is approaching their scene. As they begin to focus, they should notice what the alcoholic looks like. It might be a total stranger or it might be someone they have known or know now. Tell them to notice what the person looks like. "How is he/she dressed? How does the person seem to you? Now notice how you feel about this person entering your scene. What do you expect will happen? What do you decide to do?" Now ask them to resolve the scene and come fully back to the room and the present.

(This exercise can be expanded to include drug addicts, addicted or alcoholic colleagues, etc.)

Have a group discussion. Ask the group the following:

1. What kind of person did you see?

2. How many saw people they knew? How many saw strangers?

3. Does anyone want to share the details of how this person appeared?

4. How did you feel?

5. How many imagined a drunk?

6. How many saw men?

7. How many saw older or middle-aged people?

8. What did you anticipate would happen?

9. How did you feel?

10. What did you decide to do?

11. How did you resolve the situation?

The following **stereotypes** generally emerge:

1. The alcoholic is generally drunk, a middle-aged, disheveled male who smells bad and resembles a bum.

2. The instructor can point out statistics of how this stereotype is probably only 6–7% of the alcoholic population. The numbers of women alcoholics are growing and many alcoholics are gainfully employed, their disease much less obvious, particularly in early and middle stages.

The following **feelings** generally are discussed:

• Fear, anger, disgust, annoyance, pity, concern, confusion, wanting to run, wanting to help.

These feelings often are noted in the clinical area when an "alcoholic" is admitted.

OTHER LEARNING ACTIVITIES

Have students ask family or friends the following:

1. What is an alcoholic?

2. Is drug addiction a disease?

3. Most alcoholics can't be helped unless they want help. True or false and why?

4. The most dangerous drug is heroin. True or false?

5. The most addicting drug is heroin. True or false?

6. How do you define an addiction?

TEST QUESTIONS AND ANSWERS

TEST QUESTIONS

1. All of the following are strong influences on drug and alcohol consumption *except:*

    a. advertising.

    b. peer pressure.

    c. family history.

    d. availability.

2. Peer pressure, need to experiment, curiosity, need for relief of feelings, modeling adult behavior are all factors which influence:

    a. drug treatment choice.

    b. disclosure of drug-using patterns.

    c. adolescent drug use.

    d. attitudes of caregivers.

3. _____ is best known for describing alcoholism as a disease.

    a. Jellinek.

    b. Bill W.

    c. President Kennedy.

    d. Khantzian.

4. The Temperance movement began as:

    a. a legalistic movement.

    b. a political movement.

    c. a humanitarian movement.

    d. a moral cause.

5. List three elements essential to the concept of chemical dependency.

6. Elements essential to the concept of chemical dependency include all *except:*

    a. repeated use.

    b. adverse influence on one or more spheres of an individual's life.

    c. loss of control over use.

    d. random use.

7. Which of the following *does not* lead to negative attitudes toward the alcoholic or drug abuser?

    a. Lack of knowledge.

    b. Knowing a person active in A.A. or N.A.

    c. A family member with chemical dependency.

    d. Drinking on a regular basis.

8. A major factor which may contribute to health care professionals' vulnerability to chemical dependence is:

    a. gender.

    b. age.

    c. number of years in the profession.

    d. availability of drugs.

9. All of the following **except** _____ will aid the chemically dependent health professional:

    a. A.A. or N.A.

    b. peer intervention.

    c. the drug enforcement agency.

    d. state board regulatory agencies.

True or False:

10. Alcohol is a stimulant.

11. Caffeine is non-addicting.

12. Crack is the most rapidly addicting drug available.

13. Marijuana use can cause a motivational syndrome.

ANSWER KEY

1. d

2. c

3. a

4. c

5. Repeated use; destructive use; adverse influence on one or more spheres of an individual's life (economic, interpersonal, health, family, emotional well-being); continued use despite problematic effects; loss of control over use.

6. b

7. d

8. c

9. c

10. false

11. false

12. true

13. true

BIBLIOGRAPHY

MODULE I.1 ATTITUDES AND VALUES ABOUT DRUG AND ALCOHOL USE

Alcohol and drugs in the workplace: Costs, controls and controversies. (1986). Washington, DC: Bureau of National Affairs.

Alcohol, society and the state. (1981). Toronto, Canada: Addiction Research Foundation.

American Nurses' Association. (1984). *Addictions and psychological dysfunctions in nursing: The profession's response to the problem.* Kansas City, MO: Author.

Barber, J. G., & Grichting, W. L. (1987). Assessment of drug attitudes among university students using the short form of Drug Attitudes Scale. *International Journal of Addictions, 22*(10), 1033–1039.

Baum, C. D., Kennedy, M. F., & Jones, J. (1984). Drug use in the United States. *Journal of the American Medical Association, 251*(10), 293–297.

Bissell, L., & Haberman, P. W. (1984). *Alcoholism in the professions.* New York: Oxford University Press.

Cafiso, J., Goodstadt, M. S., & Garlington, W. K. (1982). Television portrayal of alcohol and other beverages. *Journal of Studies on Alcohol, 43,* 964–989.

Cannon, B., & Brown, J. S. (1988). Nurses' attitudes toward impaired colleagues. *Image, 24*(2), 96–101.

Chappel, J., Veach, T. L., & Krug, R. (1985). The substance abuse attitude survey: An instrument for measuring attitudes. *Journal of Studies on Alcohol, 46*(1), 48–52.

Clarke, M. D., Kachoyeanos, M., & Twadell, A. S. (1986). Educating the educators on alcoholism. *Nursing Success Today, 3*(12), 21–22.

Cohen, S. (1982). Cannabis and sex: Multifaceted paradoxes. *Journal of Psychoactive Drugs, 14*(1–2), 55–58.

Cornish, R. D., & Miller, M. V. (1976). Attitudes of registered nurses toward the alcoholic. *Journal of Psychiatric Nursing and Mental Health Services, 14*(2), 19–22.

Engs, R. C. (1978). Drinking patterns and drinking problems of college students. *Journal of Studies in Alcohol, 38*(11), 2144–2156.

Estes, N., Smith-DiJulio, K., & Heinemann, M. E. (1980). *The nursing diagnosis of the alcoholic person.* St. Louis, MO: C. V. Mosby.

Gallegos, D. V., Veir, W., Wilson, P. O., Porter, T., & Talbott, G. D. (1988). Substance abuse among health professionals. *MMJ, 37*(3), 191–197.

Green, P. (1989). The chemically dependent nurse. *Nursing Clinics of North America, 24*(1), 81–94.

Hanna, E. (1978). Attitudes toward problem drinkers. *Journal of Studies on Alcohol, 38*(1), 98–109.

Hatterer, L. (1979). *The pleasure addicts: The addictive process, food, sex, drugs, alcohol, work and more.* South Brunswick, NJ: Barnes.

Hingson, R. W. (1983). Impact on legislation raising the legal drinking age in Massachusetts from 18 to 20. *American Journal of Public Health, 73,* 163–170.

Johnston, L., O'Malley, P. M., & Bachman, J. (1989). *Drug use, drinking and smoking: National survey results from high school, college and young adult populations, 1975–1988.* University of Michigan Institute for Social Research (DHHS Publication No. (ADM) 89-1638). Rockville, MD: National Institute on Drug Abuse.

Khantzian, E. J. (1980). An ego/self theory of substance dependence: A contemporary psychoanalytic perspective. In D. J. Lettieri, M. Sayers, & H. W. Pearson (Eds.), *Theories on drug abuse: Selected contemporary perspectives* (pp. 29–33). Rockville, MD: National Institute on Drug Abuse.

Khantzian, E. J. (1985). The self-medication hypothesis of addictive disorders: Focus on heroin and cocaine dependence. *American Journal of Psychiatry, 142,* 1259–1264.

Kinney, J., & Leaton, G. (1978). *Loosening the grip: A handbook of alcohol information.* St. Louis, MO: C. V. Mosby.

Lyttle, T. (1988). Drug based religions and contemporary drug taking. *Journal of Drug Issues, 18*(2), 271–284.

Millman, R., Cushman, P., & Lowinson, J. (1981). *Research developments in drug and alcohol use.* New York: New York Academy of Sciences.

National Institute on Drug Abuse. (1988). *National household survey on drug abuse: Highlights 1988* (DHHS Publication No. (ADM) 90-1681). Rockville, MD: U. S. Department of Health and Human Services.

New York State Board for Nursing. (1986). *Annual report on the profession of nursing in New York State.* Albany, NY: New York State Education Department.

Nurco, D. N., Shaffer, J. W., Hanlon, T. E., Kinlock, T. W., Duszynski, K. R., & Stephenson, P. (1987). Attitudes toward narcotic addiction. *Journal of Nervous and Mental Disease, 175*(11), 653–660.

Peabody, R. (1936). *The common sense of drinking.* Boston: Little, Brown, & Co.

Peele, S. (1982). Love, sex, drugs and other magical solutions to life. *Journal of Psychoactive Drugs, 14*(1–2), 125–131.

Schoenborg, C. A. (1988). National health interview survey: 1985 statistics on smoking and alcohol use. In *Vital and Health Statistics, Series 10, No. 163* (DHHS Publication No. PHS 88-1591). Washington, DC: U.S. Government Printing Office.

Stephens, R. (1985). The sociocultural view of heroin use: Toward a role-theoretical model. *Journal of Drug Issues, 15*(4), 433–466.

Sullivan, E. (1989). Research update: Current studies on alcohol and other drug dependency in nurses. *Addictions Nursing Network, 1*(2), 18–20.

Sullivan, E. J., & Hale, R. E. (1987). Nurses' beliefs about the etiology and treatment of alcohol abuse: A national study. *Journal of Studies on Alcohol, 48,* 456–460.

Swanson, A., & Hurley, P. (1983). Family systems: Values and value conflicts. *Journal of Psychosocial Nursing and Mental Health Services, 21*(7), 25–30.

Szasz, T. (1974). *Ceremonial chemistry.* New York: Doubleday.

Trotter, T. (1804). An essay, medical, philosophical and chemical, on drunkenness and its effects on the human body. Excerpts in Marconi, J. T. (1959). The concept of alcoholism. *Quarterly Journal of Studies on Alcohol, 20*(2), 216–235.

Turner, T. B., Bennett, V. L., & Hernandez, H. (1981). Beneficial side of moderate alcohol use. *Johns Hopkins Medical Journal, 148*(2), 53–63.

Wechsler, H., McFadden, M., & Bohman, M. (1980). Drinking and drug use among college students in New England. *Journal of the American College Health Association, 18,* 275–279.

Werch, C. E., & Gorman, D. R. (1987). Relationship between self-control, consumption patterns and problems of college students. *Journal of Studies on Alcohol, 49*(1), 30–36.

MODULE I.2
HEALTH IMPLICATIONS OF
ALCOHOL AND OTHER DRUG USE

James P. Santomier, PhD
Patricia I. Hogan, PhD

Madeline A. Naegle, PhD, RN, FAAN
Project Director
Janet S. D'Arcangelo, MA, RN, C
Project Coordinator

Project SAEN
SUBSTANCE ABUSE
EDUCATION IN NURSING

CONTENT OUTLINE

I. Factors Which Interact to Influence Motives for, and Outcomes of, Drug Use

   A. Definitions of Addiction

   B. Individual Factors Regarding Addiction

      1. Genetic

      2. Family patterns

      3. Lifestyle

      4. Self-assessment

   C. Environmental Factors Regarding Addiction

      1. Psychosocial environment

      2. Regional patterns and accessibility

      3. Social traditions

      4. Peer activities

      5. Occupational factors

   D. Developmental Characteristics of People at Risk for Substance Abuse

      1. Identification with viable role models

      2. Identification with and responsibility for "family" processes

      3. Attitudes and values regarding problem-solving

      4. Intra-personal skills

      5. Inter-personal skills

      6. Systemic skills

      7. Judgmental skills

II. Factors Which Increase Risks of Drug Use Related to Health

   A. Dysfunctional Family Patterns

B. Drug and Alcohol Use as Coping Strategies

C. Personality Structure

D. Life Events

   1. Traumatic

   2. Developmental

   3. Health problems

III. Modalities to Promote Health in the Drug-Using Client

A. Definition of Health Promotion

B. Formulating Plans for Health Promotion/Primary Prevention

   1. Imparting information

   2. Developing and/or enriching life-coping skills

   3. Providing alternatives

C. Health Teaching to Reduce Risks and Promote Health

   1. Promotion of appropriate exercise

   2. Promotion of healthful sex practices

   3. Health promotion through support for smoking cessation

   4. Promotion of education of the health risks of drugs and alcohol

D. Strategies to Promote Relaxation, Decrease Stress, and Enhance Well-Being

   1. Therapeutic touch

   2. Relaxation techniques (i.e., guided imagery)

   3. Biofeedback

   4. Stress management

   5. Problem-solving strategies

   6. Support groups

   7. Time management

E. Use of Community and Clinical Resources through Self-Referral and Referrals of Colleagues and Clients

CONTENTS

I. FACTORS WHICH INTERACT TO INFLUENCE MOTIVES FOR, AND OUTCOMES OF, DRUG USE

A. Definitions of Addiction

Addiction can be loosely classified as:

1. Compulsion or craving.

2. Loss of control.

3. Continued use despite the adverse consequences.

Addictive behavior encompasses not only the use of drugs, tobacco, and alcohol, but food, caffeine and sugar, and compulsive behaviors such as excessive gambling, sexual activity, work, and shopping.

B. Individual Factors Regarding Addiction

1. Genetic Factors.

   a. Some researchers contend that there may be genetic determinations of susceptibility to addiction.

   b. The genetic influence does not guarantee that an individual will become addicted. However, it may predispose one to addiction as a consequence of repeated, reinforced behavior.

   c. There is some evidence to suggest that truly addicted individuals have an abnormal chromosome.

   d. Another theory suggests that certain individuals may be susceptible to addiction based on variations in intensity of the flow of neurotransmitters.

   e. Research indicates that many people, after quitting smoking, drug use, alcohol, etc., relapse because of a combination of biological, psychological, and social reasons. These include:

      (1) Troublesome personality traits.

      (2) Substitute addictions.

      (3) A narrow view of recovery.

      (4) A failure to see danger signs.

2. Family Patterns.

   a. Family factors are strongly implicated in substance abuse behaviors, especially with regard to adolescent drug use. Close family relationships, involvement, and attachment appear to discourage adolescents from substance abuse.

   b. Parental role modeling of alcohol use is positively related to adolescent alcohol use.

    c. The quality of family relationships is inversely related to the use of illicit drugs other than marijuana.

    d. Three parental factors contributing to prediction of drug use:

       (1) Drug-using behaviors.

       (2) Attitudes about drugs.

       (3) Parent-child interactions characterized by:

          (a) Lack of closeness.

          (b) Lack of maternal involvement in activities with children.

          (c) Lack of, or inconsistent parental discipline.

          (d) Low parental educational aspirations for their children.

    e. Characteristics of families of adolescent substance abusers:

       (1) Negative communication patterns (criticism, blaming, lack of praise).

       (2) Inconsistent and unclear behavioral limits.

       (3) Denial of drug use.

       (4) Unrealistic parental expectations.

       (5) Family patterns of self-medication.

3. Lifestyle.

    a. Lifestyle involves all dimensions of one's life that in any way influence how one lives. Dimensions are physical, social, intellectual/emotional, and spiritual.

    b. There is a trend in the United States toward self-fulfilling, healthier lifestyles.

    c. Those individuals living self-defeating "dysfunctional lifestyles" are likely to be involved in drug/alcohol abuse.

    d. Lifestyles of smokers revolve around cigarettes.

    e. Lifestyles of alcoholics often affect lifestyles of the entire family. Alcoholism is termed a "family disease" because every member of a family is affected by it.

4. Self-Assessment.

    a. Requires an awareness of personal attitudes toward drugs and drug users.

    b. Requires frank appraisal of personal drug use and its implications.

    c. Permits recognition of personal biases.

C. Environmental Factors Regarding Addiction

1. Psychosocial Environment.

    a. Social or psychosocial environments are made up of people and their interactions. These people create "climates" or "atmospheres," which have different "personalities."

    b. Physiological and psychological responses to stressful environments differ among different individuals.

       (1) One shaping factor is the source of distress and illness, a situation in which one attempts to function within an environment with which one is incompatible.

       (2) Most individuals are able to tolerate incompatible environments for relatively long periods of time.

    c. Evidence is strong indicating that *support* is a crucial dimension of the psychosocial environment.

    d. Drug and alcohol use are part of a complex psychoecological system; whether or not an individual will abuse a particular substance depends on a multitude of relatively complex factors.

2. Regional Patterns and Accessibility.

    a. Urban vs. rural.

       (1) The social environment of the city emphasizes noninvolvement with others, diminished social responsibility, and anonymity.

       (2) The city has an environment to which people react adaptively—one way to adapt is to become ill, or to become addicted to drugs and/or alcohol.

       (3) Rural environments, conversely, while promoting some social isolation, are also characterized by a more clearly different set of social mores in relation to drug use.

    b. As many as one out of every five people in the United States is addicted to alcohol or drugs.

3. Social Traditions.

    a. Drug use may be included or excluded in social events.

4. Peer Activities.

    a. Addiction to drugs/alcohol may result from peer pressure.

    b. At various stages of one's life, one is more vulnerable to peer pressure, especially during adolescence.

5. Occupational Factors.

    a. Occupational stress.

       (1) Type A personality related to "chronic struggle to obtain an unlimited number of relatively poorly defined things from the environment in the shortest period of time."

       (2) Rosenbaum and Friedman (1974) believe the contemporary Western environment encourages development of Type A patterns. Their view represents the interaction of environmental influences and individual susceptibilities. Research related to coronary artery disease and hypertension supports this view.

    b. Question of relative contribution of occupational stress to drug and alcohol use needs to be answered more comprehensively.

c. Pressure to perform or to succeed may cause one to feel that "one can't measure up." May lead to escape in drug/alcohol abuse.

D. Developmental Characteristics of People at Risk for Substance Abuse

According to the National Institute on Drug Abuse (1980), in general, the "high-risk" individual shows significant inadequacies in one, several, or all of the following areas:

1. *Identification with viable role models.* This refers to a person's reference group and self-concept. The vulnerable person does not see herself or himself as like (or the same as) people whose attitudes, values, and behaviors allow them to "survive" in their total environment.

2. *Identification with and responsibility for "family" processes.* In this context, "family" is used in a broad sense. It can and often does mean the traditional nuclear family (father, mother, 1.8 children, dog, cat). It is also used to mean family in the sense of broad organization, living settings, group identifications, and so forth. When this identification is poorly developed, a person does not identify strongly with things greater than herself or himself (e.g., relationships with another person, in groups, mankind, God, etc.). She or he does not see that what one does affects others. This refers to shared investment in outcomes, shared responsibility for achieving outcomes, and accountability to others for behavior.

3. *Attitudes and values regarding problem-solving.* This refers to the skills and attitudes necessary to work through problems and believe that they can be solved through application of personal resources. When poorly developed, a person believes that problems have been escaped when she or he can't feel them any more. For example, a person has faith in "miracle" solutions to problems. (This is often through the use of alcohol or drugs.) She or he does not believe that there is anything one can do about the present or future; things just happen to her or him.

4. *Intra-personal skills.* Intra-personal skills are those which a person uses to communicate with self. This refers to the skills of self-discipline, self-control, self-assessment, etc. Weaknesses in these areas express themselves as: Inability to cope with personal stresses and tensions, dishonesty with self, denial of self, inability to defer gratification, low self-esteem, etc.

5. *Inter-personal skills.* Inter-personal skills are those skills which enable a person to relate to or build a relationship with another person; e.g., sharing, trusting, etc. Weaknesses in these areas express themselves as: Dishonesty with others, lack of empathic awareness, resistance to feedback, inability to share feelings, inability to give or receive love or help, etc.

6. *Systemic skills.* These refer to the ability to respond to the limits inherent in a situation (responsibility); the ability to modify behavior according to a situation in order to get one's needs met constructively (adaptability), etc. Weaknesses in these areas express themselves as: Irresponsibility, refusal to accept consequences of behavior, scapegoating, etc. A person with low skills in these areas tends to see herself or himself as a victim of circumstances.

7. *Judgmental skills.* Judgmental skills include the ability to recognize, understand and apply relationships. Weaknesses in this area express themselves as: Crises in sexual, natural, consumer, and drug environments; repetitious self-destructive behaviors.

II. FACTORS WHICH INCREASE RISKS OF DRUG USE RELATED TO HEALTH

A. Dysfunctional Family Patterns

B. Drug and Alcohol Use as Coping Strategies

1. Drugs and alcohol are frequently used as palliative coping techniques in order to reduce negative emotions and heightened arousal levels associated with conditions of high stress.

    a. Negative palliative coping techniques, such as drug and alcohol use, may temporarily reduce the effects of stressors; however, their use often precludes individuals from learning to deal directly with stressors through healthier coping techniques.

    b. Because symptoms of stressors are often reduced through drugs and alcohol, their use is reinforced.

C. Personality Structure:

1. Addictive Personality.

    a. Addiction can be loosely classified as (1) compulsion or craving; (2) loss of control; (3) continued use despite the adverse consequences.

    b. Developmental characteristics: Similar developmental characteristics characterize addictive personalities (see previous section). Addictive behavior encompasses not only the use of drugs, tobacco, and alcohol, but food, caffeine and sugar, and compulsive behaviors such as excessive gambling, exercise, sexual activity, work, and shopping/buying.

D. Life Events

1. Traumatic.

    a. Losses.

    b. Accidents, illness, incest.

    c. Precarious financial conditions.

2. Developmental.

    a. Marriage, divorce.

    b. Frequent job changes.

    c. Stressful family relations.

3. Health problems, including HIV status, chronic mental and physical illness and poor nutritional status.

III. MODALITIES TO PROMOTE HEALTH IN THE DRUG-USING CLIENT

A. Definition of Health Promotion

Substantial variation exists relative to the meaning of "health promotion." "Health promotion is the maintenance/enhancement of existing levels of health, through the implementation of effective programs, services, and policies" (Goodstadt, Simpson & Loranger, 1987, pg. 61). *The Health Promotion Network* refers to programs, policies, and services which are targeted primarily at maintaining or increasing levels of health of those individuals who are not necessarily ill or addicted. Traditionally, the two main strategies for this approach have been risk reduction and risk avoidance.

Health promotion is dynamic, and occurs most effectively through supportive interaction among various appropriate interventions. Effective health promotion approaches usually include programs, community activities and services that assist individuals to achieve positive change, insulate and contain intractable risk, and effect positive environmental change (Goodstadt, Simpson, & Loranger, 1987).

Primary prevention, a concept closely linked to health promotion, may be defined as a proactive process utilizing an interdisciplinary approach designed to empower people with the resources to constructively confront stressful life conditions. (See HANDOUTS/OVERHEADS MASTERS for sample definitions of "primary prevention.")

B. Formulating Plans for Health Promotion/Primary Prevention

Health promotion and primary prevention programs in substance abuse generally utilize one or more of the following basic approaches: (1) disseminating information; (2) developing life-coping skills; and (3)providing alternatives to users, misusers, abusers or to nonusers. Users are individuals involved with alcohol/drugs either on a social-recreational or experimental basis. The following approaches (YWCA of the USA, 1983) represent a broad range of programming options in substance abuse prevention:]

1. Information imparted includes but is not limited to:
   a. The effects of alcohol/drugs.
   b. Prevention services and availability.
   c. Treatment services and availability.
   d. Training services and availability.
   e. Prevention approaches and strategies.
   f. Resources.
   g. Technical assistance and availability.

2. Life-coping skills developed and/or enriched are those skills necessary for positive functioning in daily living circumstances, such as:

   a. Decision-making skills.

   b. Communication techniques.

   c. Goal-setting skills.

   d. Values-clarification skills.

   e. Problem-solving techniques.

   f. Assuming responsibility for self.

   g. Developing responsible attitude toward alcohol/drugs.

3. Alternatives provided include activities that will:

   a. Contribute to use of and growth in personal skills.

   b. Create more positive self-image.

   c. Develop levels of satisfaction and self-esteem.

   d. Develop respect for individual and others.

   e. Create opportunity for positive interaction with others.

   f. Provide identification with viable role models.

   g. Alleviate boredom, unrest, apathy.

   h. Contribute to development of positive lifestyle.

C. Health Teaching to Reduce Risks and Promote Health

Nurses can promote health and reduce health risks in drug-using clients by providing information concerning, and strategies regarding, more healthy ways to deal with the problems, stresses, and frustrations of life. Nurses can make an impact by promoting and/or providing: Appropriate exercise, safer sex, appropriate stress management information and techniques, problem-solving, and other developmental skills (see I.C), honing and development, time management, information concerning smoking cessation, and information concerning support groups and community/clinical resources.

1. Promotion of Appropriate Exercise.

   a. *Psychological benefits of exercise* include, but are not limited to:

      (1) Improved mental health and well-being.

      (2) Reduction of stress emotions, such as a state of anxiety.

      (3) Decreased level of mild to moderate depression.

      (4) Reductions in traits such as neuroticism and anxiety.

      (5) May facilitate treatment of severe depression.

(6) Reductions in various stress indices, such as neuromuscular tension, resting heart rate and levels of some stress hormones.

b. *Physiological benefits of exercise* include, but are not limited to:

(1) Reduced mortality from such causes as cardiovascular disease and cancer.

(2) Enhanced management of individuals with diabetes.

(3) Reduction of blood pressure in hypertensive individuals.

(4) Maintenance of weight loss and improved body composition for obese individuals.

(5) Favorable changes in plasma triglycerides, low-density lipoprotein (LDL) and high-density lipoprotein (HDL) cholesterol.

(6) Decreased resting and exercise heart rates.

(7) Increased lung volume and oxygen utilization.

c. *Aerobic activities* are exercises or sports that develop the heart, blood vessels and lungs so that these organs are able to better supply working muscles with oxygen. Aerobic activities will also strengthen muscles specific to the chosen activity and will facilitate the expenditure of calories. Individuals engaging in aerobic activity should be concerned with four important factors:

(1) *Frequency.* Regular physical activity, in order to gain physiological and psychological benefits, should be engaged in at least three to five times per week. If weight control is also an objective, it is recommended that individuals begin exercising three to five times per week and gradually increase to six or seven times per week.

(2) *Intensity.* Intensity refers to how hard or how easily you are walking, jogging, swimming, etc. Overexercising is fatiguing and unsafe. Underexercising may not be beneficial. It is generally a good idea to start out at a low to moderate intensity and gradually increase the effort as you "get into shape."

(3) *Duration.* At each exercise session, you should attempt at least 15–45 minutes of continuous aerobic activity. At the beginning of your program, you may not be able to exercise for more than 15 minutes.

(4) *Mode.* Individuals should engage in activities that use large muscle groups (legs, back, arms), are rhythmic and aerobic in nature, and can be maintained continuously. For example, walking-hiking briskly, running, jogging, swimming, cycling, rowing, cross-country skiing, skating, aerobic-jazz dancing, etc. Sports like tennis, racquetball, squash, etc., are most beneficial as aerobic activities if played with someone of equal or greater ability.

d. *Other dimensions of physical fitness* that should be considered when developing a comprehensive fitness program are: (1) body composition; (2) muscular strength and flexibility; and (3) time flexibility. Beware, however; excessive exercise can become a substitute addiction.

2. Promotion of Healthful Sex Practices.

    a. Sexual activity and expression are seen as health-promoting if proper precautions are used.

    b. *Sexually-transmitted diseases (STDs)* have become an epidemic of national proportion in the United States. There are now over 25 known STDs, some of which are still incurable. According to the Centers for Disease Control, in 1986, more than 10 million new people were infected with STDs, including 4.6 million cases of chlamydia, 1.8 million cases of gonorrhea, 1 million cases of genital warts, 500,000 cases of herpes, 90,000 cases of syphilis, and 15,000 new cases of AIDS. The American Social Health Association indicates that 25 percent of all Americans will acquire at least one STD in their lifetime.

        (1) *Chlamydia.* A bacterial infection that can cause significant damage to the reproductive system. May occur without symptoms and is considered to be a major factor in male and female infertility. The Centers for Disease Control indicate that about 20 percent of all college students are infected with chlamydia.

        (2) *Gonorrhea.* A bacterial infection. If left untreated, leads to pelvic inflammation in women, infertility, widespread bacterial infection, heart damage, arthritis in men and women, and blindness in children born to infected women.

        (3) Other major STDs include genital warts, herpes, and syphilis.

    c. *Safer Sex: AIDS risk reduction.* The following precautions, based on reports and recommendations from U.S. Public Health Service, can help reduce the risk of contracting AIDS:

        (1) Avoid multiple and/or anonymous sexual partners.

        (2) Avoid sexual contact (including open-mouthed or French kissing—the HIV virus may be present in saliva, although no evidence exists that AIDS has been transmitted in this way) with anyone who has symptoms of AIDS or who is a member of a high-risk group for AIDS.

        (3) Avoid sexual contact with anyone who has had sex with people at risk of getting AIDS.

        (4) If you have sexual contact with someone who might be infected with the AIDS virus or whose history is unknown to you, avoid exchange of body fluids. Unless you know absolutely that your partner is not infected, a condom should be used during each sexual act, from start to finish. Use a spermicide to provide additional protection.

        (5) Avoid sex with prostitutes.

        (6) Avoid sharing toothbrushes, razors, or other implements that could become contaminated with blood with anyone who is, or who might be, infected with the HIV virus.

        (7) Use extreme caution in procedures, such as acupuncture, tattooing, ear piercing, etc., in which needles or other unsterile instruments

may be used repeatedly to pierce the skin and/or mucous membranes.

3. Health Promotion through Support for Smoking Cessation.

   a. Since 1960, the percentage of adults who smoke cigarettes has declined; however, some individuals, especially adolescents, continue to use tobacco. It is estimated that approximately 3.2 million public school students are currently smokers.

   b. It appears that for adolescents, the initial onset of cigarette smoking is related to adolescents who see themselves as risk takers and whose best friend smokes.

   c. Gender differences exist regarding intention to smoke and cigarette usage in adolescent men and women. Young women are beginning to smoke more than adolescent males. Females who smoke are more likely to have fathers who are drug users and/or are tolerant of drug use. Peer and family smoking levels are more important in predicting intention to smoke for women than for men.

   d. Research has also linked smoking cigarettes with other drug behaviors, especially alcohol use. Parental tobacco use has been linked to adolescent tobacco use, especially for individuals from single parent families.

   e. Success in smoking cessation appears to be related to parental support and other psychological variables. Smokers are more likely to participate in cessation programs if moral attitudes change, if they associate with peers who do not smoke, and if they have positive beliefs about short-term benefits of quitting smoking.

   f. Educational/prevention programs may include: (1) social skills training and parent involvement, (2) peer-led social influence programs, and (3) expert-led, teacher-led, and peer-led groups. Teacher-led groups appear to be the most effective prevention strategy, and seem to influence female adolescents more favorably than male adolescents. The peer-led approach is more effective for male adolescents.

4. Promotion of Education of the Health Risks of Drugs and Alcohol.

   a. *Health risks of alcohol use.* In moderate amounts alcohol may cause dizziness, a dulling of the senses and impairment of coordination, reflexes, memory, and judgment. Additional amounts of alcohol produce staggering, accident proneness, slurred speech, double vision, mood changes, and quite possibly, unconsciousness. Still larger amounts of alcohol may result in death. In addition, use over many years may cause damage to the liver, heart, and pancreas. Malnutrition, stomach irritation, lowered resistance to disease, and irreversible brain or nervous system damage may also result. In addition, alcohol affects the secretion of hormones, suppresses ovulation, causes changes in the menstrual cycle, and causes birth defects.

   b. *Health risks of cocaine and crack.* Cocaine and crack, a cocaine derivative, produce dilated pupils, elevated blood pressure, increased heart and respiratory rates, and elevated body temperature. They may also cause insomnia, loss of appetite, tactile hallucinations, paranoia, seizure, and death.

c. *Health risks for barbiturate use.* Although barbiturates in small doses produce calmness, relaxed muscles, and lowered anxiety, larger amounts cause slurred speech, staggering gait, and altered perception. Extremely large doses, or when taken with other central nervous system depressants like alcohol, may cause respiratory depression, coma, and in some cases death.

d. *Health risks of amphetamine use.* The use of amphetamines causes increased heart and respiratory rates, elevated blood pressure, and dilated pupils. Increased doses precipitate rapid or irregular heartbeat, tremors, and physical collapse. In the case where amphetamines are injected, a sudden increase in blood pressure may lead to stroke, high fever, heart failure, and death.

e. *Health risks for hallucinogens (PCP, LSD, Mescaline, Peyote, Psilocybin) use.* Angel dust (PCP) interrupts that part of the brain which controls the intellect and keeps impulses in check. PCP blocks pain receptors so that violent episodes, including self-inflicted injuries, may be common. Chronic users often report memory loss and speech difficulty. Extremely large doses produce convulsions, coma, heart and lung failure, and perhaps ruptured blood vessels in the brain. LSD, mescaline, peyote, etc., cause dilated pupils, elevated body temperature, increased heart rate and high blood pressure, and tremors.

f. *Health risks of narcotics (Heroin, Codeine, Morphine, Opium, Percodan) use.* Because narcotics are usually injected, the use of contaminated needles may result in the user contracting diseases such as AIDS and hepatitis. Symptoms of overdose may include shallow breathing, clammy skin, convulsions, coma, and death.

g. Approximately 60% of illegal drugs produced in the world are consumed in the United States. Americans spend over $100 billion each year on illegal drugs. According to the U.S. Department of Education, today's drugs are stronger, more addictive, and pose a greater risk than ever before.

h. Drug use modalities include snorting, injecting, ingesting, smoking.

D. Strategies to Promote Relaxation, Decrease Stress, and Enhance Well-Being

1. Therapeutic Touch.

   a. Developed from ancient practice of the laying-on of hands. Foundation of therapeutic touch is assumption of universal life energy sustaining all living organisms. Just beginning to be accepted in Western medicine.

   b. Individual's habitual and/or unconscious thinking and feeling patterns affect outcome of treatment—usually more successful with acute vs. chronic conditions.

   c. Although no data relate the efficacy of therapeutic touch in "healing" drug and alcohol addictions, it has been shown to effectively reduce anxiety.

   d. The method of therapeutic touch involves "healing"—helping the patient to re-establish open, balanced energy flow.

e. The process.

    (1) Assess quality of individual's energies, identifying areas of congestion, disorder, and deficit.

    (2) Eliminate congestion.

    (3) Transfer "life energy" into depleted areas.

    (4) Balance energy flow (Macrae, 1988).

2. Relaxation Techniques (i.e., Guided Imagery).

    a. Relaxation techniques can produce the "relaxation response" (Benson, 1976). When the body is calm and relaxed, the flow of adrenaline and other stress hormones is reduced and the body slows down.

    b. Progressive relaxation focuses on the relaxation of voluntary skeletal muscles. Individuals strive to gain control over skeletal muscles until they are able to induce low levels of tension in the muscles. Relaxation will also slow heart and breathing rates, and reduce blood pressure and hormone flow.

        (1) Practice lying down in a quiet room, remain clam, reduce anxiety, produce images.

        (2) Individuals are taught to recognize even very slight muscle contractions so that they may reduce them and reach the highest level of relaxation.

    c. Mental imagery is practiced by relaxing in a quiet, comfortable position with eyes closed. Individuals may imagine themselves to be in a serene environment such as a country field, the mountains, the coast, etc., and attempt to imagine the smells and the sounds of the environment, as well as the feel of the wind.

3. Biofeedback.

    a. Biofeedback is a way of monitoring the body's physiological responses to stressors, using sensors to determine blood pressure, heart rate, muscular tension, etc.

    b. Individuals receive auditory and/or visual feedback while practicing relaxation techniques.

    c. Biofeedback facilitates individuals to "read" or recognize bodily responses and then modify them accordingly.

    d. Biofeedback is particularly effective for individuals who require objective signs of their progress.

4. Stress Management.

    a. Stress occurs when individuals are confronted with demands which are perceived to threatened important values or goals or to exceed their capabilities to meet the demands. Stressors are those events or situations that cause individuals to have stress reactions.

    b. Many kinds of reactions to stressors may occur. Individuals may experience all, or some, of the following:

(1) Negative emotions; i.e., fear, guilt, anxiety, depression, anger.

(2) Behavioral problems; i.e., speech disturbances, muscular tension.

(3) Changes in ability to think clearly and rationally.

(4) Physiological responses such as feelings of tightness in the chest, throat, etc., or over time, the development of ulcers.

c. In severe cases of perceived loss of self-esteem, there may be potential for suicide.

d. It is important to realize that psychological stress, although usually associated with a specific event or situation (e.g., a job or school demand), occurs because of individuals' *perceptions* of how important the event or demand is to them, and how individuals feel about their abilities or capabilities to meet the demand.

e. Two categories of coping with stressors:

(1) *Palliative coping.* Coping (in the form of thoughts or behaviors) designed to temporarily relieve the emotional impact of stressors. Does not alter stressors in any way but allows individuals to reduce emotional arousal levels, feel better, and think more clearly. Examples: Relaxation, exercise, listening to music, biofeedback, etc. Primary function of palliative coping strategies is to reduce emotional arousal level and other related stress symptoms in order to facilitate second phase of coping process—instrumental or direct action phase.

(2) *Instrumental coping (direct action).* Coping designed to deal directly with demands (stressors) confronting individuals. Involves the development of skills and abilities that directly relate to the nature and characteristics of the stressor (demand). If new skills or abilities are not learned, the stressor remains significant. The phase is a critical component of stress management and is often neglected or overlooked in stress management programs.

f. Effective stress management requires a comprehensive approach which includes an educational component as well as specific palliative stress management techniques.

g. It is important for individuals to identify stress "triggers" and develop an awareness of the physical, psychological, and behavioral consequences of stressors.

h. Stress is unavoidable, but there are appropriate strategies for reducing stress.

(1) Deal with stressors and related emotions immediately by establishing positive palliative coping strategies.

(2) Remain flexible and be willing to negotiate and compromise.

(3) Attend to one problem or issue at a time.

(4) Realize that "indecision" is stressful.

(5) Discuss issues and problems with family and friends.

    (6) Be sure to take some time for thought, relaxation, and self-reinforcing activities.

5. Problem-Solving Strategies.

    a. A problem is simply the difference between what one has and what one wants. In any problem there is a desired end point, something one wants to bring about. Link up a clearly defined objective with a clearly designed starting position (de Bono, 1970).

    b. Steps to problem-solving in health promotion or primary prevention planning include:

        (1) Thinking through the problem (problem identification).

        (2) Deciding what to do (action plan).

        (3) Carrying out the plan (implementation).

        (4) Evaluation of outcomes.

    c. Strategies to address problem-solving skills and other "at risk" characteristics (intrapersonal, interpersonal skills, etc.—see section I.C) should be addressed.

6. Support Groups.

7. Time Management.

Individuals can learn to manage themselves more effectively with respect to the clock.

    a. It takes time to be more creative, initiate appropriate problem-solving methods, manage stress and conflict, and develop appropriate personal strategies.

    b. Generally, individuals choose to waste time and use what time they have in less productive ways.

    c. Individuals sometimes view time as an enemy (having deadlines and interruptions, on vacation, etc.), rather than as an asset. Individuals should learn to appreciate it and use it effectively. How time is used reflects one's values.

    d. Changing habits of time management.

        (1) Make a list of those things that you believe are wasting your time. Attempt to thoroughly understand what you are now doing—keep a time log for a week or longer.

        (2) Rank in importance and indicate which time wasters are *internally* generated and which are *externally* generated.

        (3) Initiate new time management practices as strongly as possible; tell others what you are doing.

    e. Ten points to assist in time management:

        (1) Plan (goals, objectives, action plans).

        (2) Concentrate on one task at a time.

(3) Take occasional breaks.

(4) Avoid a cluttered workspace.

(5) Avoid perfectionism.

(6) Don't hesitate to say "No."

(7) Avoid procrastination.

(8) Delegate.

(9) Avoid becoming a workaholic.

(10) Be willing to make major changes in work and personal schedules/activities.

E. Use of Community and Clinical Resources through Self-Referral and Referrals of Colleagues and Clients

1. Knowledge of community treatment resources.

2. Knowledge of community self-help groups.

3. Methods of accessing resources.

MODULE I.2
HEALTH IMPLICATIONS OF
ALCOHOL AND OTHER DRUG USE

INSTRUCTOR'S GUIDE

James P. Santomier, PhD
Patricia I. Hogan, PhD

Madeline A. Naegle, PhD, RN, FAAN
Project Director
Janet S. D'Arcangelo, MA, RN, C
Project Coordinator

Project SAEN
SUBSTANCE ABUSE
EDUCATION IN NURSING

CONTENTS

MODULE DESCRIPTION

This module presents information concerning the implications for health promotion of alcohol/drug use/misuse/abuse behaviors. It is targeted to instructors of nursing, in that it provides these instructors with information and strategies by which to empower their students to make appropriate decisions relative to alcohol/drug use and health promotion.

The following assumptions are made.

1. The decision to drink alcohol/use drugs is a personal, private one for which each individual is responsible. But alcohol/drug misuse/abuse is neither healthy nor safe and should not be sanctioned.

2. Alcohol and other drug problems are often associated with broad psychosocial, socioeconomic, and cultural issues.

3. Everyone is subject to problems, stresses, and frustrations. Although alcohol and other drugs may provide a temporary escape from them, they keep one from dealing with the sources of difficulties. There are many healthier, more effective alternatives available for reducing stress and resolving problems.

4. Through building skills in intrapersonal/interpersonal communication, self-directed learning, problem solving, and planning, individuals can be better prepared to address their health promotion needs.

TIME FRAME

3 hours

PLACEMENT

This module deals with entry-level information.

LEARNER OBJECTIVES

Upon successful completion of this module, the learner will:

1. Identify factors which interact to influence motives for and outcomes of alcohol and drug use/misuse/abuse.

2. Identify factors which increase alcohol drug use/misuse/abuse related risks to health.

3. Identify health risks for alcohol/drug use/misuse/abuse.

4. Provide a definition for health promotion.

5. Integrate information and strategies to provide nursing care to promote and maintain health/well-being for the well adult.

RECOMMENDED READINGS

FACULTY READINGS

Cummings, C. (1986). A review of the impact of nutrition on health and profits and a discussion of successful program elements. *American Journal of Health Promotion, 1*(1), 14–22.

Eckhardt, M. J., & Harford, T. C. (1981). Health hazards associated with alcohol consumption. *Journal of American Medical Association, 246*(6), 648–666.

Glenn, H. S., & Warner, J. (1977). *The developmental approach to preventing problem dependencies.* Bloomington, IN: Social Systems, Inc.

Goodstadt, M. S., Simpson, R. I., & Loranger, P. O. (1987). Health promotion: A conceptual integration. *American Journal of Health Promotion, 1*(3), 58–63.

Nurse, A. R. (1982). The role of alcohol in relationship to intimacy. *Journal of Psychoactive Drugs, 14*(1–2), 159–162.

O'Leary, D. E., O'Leary, M. R., & Donovan, D. M. (1976). Social skills acquisition and psychosocial development of alcoholics: A review. *Addictive Behaviors, 1*(2), 111–120.

Stein, J. A., Newcomb, M. D., & Bentler, P. M. (1987). Personality and drug use: Reciprocal effects across four years. *Personality and Individual Differences, 8*(3), 419–430.

STUDENT READINGS

Allen, W. A. (1987). *How drugs can affect your life.* Springfield, IL: Thomas.

Ardell, D. B. (1979). *High-level wellness.* New York: Rodale.

Clarke, M. (1984). Stress and coping: Constructs for nursing. *Journal of Advanced Nursing, 9,* 3–13.

Hafen, B. Q., Thygerson, A. L., & Frandsen, K. T. (1988). *Behavioral guidelines for health and wellness.* Englewood, CO: Morton.

Hogan, P. I., & Santomier, J. P. (1982). Stress and leisure activities. *Leisure Information Quarterly, 8*(4), 7–8.

Macrae, J. (1988). *Therapeutic touch: A practical guide.* New York: Knopf.

Wechsler, H., & Rohman, M. E. (1981). Patterns of drug use among New England college students. *American Journal of Drug and Alcohol Abuse, 8*(1), 27–37.

RECOMMENDED AUDIOVISUAL
AND
OTHER RESOURCES

BOOKLETS/PAMPHLETS/BOOKS

1. National Institute on Alcohol Abuse and Alcoholism (NIAAA)

Clearinghouse for Alcohol Information, Box 2345, Rockville, Maryland 20852, (301) 468-2600. Request handbooks (e.g., *Spectrum: Alcohol Problem Prevention for Women by Women; On the Sidelines: An Adult Leader Guide for Youth Alcohol Programs;* and *Guide to Alcohol Programs*) and other available materials.

2. ETR Associates/Network Publications

Telephone: 1-800-321-4407, P.O. Box 1830, Santa Cruz, California 95061-1830. For information (books/pamphlets) on substance abuse, sexual responsibility, life management skills and self-esteem. Request the *Family Life and Health Education 1991 Catalog of Select Educational Materials.*

DISPLAYS AND MODELS

1. ETR Associates/Network Publications (see above)

For displays/models on health and drugs and substance abuse prevention.

AUDIOVISUAL MATERIALS

1. ETR Associates/Network Publications (see above)

For information on videos on life management skills, substance abuse prevention, family life education, and HIV/AIDS prevention.

2. IBIS Media

For slide presentations on health/fitness and stress management. Telephone: (914) 747-0177, P.O. Box 308, Pleasantville, New York 10570.

Module I.2

TRAINING AND RESEARCH SERVICES

1. ETR Associates/Network Publications (see above)

For information on teacher training, trainer training, technical assistance, and research information for sexuality education; HIV/AIDS prevention education; reducing health risk behavior; and tobacco use prevention.

AUDIOVISUAL MATERIALS

Uppers, Downers, All Arounders

Effects of psychoactive drugs on the brain. Provides a general classification of drugs and reviews levels of drug-seeking behavior. 62 minutes. **Available for rent from the National Library of Medicine, Collection Access Section, 8600 Rockville Pike, Bethesda, Maryland 20894. For purchase, contact Cinmed, 2409 Sepulveda Boulevard, Manhattan Beach, California 90266.**

The Addicted Brain

This documentary takes viewers on a tour of the world's most prolific manufacturer and user of drugs—the human brain. The biochemistry of the brain is responsible for joggers' highs, for the compulsion of some people to seek thrills, for certain kinds of obsessive compulsive behavior, even for the drive to achieve power and dominance. This program explores the cutting edge of developments in the biochemistry of addiction and addictive behavior. 26 minutes. **Available from Films for the Humanities and Sciences, P.O. 2053, Princeton, New Jersey 08543. Phone: 1-800-257-5126. VHS #BD-1363, purchase ($199).**

Answers We Know

An examination of alcoholism as a medical and health issue. Dr. David Ohlms explores possible reasons why some people can drink alcohol without becoming alcoholic and others cannot. Also presented are research findings on the role heredity plays as well as a historical perspective of alcoholism as a disease. 26 minutes. **Available from New York State Council on Alcoholism, Film Library, 155 Washington Avenue, Albany, New York 12210. Phone: (518) 432-8281 or 1-800-252-2557.**

Cocaine and Heart Attacks

Young men in their twenties are appearing in hospital emergency rooms complaining of chest pains and other symptoms typical of heart attacks. But they are not having typical heart attacks: they are the victims of cocaine-induced heart attacks. 19 minutes. **Available from Films for the Humanities and Sciences, P.O. 2053, Princeton, New Jersey 08543. Phone: 1-800-257-5126. VHS #BD-1364, purchase ($199).**

Drug Profiles: The Physical and Mental Aspects

The extent of the substance abuse problem makes it more important than ever that concerned people learn how to recognize physical symptoms of abuse and understand the long- and short-term effects of drugs. The film provides detailed information about ten drugs of abuse: cocaine, heroin, methaqualone, alcohol, marijuana, barbiturates, amphetamines, tranquilizers, PCP, and LSD. This information can lead to counseling help for drug users and can influence the decisions of those who are not yet committed to the "recreational" use of drugs. 28 minutes. Available from AIMS Media, 6901 Woodley Avenue, Van Nuys, California 91406-4878. Phone: 1-800-267-2467 or (818) 785-4111. #9787, rental ($75) or purchase ($395).

Human Physiology Series

All available from AIMS Media, 6901 Woodley Avenue, Van Nuys, California 91406-4878. Phone: 1-800-367-2467 or (818) 785-4111.

1. Alcohol and Human Physiology

Most people overlook the fact that alcohol is a toxic drug. This important film explains the effects of alcohol on the human body's major organs and systems. The ill effects of alcohol on the digestive, circulatory, muscular, skeletal, urogenital, and reproductive systems are described. There are also interviews with six recovering alcoholics who briefly recount the physiological damage to their bodies. 24 minutes. #9769, rental ($50) or purchase ($375).

2. Cocaine and Human Physiology

The damage done to the body by cocaine—whether snorted, ingested or smoked—is well documented in this film. Testimonials and statistics reveal that the drug is highly addictive. Chemical dependency is established within weeks with smokable cocaine (crack or rock). The damage cocaine does to the nose, eyes, vocal cords, gums, kidneys, liver, and intestines is displayed and explained by a physician-narrator. Cocaine is shown to cause the greatest harm to the brain, the lungs, and the heart. The physical causes of cocaine-induced death and the grave effects on the new-born babies of women who used cocaine when pregnant are described. 20 minutes. #9899, rental ($75) or purchase ($350).

3. Designer Drugs and Human Physiology

"Designer" drugs are produced by drug dealers to get around anti-drug laws and to market existing drugs in new forms. The drugs include PCP, crack, amphetamines, "Ecstasy" (MDMA), and synthetic opiates. In this program, a forensic toxicologist describes the physiological and psychological damages designer drugs can cause users. The dangers of polydrug use—mixing designer drugs with alcohol or other drugs—are discussed. The effects of taking the drugs during pregnancy or while driving or working are also described. The extreme toxicity of designer drugs and their detectability in drug tests are explored. Testimonials from recovering addicts support the film's claim that designer drugs are among the most unpredictable, mind-altering, and physically debilitating substances sold on the street today.

- Crack, Cocaine, Methamphetamines. 13-1/2 minutes. #8108. 16 mm. rental ($75 for 3 days) or purchase ($335). VHS rental ($75 for 3 days) or purchase ($275).

- PCP, Ecstasy, Fentanyl. 18-½ minutes. #8113. 16 mm. rental ($75 for 3 days) or purchase ($445). VHS rental ($75 for 3 days) or purchase ($375).

4. Heroin and Human Physiology

Over five and a half million people are regular heroin users. Within five years of becoming addicted, one in six heroin addicts is dead. A physician-narrator describes the devastating effects of heroin on the body. These include infections and chronic abscesses, inflammation of the lymph glands, and swelling of the hands and tetanus. The film graphically illustrates how the drug inflicts its greatest damage on the brain, lungs, and heart. The effects of heroin on a pregnant woman's unborn child is also discussed. A major health concern today is the transmission of AIDS among intravenous heroin users. The film warns against the sharing of drug needles and shows some of the diseases contracted by IV drug users with AIDS. Depictions of heroin's effects on the body are interspersed with testimonials of recovering addicts who relate their personal experiences with this deadly drug. 22 minutes. #9961, rental ($75) or purchase ($395).

5. Marijuana and Human Physiology

Even though marijuana is the second most widely abused drug after alcohol, many people believe it offers harmless recreation. This film dispels that belief with hard facts about the drug and its effects on the body. A physician-narrator clearly describes the chemical's damaging effects on the sinuses, pharynx, uvula, lungs, heart, brain, reproductive system, and immune system. The information he provides is supported by testimonials from former marijuana users. The psychological development of the "pot personality," the hazards of driving while under the influence, and the dangers of mixing marijuana with alcohol are also discussed. 22 minutes. #9832, rental ($75) or purchase ($375).

6. Tobacco and Human Physiology

Tobacco can do tremendous harm to the body. In a university laboratory, Dr. Mark Robinson explains the physiological effects of smoke on human bodies. He covers the effects of both smoked and smokeless tobacco. Dr. Robinson shows how the human respiratory system works and how it is damaged by the particulate matter in cigarette smoke. Nicotine from chewing tobacco or dipping snuff is shown to affect the heart and the rest of the circulatory system much the way smoking tobacco does. The effect of smoking on an unborn child is also explained. 22 minutes. #9855, rental ($75) or purchase ($380).

Kick the Habit

This program focuses on the battle against cigarette smoking and its effects on the body— a battle long fought by epidemiologists and health professionals, in which the U.S. Army has now joined. But while the Army has the means to enforce its rules, the rest of society must rely on persuasion. This program shows the efforts being made to educate people to the hazards of smoking, explains the conditioning process by which people become hooked on cigarettes, and presents evidence of the dangers of secondary smoke. 19 minutes. **Available from Films for the Humanities and Sciences, P.O. 2053, Princeton, New Jersey 08543. Phone: 1-800-257-5126. VHS #BD-1370, purchase ($149).**

Living in Balance Series

All available in VHS from New York State Council on Alcoholism, Film Library, 155 Washington Avenue, Albany, New York 12210. Phone: (518) 432-8281 or 1-800-252-2557.

> **Program 1: The Overview.** With colorful animated graphics, this program explains how basic hemisphere dominance relates to alcohol/drug use, stress, adolescent/parent problems and a host of other conditions caused by imbalance. It sets the stage and challenges the viewer to explore personal balance. 20 minutes.

> **Program 2: Peer Pressure/Fear Pressure.** A class of high school students provide energy and interaction for this program, in which host John Marshall explains and demonstrates ways to take fear pressure out of peer pressure. Students demonstrate natural alternatives through exercises and role-playing. 21 minutes.

> **Program 3: Alternatives.** This program not only demonstrates ways to relax, play, interact, and have fun without alcohol or drugs, but it shows the teacher, facilitator or counselor how to make the techniques work. 28 minutes.

> **Program 4: Innercise.** This system of body-mind integration was developed by John Marshall out of a combination of Eastern and Western approaches to opening up the natural flow of energy. Unlike exercise, Innercise is done slowly for involving the right brain and bringing the whole person into balance. Balance is the recurring theme for motivating alcohol-free living. 34 minutes.

Nags

This "Young People's Special" drama is the story of one girl's efforts to help her father give up smoking. Despite all her efforts to persuade, her father resists kicking the habit that is undermining his health. It takes a near-tragedy in the family to make him realize the dangers of his habit—and finally to stop smoking. 26 minutes. Available from Films for the Humanities and Sciences, P.O. 2053, Princeton, New Jersey 08543. Phone: 1-800-257-5126. VHS #BD-1371, purchase ($249).

Safe Sex

AIDS is not just a plague that afflicts gay men—a staggering one million heterosexuals will fall victim to the virus by 1991. Just what do we need to know to protect ourselves from this sexually-transmitted disease? Most educators believe it is better to discuss safe sex frankly with teenagers and even with children, rather than risk their becoming infected with AIDS out of ignorance. Phil Donahue is joined by Safe Sex Educator Paula Van Ness from the Los Angeles AIDS Project, a brothel owner who requires the use of condoms, and several heterosexual AIDS patients. 28 minutes. Available from Films for the Humanities and Sciences, P.O. 2053, Princeton, New Jersey 08543. Phone: 1-800-257-5126. VHS #BD-1260, purchase ($149).

Smoking and Lung Cancer

Smokers are ten times as likely to develop lung cancer as nonsmokers, and the more they smoke, the higher their risk. Early detection, before cancerous cells metastasize to other vital organs, is critical to successful treatment and survival. This program profiles a man whose encounter with lung cancer gave him the motivation to quit smoking. 19 minutes. Available from Films for the Humanities and Sciences, P.O. 2053, Princeton, New Jersey 08543. Phone: 1-800-257-5126. VHS #BD-1365, purchase ($149).

Therapeutic Touch: A New Skill from an Ancient Practice

Today's highly sophisticated medical tools can diagnose and cure better than ever, but they do not replace touch, a key ingredient to healing. The therapeutic use of touch is crucially important to patients, especially as an antidote to the sterility of high-tech care. This video explores the benefits of Therapeutic Touch, a scientific use of touch, and explains its background in energy field interaction. Featuring demonstrations with actual patients, this program shows how the technique may diminish anxiety and tension and alleviate pain. The video also offers dialogue with nurses whose patients have improved with Therapeutic Touch. In today's hi-tech world of healthcare advance, this program offers a refreshing and positive look at another method of providing comfort that can be incorporated into the nurse's repertoire of skills. 28 minutes. Available from American Journal of Nursing Company, Educational Service Division, 555 West 57th Street, New York, New York 10019-2961. Phone: 1-800-223-2282 or (212) 582-8820. Rental #7538V ($60) or purchase #7538S ($275).

OVERHEAD MASTERS

MODULE I.2 HEALTH IMPLICATIONS OF ALCOHOL AND OTHER DRUG USE

1. Developmental Characteristics: Areas of Relevance in Identifying Individuals at Risk for Substance Abuse

2. Theoretical Basis of Health Promotion Based on Developmental Characteristics

3. Guidelines for Promoting Health through Developmental Theory

4. Sample Definitions of Primary Prevention from Selected Substance Abuse Agencies (4A, 4B)

5. Health Promotion Programming in Substance Abuse: Principles and Approaches

6. Programming for Information Dissemination

7. Programming for Development and Enrichment of Life-Coping Skills

8. Programming for Providing Alternatives

9. Stress Management (9A, 9B)

10. Aerobic Activities

11. Safer Sex Practices

DEVELOPMENTAL CHARACTERISTICS: AREAS OF RELEVANCE IN IDENTIFYING INDIVIDUALS AT RISK FOR SUBSTANCE ABUSE

In general, the "high risk" individual shows significant inadequacies in one, several or all of the following areas:

1. Identification with viable role models.

2. Identification with and responsibility for "family" processes.

3. Attitudes and values regarding problem-solving skills.

4. Intra-personal skills.

5. Inter-personal skills.

6. Systemic skills.

7. Judgmental skills.

Module I.2—Overhead #2

THEORETICAL BASIS OF HEALTH PROMOTION BASED ON DEVELOPMENTAL CHARACTERISTICS

Most human behavior is a composite of the seven areas described previously. Social norms define acceptable forms of behavior, and require certain levels of functioning in each of these areas. By assessing levels of functioning or development against norms, as socially and environmentally defined, these developmental characteristics are used as diagnostic indicators of "high risk" and "low risk" populations for purposes of both prevention and treatment.

At present, treatment and prevention programs have both *explicit* (expressed) and *implicit* (implied) goals which reflect the above characteristics.

Module I.2—Overhead #3

GUIDELINES FOR PROMOTING HEALTH THROUGH DEVELOPMENTAL THEORY*

An analysis of goals of programs suggests that, in virtually all current approaches to prevention, rehabilitation, and therapy, workers are attempting to establish or maintain situations in which their clients, through practice and experience can:

1. Strengthen or develop intra-personal skills (get self together); and/or

2. Strengthen or develop inter-personal skills (learn to deal effectively with others); and/or

3. Strengthen or develop systemic skills (learn to handle situations); and/or

4. Develop judgmental skills (learn to make decisions and recognize what's going on); and/or

5. Strengthen identification with and responsibility for "family" processes (become part of something greater than self and learn to carry his/her own weight); and/or

6. Strengthen identification with viable role models (learn to see self as the kind of person who is making it and identify with others who are also).

---

*From: National Institute on Drug Abuse. (1980). The developmental approach to preventing problem dependencies. In H. S. Glenn & J. W. Warner (Eds.), Community-based prevention specialist: Participant manual (pp. 133–153). Rockville, MD: NIDA.

Module I.2—Overhead #4A

SAMPLE DEFINITIONS OF PRIMARY PREVENTION FROM SELECTED SUBSTANCE ABUSE AGENCIES*

From *Planning and Prevention Programs,* National Center for Alcohol Education:

"The purpose of prevention is to increase the likelihood that individuals will develop drinking-related behaviors that are personally and socially constructive. Negatively stated, prevention programs are aimed at reducing the number of persons whose alcohol-related behavior adversely affects the way they carry on the roles and responsibilities of everyday living."

From the Center for Multicultural Awareness, a project of the National Institute on Drug Abuse's Prevention Branch:

"Primary prevention of drug abuse is a constructive process designed to promote personal, social, *economic, and political* growth of the individual toward full human potential; and thereby inhibit or reduce personal, social, *economic or political* impairment which results in or from the abuse of chemical substances."

---

*From: National Institute on Drug Abuse. (1980). The developmental approach to preventing problem dependencies. In H. S. Glenn & J. W. Warner (Eds.), *Community-based prevention specialist: Participant manual* (pp. 133–153). Rockville, MD: NIDA.

Module I.2—Overhead #4B

SAMPLE DEFINITIONS OF PRIMARY PREVENTION FROM SELECTED SUBSTANCE ABUSE AGENCIES*

From Stephen E. Goldston, Ed.D., Coordinator for Primary Prevention Programs, National Institutes of Mental Health:

"Primary prevention encompasses those activities directed at specifically identified vulnerable high-risk groups within the community who have not been labeled as psychiatrically ill and for whom measures can be undertaken to avoid the onset of emotional disturbances and/or enhance their level of positive mental health. Programs for the promotion of mental health are primarily educational rather than clinical in conception and operation, with their ultimate goal being to increase people's capacities for dealing with crises and/or taking steps to improve their own lives."

The content of the following definition of Primary Prevention was developed by the Michigan Office of Substance Abuse Services prevention staff:

"An aggregate of community education and social action programs which, within an identified length of time and for specified groups of people, are able to measurably reduce the likelihood, frequency, seriousness or duration of chemical use problems by means other than referral or recourse to the chemical dependency treatment system or correctional services."

---

*From: National Institute on Drug Abuse. (1980). The developmental approach to preventing problem dependencies. In H. S. Glenn & J. W. Warner (Eds.), *Community-based prevention specialist: Participant manual* (pp. 133–153). Rockville, MD: NIDA.

Module I.2—Overhead #5

HEALTH PROMOTION PROGRAMMING IN SUBSTANCE ABUSE: PRINCIPLES AND APPROACHES

Health promotion and primary prevention programs in substance abuse generally utilize one or more of the following basic approaches:*

1. Disseminating information.

2. Developing life-coping skills.

3. Providing alternatives to users, misusers, abusers or to nonusers. Users are individuals involved with alcohol/drugs either on a social-recreational or experimental basis.

These approaches represent a broad range of programming options in substance abuse prevention.

---

*From: YWCA of the USA. (1983). *Women as preventors: An adult-teen partnership.* New York: YWCA Printers.

Module I.2—Overhead #6

PROGRAMMING FOR INFORMATION DISSEMINATION

Information imparted includes but is not limited to:*

1. The effects of alcohol/drugs.

2. Prevention services and availability.

3. Treatment services and availability.

4. Training services and availability.

5. Prevention approaches and strategies.

6. Resources.

7. Technical assistance and availability.

---

*From: YWCA of the USA. (1983). *Women as preventors: An adult-teen partnership.* New York: YWCA Printers.

Module I.2—Overhead #7

PROGRAMMING FOR DEVELOPMENT AND ENRICHMENT OF LIFE-COPING SKILLS

Life-coping skills to be developed and/or enriched are those skills necessary for positive functioning in daily living circumstances, such as:*

1. Decision-making skills.

2. Communication techniques.

3. Goal-setting skills.

4. Values-clarification skills.

5. Problem-solving techniques.

6. Assuming responsibility for self.

7. Developing responsible attitudes toward alcohol/drugs.

---

*From: YWCA of the USA. (1983). *Women as preventors: An adult-teen partnership.* New York: YWCA Printers.

PROGRAMMING FOR PROVIDING ALTERNATIVES

Alternatives include activities that will:*

1. Contribute to the use of and growth in personal skills.
2. Create more positive self-image.
3. Develop levels of satisfaction and self-esteem.
4. Develop respect for individual and others.
5. Create opportunity for positive interaction with others.
6. Provide identification with viable role models.
7. Alleviate boredom, unrest, apathy.
8. Contribute to development of positive lifestyle.

---

*From: YWCA of the USA. (1983). *Women as preventors: An adult-teen partnership.* New York: YWCA Printers.

STRESS MANAGEMENT

Definition of Stress: Stressors (events or situations) are perceived to threaten goals or values. Stressors are also perceived to exceed the individual's capabilities to meet demands.

1. Kinds of Reactions to Stressors:
   - Negative emotions.
   - Behavioral problems.
   - Changes in ability to think clearly and rationally.
   - Physiological responses.

2. Perceptions of Stress:
   - Cause loss of self-esteem.
   - Increase potential for suicide.
   - Are a key component in the amount of stress associated with any specific event.

3. Categories of Coping:
   - Palliative coping.
   - Instrumental coping.

4. Comprehensive Approach:
   - Includes educational component.
   - Includes palliative techniques.
   - Includes identification of "triggers."
   - Includes awareness of consequences of stress.

STRESS MANAGEMENT

Strategies for reducing stress:

1. Deal with stressors immediately by establishing positive palliative coping strategies.

2. Remain flexible and be willing to negotiate and compromise.

3. Attend to one problem or issue at a time.

4. Realize that "indecision" is stressful.

5. Discuss issues and problems with family and friends.

6. Take time for thought, relaxation, and self-reinforcing activities.

AEROBIC ACTIVITIES

Aerobic Activities are exercises or sports that develop the heart, blood vessels, and lungs so that these organs are able to better supply working muscles with oxygen.

Aerobic activities will also strengthen muscles specific to the chosen activity and will facilitate the expenditure of calories.

Individuals engaging in aerobic activity should be concerned with four important factors:

1. Frequency.

2. Intensity.

3. Duration.

4. Mode.

SAFER SEX PRACTICES

AVOID:

- Multiple and/or anonymous sexual partners.

- Sexual contact, including open-mouthed (French) kissing, with a partner who has symptoms of AIDS or is a member of a high-risk group for AIDS.

- Sexual contact with anyone who has had sex with people at risk for getting AIDS.

- Sex with prostitutes.

- Sharing toothbrushes, razors, or other implements that could become contaminated with blood with anyone who is, or who might be, infected with the HIV virus.

USE EXTREME CAUTION

- If you have sexual contact with someone who might be infected with the AIDS virus or whose history is unknown to you; also avoid exchanging body fluids. Unless you know absolutely that your partner is not infected, a condom should be used during each sexual act. Use a spermicide to provide additional protection.

- In procedures such as acupuncture, tattooing, ear piercing, etc., in which needles or other unsterile instruments may be used repeatedly to pierce the skin or mucous membranes.

HANDOUT MASTERS

MODULE I.2 HEALTH IMPLICATIONS OF ALCOHOL AND OTHER DRUG USE

1. Developmental Characteristics of People at Risk for Substance Abuse (1A, 1B)

2. Theoretical Basis for Health Promotion Based on Developmental Characteristics

3. Sample Definitions of Primary Prevention (3A, 3B, 3C)

4. Health Promotion Programming: Principles and Approaches (4A, 4B)

5. Stress Management (5A, 5B)

6. Aerobic Activities

7. Safer Sex Practices

Module I.2—Handout #1A

DEVELOPMENTAL CHARACTERISTICS OF
PEOPLE AT RISK FOR SUBSTANCE ABUSE*

In general, the "high-risk" individual shows significant inadequacies in one, several, or all of the following areas:

1. *Identification with viable role models.* This refers to a person's reference group and self-concept. The vulnerable person does not see herself or himself as like (or the same as) people whose attitudes, values, and behaviors allow them to "survive" in their total environment.

2. *Identification with and responsibility for "family" processes.* In this context, "family" is used in a broad sense. It can and often does mean the traditional nuclear family (father, mother, 1.8 children, dog, cat). It is also used to mean family in the sense of broad organization, living settings, group identifications, and so forth. When this identification is poorly developed, a person does not identify strongly with things greater than herself or himself (e.g., relationships with another person, in groups, mankind, God, etc.). She or he does not see that what one does affects others. This refers to shared investment in outcomes, shared responsibility for achieving outcomes, and accountability to others for behavior.

3. *Attitudes and values regarding problem-solving.* This refers to the skills and attitudes necessary to work through problems and believe that they can be solved through application of personal resources. When poorly developed, a person believes that problems have been escaped when she or he can't feel them any more. For example, a person has faith in "miracle" solutions to problems. (This is often through the use of alcohol or drugs.) She or he does not believe that there is anything one can do about the present or future; things just happen to her or him.

4. *Intra-personal skills.* Intra-personal skills are those which a person uses to communicate with self. This refers to the skills of self-discipline, self-control, self-assessment, etc. Weaknesses in these areas express themselves as: inability to cope with personal stresses and tensions, dishonesty with self, denial of self, inability to defer gratification, low self-esteem, etc.

*From: National Institute on Drug Abuse. (1980). The developmental approach to preventing problem dependencies. In H. S. Glenn & J. W. Warner (Eds.), *Community-based prevention specialist: Participant manual* (pp. 133–153). Rockville, MD: NIDA.

Module I.2—Handout #1B

DEVELOPMENTAL CHARACTERISTICS OF
PEOPLE AT RISK FOR SUBSTANCE ABUSE*

5. *Inter-personal skills.* Inter-personal skills are those skills which enable a person to relate to or build a relationship with another person; e.g., sharing, trusting, etc. Weaknesses in these areas express themselves as: dishonesty with others, lack of empathic awareness, resistance to feedback, inability to share feelings, inability to give or receive love or help, etc.

6. *Systemic skills.* These refer to the ability to respond to the limits inherent in a situation (responsibility); the ability to modify behavior according to a situation in order to get one's needs met constructively (adaptability), etc. Weaknesses in these areas express themselves as: irresponsibility, refusal to accept consequences of behavior, scapegoating, etc. A person with low skills in these areas tends to see herself or himself as a victim of circumstances.

7. *Judgmental skills.* Judgmental skills include the ability to recognize, understand and apply relationships. Weaknesses in this area express themselves as: crises in sexual, natural, consumer, and drug environments; and repetitive self-destructive behaviors.

*From: National Institute on Drug Abuse. (1980). The developmental approach to preventing problem dependencies. In H. S. Glenn & J. W. Warner (Eds.), *Community-based prevention specialist: Participant manual* (pp. 133–153). Rockville, MD: NIDA.

THEORETICAL BASIS FOR HEALTH PROMOTION BASED ON DEVELOPMENTAL CHARACTERISTICS*

Most human behavior is a composite of the seven areas described previously. Social norms define acceptable forms of behavior, and require certain levels of functioning in each of these areas. By assessing levels of functioning, developmental characteristics are used as diagnostic indicators of "high-risk" and "low-risk" populations for purposes of both prevention and treatment. At present, treatment and prevention programs have both explicit (expressed) and implicit (implied) goals which reflect the above characteristics. An analysis of these goals suggests that, *in virtually all current approaches to prevention, rehabilitation, and therapy, workers are attempting to establish or maintain situations in which their clients, through practice and experience, can:*

- Strengthen or develop intra-personal skills (get self together); and/or

- Strengthen or develop inter-personal skills (learn to deal effectively with others); and/or

- Strengthen or develop systemic skills (learn to handle situations); and/or

- Develop judgmental skills (learn to make decisions and recognize what's going on); and/or

- Strengthen identification with and responsibility for "family" processes (become part of something greater than self and learn to carry one's own weight); and/or

- Strengthen identification with viable role models (learn to see self as the kind of person who is making it and identify with others who are also making it).

*From: National Institute on Drug Abuse. (1980). The developmental approach to preventing problem dependencies. In H. S. Glenn & J. W. Warner (Eds.), *Community-based prevention specialist: Participant manual* (pp. 133–153). Rockville, MD: NIDA.

Module I.2—Handout #3A

SAMPLE DEFINITIONS OF PRIMARY PREVENTION*

1. "Primary drug abuse prevention is a constructive process designed to promote personal and social growth of the individual toward full human potential and thereby inhibit or reduce physical, emotional, or social impairment which results in or from abuse of chemical substances."

    —NIDA Drug Abuse Prevention Delphi, 1975.

2. "The purpose of prevention is to increase the likelihood that individuals will develop drinking-related behaviors that are personally and socially constructive. Negatively stated, prevention programs are aimed at reducing the number of persons whose alcohol-related behavior adversely affects the way they carry on the roles and responsibilities of everyday living."

    —Planning Prevention Programs,
    National Center for Alcohol Education.

3. "Primary prevention of drug abuse is a constructive process designed to promote personal, social, *economic and political* growth of the individual toward full human potential; and thereby inhibit or reduce personal, social, *economic or political* impairment which results in or from the abuse of chemical substances."

    —Center for Multicultural Awareness,
    a project of NIDA's Prevention Branch.

4. "Primary prevention encompasses those activities directed at specifically identified, vulnerable high-risk groups within the community who have not been labeled as psychiatrically ill and for whom measures can be undertaken to avoid the onset of emotional disturbances and/or to enhance their level of positive mental health. Programs for the promotion of mental health are primarily educational rather than clinical in conception and operation, with their ultimate goal being to increase people's capacities for dealing with crises and for taking steps to improve their own lives."

    —Stephen E. Goldston, Ed.D.,
    Coordinator for Primary Prevention Programs,
    National Institutes of Mental Health.

*From: National Institute on Drug Abuse. (1980). The developmental approach to preventing problem dependencies. In H. S. Glenn & J. W. Warner (Eds.), *Community-based prevention specialist: Participant manual* (pp. 29–30). Rockville, MD: NIDA.

SAMPLE DEFINITIONS OF PRIMARY PREVENTION*

5. "The Alcohol, Drug Abuse and Mental Health Administration (ADAMHA) requires the description of two types of behavior—behavioral antecedents and consequences—which are useful in designing primary prevention activities, particularly with regard to health promotion and disease prevention.

   • Prevention of behavioral antecedents refers to interventions to reduce high-risk behaviors, such as teenage drinking, smoking and experimental drug use, which increase the probability of developing physical, emotional and behavioral problems.

   • Prevention of behavioral consequences refers to interventions to prevent the deleterious effects (consequences) of high-risk behavior, such as accidents resulting from drinking while driving, or suicides or homicides resulting from emotional disorders, excessive drinking or substance abuse."

   —ADAMHA Prevention Policy Paper,
   August 17, 1979.

6. "An aggregate of community education and social action programs which, within an identified length of time and for specified *groups* of people, are able to measurably reduce the likelihood, frequency, seriousness or duration of chemical use problems by means other than referral or recourse to the chemical dependency treatment system or correctional services."

   —The content of this definition was developed
   by the Michigan Office of Substance
   Abuse Services prevention staff.

7. "Primary prevention of social and behavioral problems is accomplished through ongoing processes that provide opportunities for individuals, small groups and organizations to increase: (1) knowledge or awareness of personal and collective potentials; (2) skills necessary to attain those potentials; and (3) creative use of resources to the end that all people have the ability to effectively cope with *typical* life problems and recognize, reduce or eliminate *unnecessary* or debilitating stress in the community without abusing themselves or others and prior to the onset of incapacitating individual, group or organizational problems."

   —The content of this definition was developed by
   the Human Services Training Institute,
   Michael B. Winer, Associate Director,
   Spokane, Washington.

*From: National Institute on Drug Abuse. (1980). The developmental approach to preventing problem dependencies. In H. S. Glenn & J. W. Warner (Eds.), *Community-based prevention specialist: Participant manual* (pp. 29–30). Rockville, MD: NIDA.

SAMPLE DEFINITIONS OF PRIMARY PREVENTION*

8. "Prevention includes purposeful activities designed to promote personal (emotional, intellectual, physical, spiritual and social) growth of individuals and strengthen the aspects of the community environment which are supportive to them, in order to preclude, forestall or impede the development of alcohol and other drug abuse problems."

    —Wisconsin State Drug Abuse Plan.

9. "Another way to break down the concept of health promotion is to consider the community as well as the individual. We are accustomed to think of an individual's health, both in terms of treatment and building resistance, but we can extend this to the community. Often people succumb to ill health in part as a result of forces in the social context. Such could include unemployment, insensitive institutions, including schools, or prevalent attitudes which reinforce unhealthy behaviors. If this is the case, then it makes sense to design programs which deal with these factors."

    —Vermont Alcohol and Drug Abuse Division.

10. Primary prevention is "a proactive process utilizing an interdisciplinary approach designed to empower people with their resources to constructively confront stressful life conditions."

    —National Association of Prevention Professionals.

---

*From: National Institute on Drug Abuse. (1980). The developmental approach to preventing problem dependencies. In H. S. Glenn & J. W. Warner (Eds.), *Community-based prevention specialist: Participant manual* (pp. 29–30). Rockville, MD: NIDA.

Module I.2—Handout #4A

HEALTH PROMOTION PROGRAMMING: PRINCIPLES AND APPROACHES*

Health promotion and primary prevention programs in substance abuse generally utilize one or more of the following basic approaches: (1) disseminating information; (2) developing life-coping skills; and (3) providing alternatives to users, misusers, abusers, or to nonusers. Users are individuals involved with alcohol/drugs either on a social-recreational or experimental basis.

The following three approaches represent a broad range of programming options in substance abuse prevention:

1. Information imparted includes but is not limited to:

   - The effects of alcohol/drugs.

   - Prevention services and availability.

   - Treatment services and availability.

   - Training services and availability.

   - Prevention approaches and strategies.

   - Resources.

   - Technical assistance and availability.

2. Life-coping skills developed and/or enriched are those skills necessary for positive functioning in daily living circumstances, such as:

   - Decision-making skills.

   - Communication techniques.

   - Goal-setting skills.

   - Values-clarification skills.

   - Problem-solving techniques.

   - Assuming responsibility for self.

   - Developing responsible attitudes toward alcohol/drugs.

*From: YWCA of the USA. (1983). *Women as preventors: An adult-teen partnership*. New York: YWCA Press.

124

HEALTH PROMOTION PROGRAMMING:
PRINCIPLES AND APPROACHES*

3. Alternatives provided include activities that will contribute to use of and growth in personal skills.

   • Create more positive self-image.

   • Develop levels of satisfaction and self-esteem.

   • Develop respect for individual and others.

   • Create opportunity for positive interaction with others.

   • Provide identification with viable role models.

   • Alleviate boredom, unrest, apathy.

   • Contribute to development of positive lifestyle.

*From: YWCA of the USA. (1983). Women as preventors: An adult-teen partnership. New York: YWCA Press.

STRESS MANAGEMENT

1. Stress occurs when individuals are confronted with demands which are perceived to threaten important values or goals, or to exceed their capabilities to meet the demands. Stressors are those events or situations that cause individuals to have stress reactions.

2. Many kinds of reactions to stressors may occur. Individuals may experience all, or some of, the following:

    a. Negative emotions; i.e., fear, guilt, anxiety, depression, anger.

    b. Behavioral problems; i.e., speech disturbances, muscular tension.

    c. Changes in ability to think clearly and rationally.

    d. Physiological responses, such as feelings of tightness in the chest, throat, etc., or over time, the development of ulcers.

3. In severe cases of perceived loss of self-esteem, there may be potential for suicide.

4. It is important to realize that psychological stress, although usually associated with a specific event or situation (for example, a job or school demand), occurs because of individuals' *perceptions* of how important the event or demand is to them; and how individuals feel about their abilities or capabilities to meet the demand.

5. Two categories of coping with stressors:

    a. Palliative coping—coping (in the form of thoughts or behaviors) designed to temporarily relieve the emotional impact of stressors. Does not alter stressors in any way but allows individuals to reduce emotional arousal levels, feel better, and think more clearly. Examples: relaxation, exercise, listening to music, biofeedback, etc. Primary function of palliative coping strategies is to reduce emotional arousal level and other related stress symptoms in order to facilitate second phase of coping process—instrumental or direct action phase.

    b. Instrumental coping—coping (direct action) designed to deal directly with demands (stressors) confronting individuals. Involves the development of skills and abilities that directly relate to the nature and characteristics of the stressor (demand). If new skills or abilities are not learned, the stressor remains significant. The phase is a critical component of stress management and is often neglected or overlooked in stress management programs.

Module I.2—Handout #5B

STRESS MANAGEMENT

6. Effective stress management requires a comprehensive approach which includes an educational component, as well as specific palliative stress management techniques.

7. Important for individuals to identify stress "triggers" and develop an awareness of the physical, psychological and behavioral consequences of stressors.

8. Stress is unavoidable, but there are appropriate strategies for reducing stress:

   a. Deal with stressors and related emotions immediately by establishing positive palliative coping strategies.

   b. Remain flexible and be willing to negotiate and compromise.

   c. Attend to one problem or issue at a time.

   d. Realize that "indecision" is stressful.

   e. Discuss issues and problems with family and friends.

   f. Be sure to take some time for thought, relaxation, and self-reinforcing activities.

AEROBIC ACTIVITIES

Aerobic activities are exercises or sports that develop the heart, blood vessels, and lungs, so that these organs are able to better supply working muscles with oxygen. Aerobic activities will also strengthen muscles specific to the chosen activity and will facilitate the expenditure of calories. Individuals engaging in aerobic activity should be concerned with four important factors:

1. *Frequency.* Regular physical activity, in order to gain physiological and psychological benefits, should be engaged in at least three to five times per week. If weight control is also an objective, it is recommended that individuals begin exercising three to five times per week and gradually increase to six or seven times per week.

2. *Intensity.* Intensity refers to how hard or how easily you are walking, jogging, swimming, etc. Overexercising is fatiguing and unsafe. Underexercising may not be beneficial. It is generally a good idea to start out at a low to moderate intensity and gradually increase the effort as you "get into shape."

3. *Duration.* At each exercise session, you should attempt at least 15–45 minutes of continuous aerobic activity. At the beginning of your program, you may not be able to exercise for more than 15 minutes.

4. *Mode.* Individuals should engage in activities that use large muscle groups (legs, back, arms), are rhythmic and aerobic in nature, and can be maintained continuously. For example, walking-hiking briskly, running, jogging, swimming, cycling, rowing, cross-country skiing, skating, aerobic-jazz dancing, etc. Sports like tennis, racquetball, squash, etc., are most beneficial as aerobic activities if played with someone of equal or greater ability.

Module I.2—Handout #7

SAFER SEX PRACTICES

1. Avoid multiple and/or anonymous sexual partners.

2. Avoid sexual contact (including open-mouthed or French kissing—the HIV virus may be present in saliva, although no evidence exists that AIDS has been transmitted in this way) with anyone who has symptoms of AIDS or who is a member of a high-risk group for AIDS.

3. Avoid sexual contact with anyone who has had sex with people at risk of getting AIDS.

4. If you have sexual contact with someone who might be infected with the AIDS virus or whose history is unknown to you, avoid exchange of body fluids. Unless you know absolutely that your partner is not infected, a condom should be used during each sexual act, from start to finish. Use a spermicide to provide additional protection.

5. Avoid sex with prostitutes.

6. Avoid sharing toothbrushes, razors or other implements that could become contaminated with blood with anyone who is, or who might be infected with the HIV virus.

7. Use extreme caution in procedures, such as acupuncture, tattooing, ear piercing, etc., in which needles or other unsterile instruments may be used repeatedly to pierce the skin and/or mucous membranes.

RECOMMENDED TEACHING STRATEGIES AND SAMPLE ASSIGNMENTS

RECOMMENDED TEACHING STRATEGIES

ACTIVITY 1

Attitudes Continuum*

Objectives:

- To illustrate the concept that more than facts are involved in alcohol- and drug-related decisions.

- To examine individual attitudes concerning use and abuse of alcohol and other drugs.

- To provide a structure for the sharing of various attitudes, feelings and/or opinions concerning the issues of alcohol and drug use.

Time: 45–60 minutes.

Materials: "Attitudes Continuum" handouts, pencils, newsprint, magic markers.

Detailed Procedural Steps:

1. Tell the participants that they are about to engage in an exercise of attitude exploration. Explain the use of the continuum: As each statement is read aloud, participants should mark the statement indicator at the point on the continuum that corresponds to how they feel about that statement. It is important to note that there are no right or wrong answers. Feelings are real for each individual and reactions to the statements need to be made on a feeling level. Read the following statements and have the participants mark on a continuum sheet their reactions to a:

   a. Person who takes aspirin for the slightest ache.

   b. Person who has drinks before going to a party in order to get into a "social" mood.

From: Pennsylvania State University, Addictions Prevention Laboratory. (1977). *Instructor's manual in developing life skills through guidance in the classroom* (pp. 147–148). University Park, PA: Pennsylvania State University. (Funded by Governor's Council on Drug and Alcohol Abuse for the Commonwealth of Pennsylvania.)

   c. Person who drinks a case of beer every weekend.

   d. Person who has a cigarette and/or coffee first thing every morning to get started.

   e. Person who takes 25 mg of Valium a day to tolerate back pain.

   f. Person who has a couple of drinks before supper nightly to "unwind."

   g. Person who smokes a pack of cigarettes daily.

   h. Person who smokes a marijuana joint with friends a couple of times a week.

   i. Person who frequently goes to happy hours with friends after work.

   j. Person who frequents happy hours to delay arriving home.

2. After each participant has finished, discussion groups of four or five can be formed to attempt to arrive at a consensus about individual attitudes. Groups can report to the whole group regarding their consensus and attitudes, as well as personal reactions to the exercise. The types of processing questions relative to this exercise are:

   a. Emphasis on facts alone is not enough when dealing with the area of alcohol/drugs. Can you remember how you felt during the exercise?

   b. What determines your personal decision about placement on the continuum?

   c. What will change your placement on the continuum?

   d. What are your reactions to people who have different ratings?

   e. Does knowledge change minds?

   f. Do reactions vary depending on sex? Age?

Additional Facilitation Suggestions and Activities:

1. A discussion relating to the terms "user" and "abuser" may be appropriate prior to the exercise. Such a discussion is not likely to change the participants' attitudes about these terms, but it will be important in helping participants understand that individual attitudes differ.

2. Two other ways of conducting this exercise could be:

   a. Using a forced choice format where participants must rank statements according to the strength of their feelings from positive to negative.

   b. Having participants physically place themselves on an imaginary continuum in the room so they can see each other's reactions to the statements.

3. The following alternate method can be used to allow participants the opportunity of experiencing how social roles (i.e., sex roles) affect attitudes about specific situations:

   a. Prepare four different master copies of the 10 statements. Each of the four sets of 10 statements will begin with a different subject. The first set should read "A person who . . ."; the second set "A woman who . . ."; the third set "A man who . . ."; and the fourth set "A youth who . . .".

b. Each participant will receive only one of the four sets of statements as a handout. Prepare copies of each set equal to one-fourth of the total participants (e.g., for 20 participants, make five copies of each of the four sets of statements).

c. Without acknowledging differences, randomly distribute handouts and the continuums. Instruct participants to individually complete the continuum by placing the number of the statement at the point on the continuum where their feelings indicate its appropriateness.

d. When continuums are completed, state that the handouts are slightly different and that groups of four will be formed according to the handout received. (Each group should have a participant representing each type of handout; i.e., person, man, woman, youth).

e. Form small groups and instruct participants first to discuss their continuum individually and then to consider whether a different handout would have affected their rankings on the continuum. If so, why?

f. Process as in the other method.

Instructor's Guide

ACTIVITY 2

ATTITUDES CONTINUUM

USER   **ABUSER**

Values Clarification—Alcohol

Objectives:

- To help participants examine individual attitudes concerning use and abuse of alcohol and other drugs.

- To demonstrate that more than facts are involved in alcohol- and other drug-related decisions.

Time: 45–60 minutes.

Materials: "Alcohol Opinion Poll" handouts, pencils.

Detailed Procedural Steps:

1. Distribute the "Alcohol Opinion Poll" handouts and ask participants to answer each question by circling the answer that best represents their thinking.

2. Assure participants that there are no right or wrong answers. Feelings are real for each individual and reactions to the statements need to be made on a feeling level.

3. After individual completion of sheets, conduct an unstructured group discussion revolving around responses and feelings generated by issues in the exercise.

4. Depending on time allowances, you may also want to use the "Optional Opinion Poll" or substitute it for the "Alcohol Opinion Poll."

ALCOHOL OPINION POLL*

For each question, circle the *one* answer that best represents your thinking.

1. Ogden Nash once wrote, regarding getting people to "mix" at parties: "Candy is dandy, but liquor is quicker." For a successful party, liquor is:

   a. necessary.

   b. helpful.

   c. not needed.

From: Pennsylvania State University, Addictions Prevention Laboratory. (1977). *Instructor's manual in developing life skills through guidance in the classroom* (pp. 147–148). University Park, PA: Pennsylvania State University. (Funded by Governor's Council on Drug and Alcohol Abuse for the Commonwealth of Pennsylvania.)

133

2. While they are drinking, people are:

    a. more likeable than usual.

    b. less likeable.

    c. neither more nor less likeable.

3. It is:

    a. more acceptable for males to drink.

    b. more acceptable for females to drink.

    c. equally acceptable for males and females to drink.

4. Teenagers who drink are:

    a. more socially sought after.

    b. less socially sought after.

    c. equally sought after socially.

5. Most teenagers who drink are:

    a. very dependent on alcohol.

    b. somewhat dependent on alcohol.

    c. not dependent on alcohol.

6. Most teenagers who use alcohol are considered by their peers to be:

    a. very mature.

    b. somewhat mature.

    c. somewhat immature.

    d. very immature.

    e. same as teenagers who abstain.

7. Most teenagers who use alcohol:

    a. brag about it openly.

    b. tell only close friends.

    c. conceal this activity.

    d. other.

8. Most teenagers who drink do so because:

    a. they want to escape problems.

    b. they want to be considered "adult."

    c. they want to be considered "one of the group."

    d. other.

9. While teenagers are drinking, they feel:

   a. more self-confident.

   b. less self-confident.

   c. equally as self-confident as they do when not drinking.

10. Teenagers who use alcohol are more likely than nondrinkers:

    a. to engage in premarital sex.

    b. to avoid premarital sex.

    c. equally as likely to participate in premarital sex as when they do not drink.

11. If teenagers are going to drink, they should do so:

    a. out-of-doors at the beach, parks, etc.

    b. at home.

    c. in bars.

    d. in cars.

    e. other.

12. Teenagers should:

    a. avoid alcohol altogether.

    b. sample it when they can do so safely.

    c. use alcohol all they want.

13. The legal age for using alcohol should be:

    a. 21.

    b. 18.

    c. 16.

    d. 14.

14. On which of the following media should whiskey advertising be permitted? (More than one choice is okay.)

    a. television.

    b. magazines.

    c. newspapers.

    d. signboards.

    e. none of these.

Module I.2

OPTIONAL OPINION POLL*

In this section, please rank each set of responses. The response that most closely represents your thinking will be #1, your second choice #2, and so forth. Rank the responses in this manner even if you do not fully agree with any of the choices.

1. Use of alcohol should be considered as a:

    _____ moral issue

    _____ social issue

    _____ religious issue

    _____ personal issue

    _____ health issue

2. At my school, the biggest problem is:

    _____ marijuana

    _____ alcohol

    _____ misbehavior

    _____ boredom

3. If people are going to use alcohol, they should:

    _____ use it at meals

    _____ use it alone

    _____ use it socially with others

4. Society suffers most from public use of:

    _____ alcohol

    _____ marijuana

    _____ cigarettes

5. Which of the following is most dangerous to one's own mental and physical health?

    _____ alcohol

    _____ marijuana

    _____ cigarettes

6. Which is most dangerous for society? A teenager who is:

    _____ driving while intoxicated

    _____ driving while emotionally upset

    _____ driving fast to show off for peers

*From: Boys' Clubs of America. (1978). *Alcohol abuse prevention: A comprehensive guide for youth organizations* (pp. 46–47). New York: Boys' Clubs of America.

136

7. Teenagers who drink:

_____ use alcohol to have fun

_____ use alcohol to be accepted by those who also drink

_____ use alcohol to face or get away from their problems

_____ other

8. What would you least like your best friend to do the next time you are together?

_____ be drunk

_____ be high on pills

_____ be high on marijuana

9. Which would you least like to be?

_____ an alcoholic

_____ addicted to heroin

_____ addicted to uppers

10. Which would be hardest for you to admit to your friends?

_____ that you cheated on a test

_____ that you had shoplifted a valuable article

_____ that you had gotten drunk the night before

_____ that you had engaged in premarital sex

11. Which would be hardest for you to admit to your parents?

_____ that you cheated on a test

_____ that you had shoplifted a valuable article

_____ that you had gotten drunk the night before

_____ that you had engaged in premarital sex

12. Which is the worst news you could learn about *your own* teenager?

_____ that he/she was using alcohol

_____ that he/she was using marijuana

_____ that he/she was shoplifting

_____ that he/she was engaging in premarital sex

13. If *your own* teenager were to come home drunk, which of the following would you do?

_____ call a youth agency for help

_____ punish him/her severely

_____ order him/her never to drink again

———— "laugh it off" as part of growing up

———— other

Complete each of the following sentences:

14. A person is abusing alcohol when . . .

15. If I drink too much . . .

16. When my friends drink . . .

17. I would drink if . . .

18. I wouldn't drink if . . .

ACTIVITY 3

Primary Prevention Messages*

Objectives:

- To provide an experiential perspective on primary prevention.
- To examine the social messages that can influence drinking decisions or promote problem drinking.
- To begin to explore ways prevention messages can counter social messages.

Time: 70 minutes.

Materials: Magazines and other advertisements for alcohol, newsprint or blackboard.

Detailed Procedural Steps:

1. As preparation for this session, collect several examples of advertisements for alcohol.

2. At the start of this session, explain that the purpose of the session is to illustrate the kinds of social messages that can influence drinking decisions, and to suggest prevention messages that promote healthy decisions about drinking.

3. Pass out the advertisements to participants. Give participants a few minutes to read the advertisements.

4. Ask participants to point out the messages in the advertisements. For example: "I'm cool when I drink."

*From: YWCA of the USA (1983). *Women as preventors: An adult-teen partnership.* New York: YWCA Press.

5. List messages on newsprint or blackboard.

6. Questions that may be relevant to this discussion are as follows:

   a. How do you think most people (women, teens, children, etc.) view these advertisements? What do you observe about the age of people in these advertisements?

   b. What messages do these advertisements give to adolescent females?

   c. Do these advertisements influence our thoughts and decisions about drinking? How?

   d. How do television commercials also influence attitudes and feelings about drinking?

7. Sum up by having participants voice their feelings about the various ways people are influenced to use alcohol or drugs.

ACTIVITY 4

Force Field Analysis*

Force Field Analysis is a problem-solving technique based on the writings of Kurt Lewin and originally designed for laboratory training experiences by the National Training Laboratory (NTL) Institute.

This technique provides a method for analyzing a situation participants would like to change and for learning how to go about making the change in a structured, uncomplicated manner. The steps for problem-solving are as follows:

1. Identify the problem situation to be solved. Select a realistic and practical problem to approach. For example, you may choose to work within the school system trying to eliminate teenage drinking on school property.

2. Define the problem situation, indicating the direction of the change you desire, such as eliminating all drinking on school property.

3. Look at your problem situation in terms of what forces will help toward improvement of the problem (driving forces), and what forces will resist improvement of the problem (restraining forces).

4. Define the driving and restraining forces affecting your problem situation—don't be selective or critical; remember such issues as physical resources and restraints, feelings, social pressures and personalities.

5. Identify the forces (both driving and restraining) that appear to be most important. Try to limit your choices to two or three in each category.

6. Take each of the restraining forces and think of a few practical methods to reduce or eliminate the force.

*From: YWCA of the USA (1983). *Women as preventors: An adult-teen partnership.* New York: YWCA Press.

7. Follow the same process as stated above for the driving forces. The goal is to increase the effect of the driving force.

8. Identify the materials, people and resources that can assist in reducing the restraining forces and those that can increase the effect of the driving forces.

9. Look at your accumulated information, eliminate the impractical and focus on the possibilities for positive action.

10. Devise an implementation plan from information generated.

11. Devise an evaluation plan.

ACTIVITY 5

Primary Prevention Planning*

Objectives:

- To help participants identify alcohol problems.

- To introduce problem-solving techniques applicable to prevention planning.

Time: 90 minutes.

Materials: "Primary Prevention Planning Flow Chart," pencils.

Detailed Procedural Steps:

1. Point out that in this activity, participants will practice prevention planning skills that can be used not only for alcohol issues but for dealing with everyday life situations and planning community prevention projects.

2. Explain Primary Prevention Planning (PPP):

   a. Pass out copies of the "Primary Prevention Planning Flow Chart" to all participants and explain that the chart will be a resource for this session. Briefly go over steps 1 and 2, which will be used in this session.

   b. Review the steps to PPP:

      (1) Think through the problem (problem identification).

      (2) Decide what to do (action plan).

      (3) Carry out the plan (implementation).

      (4) Evaluate.

   c. Comment that "We encounter and solve problems on a daily basis. More often than not, we practice PPP already. This activity is designed to make us

From: Pennsylvania Governor's Council on Drug and Alcohol Abuse. (1977). In J. D'Angelli, & J. Weener, *Communication and parenting skills.* University Park, PA: Governor's Council on Drug and Alcohol Abuse.

conscious of skills we already use, to demonstrate how these skills can be applied in any situation, and to allow practice in acting as preventors and health promoters."

3. Introduce a problem-solving activity related to alcohol/drug using behavior.

4. Divide group into triads and have each triad read through the problem/issues and, as a group, proceed through steps 1 and 2 on the planning flow chart. The task of each triad is to agree on a potential program plan for the situation that is based on the sketchy information given. Participants may need to be reminded to draw upon their own experiences and their own knowledge to fill in gaps that require more information relative to the problem.

5. After steps 1 and 2 have been completed, have triads return to defining the problem. Their task is to come to a consensus and define their perception of the problem as specifically as possible.

6. Have groups share with each other any discoveries and reactions they had during the preceding task assignments.

Facilitation Hints: Those leaders familiar with brainstorming techniques may want to employ brainstorming as a means of accomplishing step 2 on the "Primary Prevention Planning Flow Chart."

PRIMARY PREVENTION PLANNING FLOW CHART*

Step 1: Problem Identification.

1. Define the problem(s) or potential problem(s).

2. Identify your own feelings and expectations about the problem.

3. Define the target group—whether the community, peers, teens or others; think about and try to identify this target group's feelings and needs.

4. Assess and identify possible resources.

Step 2: Action Planning.

Environmental Control		
Approaches	Advance Planning	Individual Approaches
Think of all the possibilities for modifying the environment.	Think of all possibilities to head off the problem.	Think of all possibilities to meet the goals through alternatives/education.
Redefine problem statement specifically.	Redefine problem statement specifically.	Redefine problem statement specifically.

*From: Pennsylvania Governor's Council on Drug and Alcohol Abuse. (1977). In J. D'Angelli, & J. Weener, *Communication and parenting skills*. University Park, PA: Governor's Council on Drug and Alcohol Abuse.

Step 3:   Program Implementation.

1.   Conduct force field analysis (problem-solving technique).

2.   Agree on tasks and responsibilities.

3.   Plan a schedule.

4.   Implement program.

Step 4:   Assessment/Evaluation.

1.   Document program tasks, programs, participants, etc.

2.   Arrange support and reinforcement for program.

TEST QUESTIONS AND ANSWERS

TEST QUESTIONS

1. Three factors which interact to influence motives for and outcomes of alcohol/ drug use/misuse/abuse are:

   a. Individual, environmental, developmental.

   b. Individual, peer, socioeconomic status.

   c. Family patterns, lifestyle, genetic.

   d. None of the above.

   e. All of the above.

2. Inadequacies in which of the following is *not* associated with "high risk" for addictive behaviors?

   a. Identification with viable role models.

   b. Identification with and responsibility for family processes.

   c. Intra-personal skills.

   d. Inter-personal skills.

   e. Nutrition knowledge.

3. Health promotion is:

   a. The maintenance/enhancement of existing levels of health through the implementation of effective programs, services and policies.

   b. Being physically fit.

   c. The absence of disease.

   d. Eating properly.

   e. Safe dieting.

4. Factors which increase drug use/misuse/abuse related risks to health include:

   a. Dysfunctional family patterns.

   b. Drug/alcohol use as coping strategies.

   c. Personality structure.

   d. Life events.

   e. All of the above.

5. Which of the following are considered when prescribing appropriate exercise?

   a. Frequency, intensity, duration, mode of exercise.

   b. Frequency, intensity, duration, time of exercise.

   c. Intensity, duration, mode.

   d. Intensity only.

   e. Duration only.

6. Which of the following are psychological benefits of appropriate exercise?

   a. Improved general mental health and well-being.

   b. Improved nutrition.

   c. Reduced stress.

   d. All of the above.

   e. None of the above.

7. Which of the following are physiological benefits of appropriate exercise?

   a. Decreased incidences of cardiovascular disease.

   b. Decreased incidences of cancer.

   c. Reduction of blood pressure in hypertensives.

   d. Improved nutrition.

   e. All of the above.

8. Which of the following are health risks for alcohol abuse?

   a. Death.

   b. Damage to liver, heart and pancreas.

   c. Malnutrition.

   d. Lowered resistance to disease.

   e. All of the above.

9. Which are strategies used as palliative coping techniques to reduce stress?

   a. Exercise.

   b. Alcohol use.

   c. Drug use.

   d. Biofeedback.

   e. All of the above.

10. Palliative coping:

   a. Alters stressors.

   b. Temporarily relieves the emotional impact of stressors.

   c. Increases emotional arousal levels.

   d. Enhances the emotional impact of stressors.

   e. All of the above.

ANSWER KEY

1. e
2. e
3. a
4. e
5. a
6. a and c
7. a, b, and c
8. e
9. e
10. b

BIBLIOGRAPHY

MODULE I.2 HEALTH IMPLICATIONS OF ALCOHOL AND OTHER DRUG USE

Allen, R. F., & Allen, J. (1987). A sense of community, a shared vision and a positive culture: Core enabling factors in successful culture-based health promotion. *American Journal of Health Promotion, 1*(3), 40–47.

Allen, W. A. (1987). *How drugs can affect your life.* Springfield, IL: Thomas.

American Nurses' Association, Drug and Alcohol Nurses Association, & National Nurses Society on Addictions. (1987). *The care of clients with addiction: Dimensions of nursing practice.* Kansas City, MO: Author.

American Nurses' Association, & National Nurses Society on Addictions. (1988). *Standards of addictions nursing practice with selected diagnoses and criteria.* Kansas City, MO: Author.

Ardell, D. B. (1979). *High-level wellness.* New York: Rodale.

Barresi, C. M., & Gigliotti, R. S. (1975). Are drug education programs effective? *Journal of Drug Education, 5*(4), 301.

Bellingham, R., Cohen, B., Jones, J., & Spaniol, L. (1989). Connectedness: Some skills for spiritual health. *American Journal of Health Promotion, 4*(1), 18–24.

Benson, H. B. (1976). *The relaxation response.* New York: Avon.

Blair, S. N., Kohl, H. W., Paffenbarger, R. S., Clark, D. G., Cooper, K. H., & Gibbons, L. W. (1989). Physical fitness and all-cause mortality: A prospective study of healthy men and women. *Journal of American Medical Association, 262*(17), 2395–2401.

Bonaguro, E. W., & Bonaguro, J. A. (1989). Tobacco use among adolescents: Directions for research. *American Journal of Health Promotion, 4*(1), 37–41.

Boys' Clubs of America. (1978). *Alcohol abuse prevention: A comprehensive guide for youth organizations* (pp. 46–47). New York: Boys' Clubs of America.

Branca, M., D'Angelli, J., & Evans, K. (1974). *Development of a decision-making skills education program: Study 1: A research report.* University Park, PA: Addictions Prevention Laboratory, Pennsylvania State University.

Burke, E. L. (1970). Patient values on an adolescent drug unit. *American Journal of Psychotherapy, 24*(3), 400–410.

Childress, A. R., McLellan, A. T., & O'Brien, C. P. (1985). Behavioral therapies for substance abuse. *International Journal of Addictions, 20*(6–7), 947–969.

Clarke, C. (1986). *Wellness: Concepts, theory, research and practice.* New York: Springer.

Clarke, M. (1984). Stress and coping: Constructs for nursing. *Journal of Advanced Nursing, 9,* 3–13.

Crosby, J. F. (1971, April). The effects of family life education on the values and attitudes of adolescents. *Family Coordinator,* 137–140.

Cummings, C. (1986). A review of the impact of nutrition on health and profits and a discussion of successful program elements. *American Journal of Health Promotion, 1*(1), 14–22.

Curran, F. J. (1971). Child psychiatrist looks at the drug problem. *New York State Journal of Medicine, 71*(13), 639–650.

de Bono, E. (1970). *Lateral thinking: Creativity step by step.* New York: Harper & Row.

Eckhardt, M. J., & Harford, T. C. (1981). Health hazards associated with alcohol consumption. *Journal of American Medical Association, 246*(6), 648–666.

Eldred, C. A., & Washington, M. N. (1976). Interpersonal relationships in heroin use by men and women and their role in treatment outcome. *International Journal of Addictions, 11*(1), 117–130.

Eng, R., & Hanson, D. J. (1989). *College Student Journal, 23*(1), 82–88.

Glenn, H. S. (1975). Education for alternative behavior (keynote address). *Proceedings from First Annual Southeast Drug Conference.* Atlanta, GA: Georgia State University.

Glenn, H. S., & Warner, J. (1977). *The developmental approach to preventing problem dependencies.* Bloomington, IN: Social Systems, Inc.

Goodspeed, R. B., & DeLucia, A. G. (1990). Stress reduction at the worksite: An evaluation of two methods. *American Journal of Health Promotion, 4*(5), 333–337.

Goodstadt, M. S., Simpson, R. I., & Loranger, P. O. (1987). Health promotion: A conceptual integration. *American Journal of Health Promotion, 1*(3), 58–63.

Gotestam, K. G., Melin, L., & Ost, L. G. (1976). Behavioral techniques in the treatment of drug abuse: An evaluative review. *Addictive Behaviors, 1*(3), 205–225.

Haack, M. R., & Harford, T. C. (1984). Drinking patterns among student nurses. *International Journal of the Addictions, 19*(5), 577–583.

Haberman, P. W. (1987). Alcohol use and alcoholism among motor vehicle driver fatalities. *International Journal of the Addictions, 22*(11), 1119–1128.

Hafen, B. Q., Thygerson, A. L., & Frandsen, K. T. (1988). *Behavioral guidelines for health and wellness.* Englewood, CO: Morton.

Hart, H. (1923). What is a social problem? *American Journal of Sociology, 29,* 350.

Hilton, M. E. (1987). *Regional diversity of U.S. drinking patterns.* Berkeley, CA: Institute of Epidemiology and Behavioral Science.

Hoeger, W. W. K. (1989). *Principles and labs for physical fitness and wellness* (2nd ed.). Englewood, CO: Morton.

Hogan, P. I., & Santomier, J. P. (1982). Stress and leisure activities. *Leisure Information Quarterly, 8*(4), 7–8.

Hutchinson, S. (1988). Self-care and job stress. *Image, 19,* 192–196.

Insel, P. M., & Moos, R. H. (1974). *Health and the social environment.* Lexington, MA: D. C. Heath.

Jensen, M. A. (1987). Understanding addictive behaviors: Implications for health promotion programming. *American Journal of Health Promotion, 1*(3), 48–57.

Johnson, K. G., Abbey, J., Schebel, R., & Weitman, M. (1972). Survey of adolescent drug use: Social and environmental factors. *American Journal of Public Health, 2*(3), 164–170.

Knipping, P., & Maultsby, M. (1977). Rational self-counseling: Primary prevention for alcohol abuse. *Alcohol Health and Research World, 2*(1), 31–35.

Knox, J. M. (1988). *Drinking, driving and drugs.* New York: Chelsea House Publishers.

Levy, S. (1983). *Managing the drugs in your life: A personal guide to the responsible use of drugs, alcohol, medicine.* New York: McGraw Hill.

Macrae, J. (1988). *Therapeutic touch: A practical guide.* New York: Knopf.

McArdle, W. D., Katch, F. I., & Katch, V. L. (1986). *Exercise physiology: Energy, nutrition, and human performance* (2nd ed.). Philadelphia, PA: Lea & Febiger.

National Institute on Drug Abuse. (1980). The developmental approach to preventing problem dependencies. In H. S. Glenn & J. W. Warner (Eds.), *Community-based prevention specialist: Participant manual* (pp. 133–153). Rockville, MD: NIDA.

Nurse, A. R. (1982). The role of alcohol in relationship to intimacy. *Journal of Psychoactive Drugs, 14*(1–2), 159–162.

O'Leary, D. E., O'Leary, M. R., & Donovan, D. M. (1976). Social skills acquisition and psychosocial development of alcoholics: A review. *Addictive Behaviors, 1*(2), 111–120.

Pennsylvania Governor's Council on Drug and Alcohol Abuse. (1977). In J. D'Angelli, & J. Weener, *Communication and parenting skills.* University Park, PA: Governor's Council on Drug and Alcohol Abuse.

Pennsylvania State University, Addictions Prevention Laboratory. (1977). *Instructor's manual in developing life skills through guidance in the classroom* (pp. 147–148). University Park, PA: Pennsylvania State University. (Funded by Governor's Council on Drug and Alcohol Abuse for the Commonwealth of Pennsylvania.)

Pinto, R. P., Abrams, D. B., Monti, P. M., & Jacobus, S. I. (1987). Nicotine dependence and likelihood of quitting smoking. *Addictive Behaviors, 12*(4), 371–374.

Pollock, S. E., & Duffy, M. E. (1990). The Health-Related Hardiness Scale: Development and psychometric analysis. *Nursing Research, 39*(4), 218–222.

Prendergast, T. J., Jr. (1974). Family characteristics associated with marijuana use among adolescents. *International Journal of the Addictions, 9,* 827–839.

Rosenbaum, R. H., & Friedman, M. (1974). *Type A behavior and the heart.* New York: Knopf, Inc.

Sanchez-Craig, M. (1985). Patterns of alcohol use associated with self-identified problem drinking. *American Journal of Public Health, 75*(2), 178–180.

Santomier, J. P. (1989). Exercise: A neglected component in treatment. *Addictions Nursing Network, 1*(4), 10–44.

Schaps, E., Cohen, A. Y., & Resnik, H. S. (Eds.). (1975). *Balancing head and heart: Sensible ideas for the prevention of drug and alcohol abuse* (books 1–2). Lafayette, CA: Prevention Materials Institute Press.

Scott, C., & Hawk, J. (1986). *Heal thyself: The health of health care professionals.* New York: Brunner/Mazel.

Segall, M. E., & Wynd, C. A. (1990). Health conception, health locus of control, and power as predictors of smoking behavior change. *American Journal of Health Promotion, 4*(5), 338–344.

Siegel, R. K. (1982). Cocaine and sexual dysfunction: The course of mama coca. *Journal of Psychoactive Drugs, 14*(1–2), 17–74.

Solomon, K. E., & Annis, H. M. (1990). Outcome and efficacy expectancy in the prediction of post-treatment drinking behavior. *British Journal of Addiction, 85*, 659–665.

Stein, J. A., Newcomb, M. D., & Bentler, P. M. (1987). Personality and drug use: Reciprocal effects across four years. *Personality and Individual Differences, 8*(3), 419–430.

Wechsler, H., & Rohman, M. E. (1981). Patterns of drug use among New England college students. *American Journal of Drug and Alcohol Abuse, 8*(1), 27–37.

YWCA of the USA. (1983). *Women as preventors: An adult-teen partnership.* New York: YWCA Press.

MODULE I.3
ASSESSMENT OF THE ADULT CLIENT FOR DRUG AND ALCOHOL USE

Phyllis Lisanti, PhD, RN

Madeline A. Naegle, PhD, RN, FAAN
Project Director
Janet S. D'Arcangelo, MA, RN, C
Project Coordinator

Project SAEN
SUBSTANCE ABUSE
EDUCATION IN NURSING

CONTENT OUTLINE

I. Components of the Nursing Assessment with Particular Relevance to Alcohol and Drug Use in the Adult Client

    A. Signs Commonly Observed in Association with Drug Use and Abuse

    B. Signs and Symptoms Suggesting Dependence on Drugs and/or Alcohol

II. History-Taking and Client Evaluation Related to Drug and Alcohol Use

    A. Use of Direct Communication Techniques to Elicit Relevant Drug-Taking Information

    B. Use of Observation and Inspection Skills to Corroborate Client History

    C. Identification of Family and Significant Others as Important Informants

    D. Identification of Health Implications of Drug Use by Family Members and Significant Others, Including Seropositive Status

III. Drug-Using Patterns

    A. Classifications

        1. Social use

        2. Maladaptive use or abuse

        3. Interactional drug-using patterns

        4. Drug misuse

        5. Dependence

    B. Impact on Patterns of Human Relationships

IV. Nursing Diagnoses Associated with Substance Abuse

    A. Biological Responses

    B. Cognitive Responses

C. Psychosocial Responses

D. Spiritual Responses

V. Communication Skills Basic to Assessment

   A. Client Behaviors Which Influence History-Taking

   B. Facilitating Self-Disclosure

   C. Establishing a Short-Term Trusting Relationship

   D. Presenting Diagnoses

   E. Use of Findings to Educate Clients and Families

CONTENTS

I. **COMPONENTS OF THE NURSING ASSESSMENT WITH PARTICULAR RELEVANCE TO ALCOHOL AND DRUG USE IN THE ADULT CLIENT**

    A. **Observed Signs Commonly Associated with Drug Use and Abuse**

       1. General survey: Physical signs/objectives.

         a. Neglect of health and personal care.

           (1) Undernutrition or malnourishment.

           (2) Dental caries, bad breath, gingivitis.

           (3) Poor muscle tone.

           (4) Trench mouth.

           (5) Unkempt appearance.

         b. Specific route of administration: *Inhalation.*

           (1) Destruction of nasal mucosa; cartilaginous structures.

           (2) Irritation of nasal mucosa and bleeding.

           (3) Depression of respiration.

           (4) Seizure activity.

         c. Specific route of administration: *Intravenous.*

           (1) Contact dermatitis.

           (2) Scarring of veins—needlemarks.

           (3) Skin infections, cellulitis.

           (4) Abscesses, ululations.

           (5) Sepsis.

           (6) Enlarged lymph nodes.

           (7) Hematomas, ecchymosis.

         d. Specific route of administration: *Ingestion.*

           (1) Presence of acne rosacea.

           (2) Spider angioma.

           (3) Palmar erythema.

           (4) Enlarged abdomen, ascites.

           (5) Alcohol on breath.

           (6) Nystagmus.

e. Cardiovascular.

   (1) Heart rate and systolic blood pressure rise with hallucinogen.

   (2) Chest pains, myocardial ischemia.

   (3) Dysrhythmias, palpitation.

f. Pulmonary.

   (1) Chronic cough producing brown to black sputum.

   (2) Inflamed throat.

   (3) Rapid, deep respirations or respiratory depressions.

   (4) Shortness of breath.

   (5) Crackles and wheezes.

g. Neuromuscular.

   (1) Dilated pupils or pinpoint pupils.

   (2) Elevated temperature—hyperthermia.

   (3) Generalized seizures—coma.

   (4) Loss of sense of smell and taste.

   (5) Tremors.

   (6) Slurred speech, garbled speech.

   (7) Lack of coordination.

   (8) Flaccid muscles.

   (9) Hyperactive reflexes.

   (10) Extremity weakness.

h. Genitourinary.

   (1) Decreased urine production.

   (2) Frequent episodes of sexually transmitted diseases (STD's).

i. Integumentary.

   (1) Sweating, pale, clammy.

   (2) Flushing.

   (3) Jaundice.

   (4) Reddened eyes.

   (5) Acne.

   (6) Burned skin.

   (7) Loss of eyelashes and eyebrows.

   (8) Dehydration, dry skin.

      j. Gastrointestinal.

         (1) Nausea.

         (2) Vomiting.

         (3) Constipation or diarrhea.

         (4) Pain.

2. Subjective signs.

    a. Relaxation, decreased tension.

    b. Release of inhibition.

    c. Euphoria/grandiosity.

    d. Headache.

    e. Giddiness.

    f. Fatigue.

    g. Increased sense of strength/illusions of strength.

    h. Stimulation.

    i. Decreased sensory awareness.

    j. Depression.

    k. Wakefulness, sleep disturbance.

    l. Suppression of appetite.

    m. Aggressive, violent, and/or combative behavior.

    n. Paranoia, anxiety, panic.

    o. Altered perceptions.

    p. Dizziness.

    q. Failure in judgment, emotional lability.

    r. Analgesia.

    s. Sedation, sleepiness, drowsiness.

    t. Dysphagia.

    u. Memory loss.

    v. Hallucinations.

    w. Heightened sexual desire (usually associated with early use).

    x. Loss of sexual desires, delayed orgasm, anorgasmia, erectile dysfunction, retarded ejaculation (usually associated with continued use).

    y. Unexplained mood changes and mood swings.

    z. Personality changes.

    aa. Changes in intellectual function.

bb. Sexual promiscuity.

cc. Dishonesty.

dd. Unreliability in social and job performance.

ee. Anorexia.

B. Signs and Symptoms Suggesting Dependence on Drugs and/or Alcohol

1. Trauma secondary to falls, auto accidents, fights.

2. Fatigue.

3. Insomnia.

4. Headaches.

5. Vague physical complaints.

6. Sexual dysfunction, loss of libido, erectile dysfunction.

7. Anorexia—weight loss.

8. Seizure disorders and convulsions.

9. Appears older than stated age.

10. Problems in areas of life function.

    a. Frequent job changes.

    b. Marital conflict, separation, and/or divorce.

    c. Work-related accidents, lateness, absenteeism.

    d. Legal problems, including arrest.

    e. Social isolation, estrangement from friends and/or family.

11. Driving while intoxicated (more than one incident suggests dependence).

12. Leisure activities that involve alcohol and/or other drugs.

13. Financial problems, including those related to spending for drugs.

II. HISTORY-TAKING AND CLIENT EVALUATION RELATED TO DRUG AND ALCOHOL USE

A. Use of Direct Communication Techniques to Elicit Relevant Drug-Taking Information

1. Commonly used screening tools.

   a. C A G E: Four-question screening tool for alcoholism which can be integrated into the interview.

   b. M A S T (Michigan Alcohol Screening Test).

      (1) 25 questions about drinking behavior.

      (2) Brief M A S T available.

   c. **D A S T** (Drug Abuse Screening Test): 28 questions about drug use and related behavior.

   d. **Trauma Scale:** Five questions about history of trauma since 18th birthday.

2. Alternate approach to screening tools:

The following questions about alcohol/drug use may be incorporated into a routine, non-threatening inquiry about other habits such as smoking or coffee drinking:

   a. *How often do you use alcohol/drugs?*

     (1) Include names of groups; i.e., over-the-counter drugs (OTC's), prescription drugs, street drugs.

   b. *How much do you usually use?*

     (1) Give amounts: number of joints, ounces per glass, number of pills at what dosage.

   c. *Have you ever used alcohol/drugs more than you use them now?*

     (1) *When?*

     (2) *Under what circumstances did you use drugs more heavily?*

B. Use of Observation and Inspection Skills to Corroborate Client History

1. See Sections I.A and I.B (above) for signs and symptoms associated with or suggesting drug or alcohol use and/or abuse. These signs and symptoms can corroborate information from interview/screening tools.

2. Body language: Signs of discomfort or denial.

   a. Uncomfortable posture.

   b. Avoiding eye contact.

   c. Long pauses before answering.

3. Frank denial.

C. Identification of Family and Significant Others as Important Informants

1. Confidentiality may be an overriding issue with illicit drug use or under age alcohol use.

2. Denial compromises the informant's accurate reporting.

D. Identification of Health Implications of Drug Use by Family Members and Significant Others, Including Seropositive Status

1. Physical health problems.

   a. Malnutrition.

   b. Dental caries.

     c. Respiratory infections.

     d. Skin infections.

     e. Hepatitis and/or cirrhosis.

     f. Endocarditis.

     g. HIV, ARC, AIDS.

2. Psychosocial.

     a. Antisocial behavior.

     b. Aggression, hostility.

     c. Depression.

     d. Fear, anxiety, panic.

     e. Self-destruction behaviors.

     f. Mental deterioration.

III. DRUG-USING PATTERNS

A. Classifications

1. *Social Use:* A psychoactive drug or substance is used in a social setting to join in with others who are enjoying themselves. The drug or substance enables the individual to express feelings more easily.

2. *Maladaptive use or abuse:* A psychoactive drug or substance is being abused if it is regularly taken indiscriminately in excessive quantities to the extent that physiological, psychological, or social functioning is impaired. The substance is used:

     a. Recurrently in situations in which use is physically hazardous (e.g., driving while intoxicated).

     b. Use continues despite knowledge of having persistent or recurrent social, occupational, psychosocial, or physical problems that are caused or exacerbated by use of the substance.

3. *Interactional drug-using patterns:* Drugs are used by the individual with personality problems who finds the effects of drugs assist with adjustment to personality deficiencies. The euphoria perceived or other experienced drug effect provides an immediate sense of gratification and promotes more positive feelings about the self.

4. *Drug misuse:* A drug or substance is misused if taken indiscriminately, whether as prescribed or self-administered as an over-the-counter medication, or taken improperly by a client who does not clearly understand the correct use and dosage.

5. *Dependence:* On a psychoactive drug, includes both psychological and physiological dependence and is diagnosed when three or more of the following symptoms are present for at least a month at a time:

a. Substance often taken in larger amounts or over a longer period than the person intended.

b. Persistent desire or one or more unsuccessful efforts to cut down or control substance use.

c. A great deal of time spent in activities necessary to get the substance (e.g., theft), taking the substance (e.g., chain smoking), or recovering from its effects.

d. Frequent intoxication or withdrawal symptoms when expected to fulfill major role obligations at work, school, or home (e.g., does not go to work because hung over, goes to school or work "high," intoxicated while taking care of his or her children), or when substance use is physically hazardous (e.g., drives when intoxicated).

e. Important social, occupational, or recreational activities given up or reduced because of substance use.

f. Continued substance use despite knowledge of having a persistent or recurrent social, psychological, or physical problem that is caused or exacerbated by the use of the substance (e.g., keeps using heroin despite family arguments about it, cocaine-induced depression, or having an ulcer made worse by drinking).

g. Marked tolerance: Need for markedly increased amounts of the substance (i.e., at least 50% increase) in order to achieve intoxication or desired effect, or markedly diminished effect with continued use of the same amount.

Note: The following items may not apply to cannabis, hallucinogens, or phencyclidine (PCP):

h. Characteristic withdrawal symptoms (see specific withdrawal syndromes under: Psychoactive substance-induced organic mental disorders in American Psychiatric Association (1987), *DSM-III-R*. Washington, DC: Author).

i. Substance often taken to relieve or avoid withdrawal symptoms.

j. Some symptoms of the disturbance have persisted for at least one month, or have occurred repeatedly over a longer period of time.

B. Impact on Patterns of Human Relationships

1. Impact on socialization.

   a. Jobs are lost or job performance is poor.

   b. Quality of family life deteriorates; families become dysfunctional or estranged.

   c. Children are neglected or abused.

   d. Dependent persons are at risk for victimization.

2. Impact on family.

   a. Substance abuse involves all aspects of relationship and life with spouse, including anger and resentment of spouse.

Module I.3

b. Children of substance abusers have problems with trust, lack of self-esteem, and conflicts over dependency/independence.

c. Emotional and physical abuse and/or neglect of children occur.

d. Family conflict and violence are common.

e. Children are at risk for sexual abuse.

f. Role reversal of children often occurs.

g. Children lack good role models.

h. Children have altered relationships with peers.

i. Children may manifest poor academic performance.

j. Children of substance abusers are at greater risk for becoming substance abusers themselves.

IV. NURSING DIAGNOSES ASSOCIATED WITH SUBSTANCE ABUSE

A. Biological Responses

1. Alteration in nutrition: Less than body requirements.
2. Self-care deficit.
3. Sensory-perceptual alteration.
4. Potential for injury.
5. Sleep pattern disturbance.
6. Potential for infection.
7. Sexual dysfunction.
8. Alteration in comfort: Pain.
9. Altered growth and development: Biological.
10. Activity intolerance.
11. Mobility: Impaired physical.
12. Substance withdrawal.
13. Fluid volume excess.

B. Cognitive Responses

1. Knowledge deficit.
2. Alteration in thought processes.
3. Noncompliance.

C. Psychosocial Responses

1. Impaired communication.
2. Ineffective individual coping.
3. Alteration in self-concept.

    4. Anxiety.

    5. Fear.

    6. Social isolation.

    7. Dysfunctional family process.

    8. Altered parenting.

    9. Altered growth and development: Psychosocial.

  10. Potential for violence.

D. Spiritual Responses

    1. Spiritual distress.

    2. Powerlessness.

    3. Hopelessness.

    4. Grief.

V. COMMUNICATION SKILLS BASIC TO ASSESSMENT

A. Client Behaviors Which Influence History-Taking

    1. Manipulation.

    2. Denial.

    3. Impulsiveness.

    4. Avoidance.

    5. Underreporting or minimizing substance use and giving inaccurate information.

    6. Accuracy of self-report may be affected by level of sobriety.

    7. Test data are obtained when asking about specific use on a specific day.

B. Facilitating Self-Disclosure

    1. Self-awareness of nurse.

    2. Ability to self-disclose on part of nurse.

    3. Openness, honesty.

    4. Empathy.

    5. Heightened awareness and perceptions of nurse.

    6. Nonjudgmental attitude.

    7. Facilitate privacy.

    8. Avoid or minimize interruptions.

    9. Communicate caring.

10. Provide client support.

11. Explanations should be concrete, direct, and specific.

C. Establishing a Short-Term Trusting Relationship

1. Empathy.

2. Warmth.

3. Respect.

4. Genuineness.

5. Nonjudgmental attitude.

6. Concreteness.

7. Confrontation.

8. Immediacy of relationship.

9. Limit-setting.

10. Caring (Haber, Leech, Scheedy, & Sideleau, 1982).

D. Presenting Diagnoses

1. Empathy.

2. Communicate hope in relation to treatment.

3. Confrontation.

4. Concreteness.

5. Avoid arguments.

6. Acknowledge positive aspects of substance use.

7. Provide learning opportunities.

8. Be realistic.

9. Offer care options.

E. Use of Findings to Educate Clients and Families

1. Provide learning opportunities.

2. Provide role-modeling.

3. Refer client to Twelve Step self-help programs; e.g., Alcoholics Anonymous, Cocaine Anonymous.

4. Refer family members to Twelve Step programs for self-help; e.g., Al-Anon, Alateen.

5. Refer to treatment agencies which specifically address alcohol and drug problems.

6. Introduce notion of HIV testing and counseling as appropriate; refer as necessary.

MODULE I.3
ASSESSMENT OF THE ADULT CLIENT FOR DRUG AND ALCOHOL USE

INSTRUCTOR'S GUIDE

Phyllis Lisanti, PhD, RN

Madeline A. Naegle, PhD, RN, FAAN
Project Director
Janet S. D'Arcangelo, MA, RN, C
Project Coordinator

Project SAEN
SUBSTANCE ABUSE
EDUCATION IN NURSING

CONTENTS

MODULE DESCRIPTION

This module assists the student in the development of beginning knowledge and basic skills in assessing patterns of drug and alcohol use, and their health implications for adult clients.

TIME FRAME

3 hours

PLACEMENT

Fundamentals of Nursing; Adult Health

LEARNER OBJECTIVES

Upon successful completion of this module, the learner will:

1. Perform basic drug and alcohol assessment of the adult client, including a short-form drug and alcohol history.

2. Identify patterns of drug use in the adult client.

3. Identify drug-using modes and patterns and their effects on health.

4. Propose nursing diagnoses, related to alcohol and drug use, based on data gathered.

RECOMMENDED READINGS

FACULTY READINGS

Brown, S. A., Christiansen, B. A., & Goldman, M. S. (1987). Alcohol expectancy questionnaire: An instrument for assessment and adult alcohol expectancies. *Journal of Studies on Alcohol, 48*(5), 483–491.

Cohen, S., & Gallant, D. M. (1981). Diagnosis of drug and alcohol abuse. *Medical Monograph Series, 1*(Serial No. 6).

Gallant, D. (1987). *Alcoholism: A guide to diagnostic intervention and treatment.* New York: W. W. Norton & Co.

Schuckit, M. (1979). *Drug and alcohol abuse: A clinical guide to diagnosis and treatment.* New York: Plenum Press.

STUDENT READINGS

American Nurses' Association, Drugs and Alcohol Nursing Association, & National Nurses Society on Addictions. (1987). *The care of clients with addictions: Dimensions of nursing practice.* Kansas City, MO: Author.

American Nurses' Association & National Nurses Society on Addictions. (1988). *Standards of addictions nursing practice with selected diagnoses and criteria.* Kansas City, MO: Author.

Babb, D., & Jenkins, B. (1990). Action stat!: Alcohol withdrawal syndrome. *Nursing, 20*(10), 33.

Burgess, A. (1990). *Psychiatric Nursing* (5th ed., pp. 634–698). Norwalk: Appleton & Lange.

Cohn, L. (1982). The hidden diagnosis. *American Journal of Nursing, 82,* 1862–1864.

Dubiee, D. (1990). Action stat!: Cocaine overdose. *Nursing, 20*(3), 33.

Podrosky, D. L., & Sexton, D. L. (1988). Nurses' reaction to difficult patients. *Image, 26,* 16–20.

Potter, P., & Perry, A. (1989). *Fundamentals of nursing concepts, process and practice* (2nd ed., pp. 1323–1343). St. Louis, MO: C. V. Mosby.

Povenmire, K., & House, M. A. (1990). Recognizing the cocaine addict. *Nursing, 20*(5), 46–48.

Zahourek, R. (1986). Identification of the alcoholic in the acute care setting. *Critical Care Quarterly, 8*(4), 1–10.

RECOMMENDED AUDIOVISUAL
AND
OTHER RESOURCES

MODELS, POSTERS, CHARTS

Materials for a wide variety of purposes are available through the following catalogs:

1. **Health Edco**

   A Division of WRS Groups, Inc.
   P.O. Box 21207
   Waco, Texas 76702-1207
   Telephone: 1-800-433-2677

2. **Anatomical Chart Company**

   8221 North Kimball
   Skokie, Illinois 60076
   Telephone: 1-800-621-7500

3. **Hazelden Educational Materials**

   Pleasant Valley Road
   P.O. Box 176
   Center City, Minnesota 55012-0176

VIDEOS

Videos featuring the assessment process:

1. **Drug Profiles: The Physical and Mental Aspects**

   The extent of the substance abuse problem makes it more important than ever that concerned people learn how to recognize physical symptoms of drug abuse and understand the long- and short-term effects of drugs. The film provides detailed information about 10 drugs of abuse: cocaine, heroin, methaqualone, alcohol, marijuana, barbiturates, amphetamines, tranquilizers, PCP, and LSD. This information can lead to counseling help for drug users and can influence the decisions of those who are not yet committed to the "recreational" use of drugs.

28 minutes. Available from AIMS Media, 6901 Woodley Avenue, Van Nuys, California 91406-4878. Phone: 1-800-267-2467 or (818) 785-4111. #9787, rental ($75) or purchase ($395).

2. **Recovery Starts with Us**

Designed for staff development, this video dramatically illustrates eight diagnostic situations. It addresses the problems of denial, hostility, and rationalization as well as other typical behaviors which may occur during assessment interviews. Co-dependency and the roles of significant others are also portrayed and analyzed. 33 minutes. Available from New York State Council on Alcoholism, Film Library, 155 Washington Avenue, Albany, New York 12210. Telephone: (518) 432-8281 or 1-800-252-2557.

OVERHEAD MASTERS

MODULE I.3 ASSESSMENT OF THE ADULT CLIENT FOR DRUG AND ALCOHOL USE

1. Steps in Early Identification
2. Addictions Nursing Diagnoses—Biological Responses
3. Addictions Nursing Diagnoses—Cognitive Responses
4. Addictions Nursing Diagnoses—Psychosocial Responses
5. Addictions Nursing Diagnoses—Spiritual Responses
6. Nursing Diagnostic Class—Substance Abuse
7. Medical Diagnostic Class—Psychoactive Substance Abuse Disorders
8. C A G E Screening Tool
9. M A S T (9A, 9B)
10. Brief M A S T
11. D A S T (11A, 11B)
12. Trauma Scale Screening Tool
13. Short Drug and Alcohol History (13A, 13B, 13C)
14. Laboratory Screening
15. Laboratory Values That May Be Abnormal in Alcoholics
16. The SMA-20 and C.B.C. in Alcoholism
17. Blood Alcohol Level (BAL/BAC)
18. Urine Screening
19. Decision Tree for Primary Care Alcohol Screening
20. Sample Referral Form

STEPS IN EARLY IDENTIFICATION

- Take careful routine history.
- Know early behavioral and physical signs.
- Know lab values.
- Know high-risk populations.
- Know addictive diseases and effects on family.
- Learn community resources and necessity of referrals.

ADDICTIONS NURSING DIAGNOSES—BIOLOGICAL RESPONSES

1. Alteration in nutrition: Less than body requirement.
2. Self-care deficit.
3. Sensory-perceptual alteration.
4. Potential for injury.
5. Sleep pattern disturbance.
6. Potential for infection.
7. Sexual dysfunction.
8. Alteration in comfort: Pain.
9. Altered growth and development: Biological.
10. Activity intolerance.
11. Mobility: Impaired physical.
12. Substance withdrawal.
13. Fluid volume excess.

ADDICTION NURSING DIAGNOSES—COGNITIVE RESPONSES

1. Knowledge deficit related to:
   - Learning needs.
   - Agitation.
   - Cognitive distortion.
2. Alteration in thought processes.
3. Noncompliance.

ADDICTIONS NURSING
DIAGNOSES—PSYCHOSOCIAL RESPONSES

1. Impaired communication.

2. Ineffective individual coping.

3. Alteration in self-concept related to:

   - Body image.

   - Self-esteem.

   - Role performance.

   - Personal identity.

4. Anxiety.

5. Fear.

6. Social isolation.

7. Dysfunctional family process.

8. Altered parenting.

9. Altered growth and development: Psychosocial.

10. Potential for violence.

ADDICTIONS NURSING DIAGNOSES—SPIRITUAL RESPONSES

1. Spiritual distress.
2. Powerlessness.
3. Hopelessness.
4. Grief.

NURSING DIAGNOSTIC CLASS—SUBSTANCE ABUSE

Related Nursing Diagnoses (NANDA):

1. Anxiety.
2. Ineffective individual coping.
3. Impaired adjustment.
4. Impaired social interaction.
5. Potential for injury.
6. Disturbances in self-concept.
7. Potential for violence.
8. Alteration in thought process.
9. Sleep pattern disturbance.
10. Sensory-perceptual alteration.

MEDICAL DIAGNOSTIC CLASS—PSYCHOACTIVE SUBSTANCE ABUSE DISORDERS

Related Medical Diagnoses (DSM-IIIR):

1. Alcohol intoxication.
2. Alcohol withdrawal.
3. Alcohol withdrawal delirium.
4. Alcohol hallucinosis.
5. Barbiturate or similarly acting sedative or hypnotic intoxication.
6. Barbiturate or similarly acting sedative or hypnotic withdrawal.
7. Opioid intoxication.
8. Opioid withdrawal.
9. Cocaine intoxication.
10. Cocaine withdrawal.
11. Amphetamine or similarly acting sympathomimetic intoxication.
12. Amphetamine or similarly acting sympathomimetic withdrawal.
13. Phencyclidine or similarly acting arylcyclohexylamine intoxication.
14. Hallucinogen hallucinosis.
15. Psychoactive substance dependance.

C A G E SCREENING TOOL

1. C—Have you ever felt you ought to *cut down* on your drinking?

2. A—Have people *annoyed* you by criticizing your drinking?

3. G—Have you ever felt bad or *guilty* about your drinking?

4. E—Have you ever had a drink first thing in the morning—*Eye-Opener*—to steady your nerves or get rid of a hangover?

M A S T—MICHIGAN ALCOHOL SCREENING TEST

Points			Yes	No
0		Do you enjoy a drink now and then?	_____	_____
2	1	Do you feel you are a normal drinker? (Normal means you drink less or no more than other people.)	_____	_____
2	2	Have you ever wakened the morning after drinking the night before and found you could not remember part of the evening?	_____	_____
1	3	Does your spouse, parent or other close person ever complain or worry about your drinking?	_____	_____
2	4	Can you stop drinking without a struggle after one or two drinks?	_____	_____
1	5	Do you ever feel guilty about your drinking?	_____	_____
2	6	Do friends or relatives think you are a normal drinker?	_____	_____
2	7	Are you able to stop drinking when you want to?	_____	_____
5	8	Have you ever attended a meeting of AA (Alcoholics Anonymous)?	_____	_____
1	9	Have you gotten into physical fights when drinking?	_____	_____
2	10	Has your drinking ever created problems with your spouse, a parent, or other close relative(s) or person(s)?	_____	_____
2	11	Has your spouse or any family member ever sought help from anyone about your drinking?	_____	_____
2	12	Have you ever lost friends because of your drinking?	_____	_____

M A S T—MICHIGAN ALCOHOL SCREENING TEST

Points			Yes	No
2	13	Have you ever gotten in trouble at work or school because of your drinking?	_____	_____
2	14	Have you ever lost a job because of drinking?	_____	_____
2	15	Have you ever neglected obligations, family, or work for two or more days in a row because of drinking?	_____	_____
1	16	Do you drink before noon fairly often?	_____	_____
2	17	Have you ever been told you have liver trouble (cirrhosis)?	_____	_____
5	18	After heavy drinking have you ever had delirium tremens, the "shakes," seen or heard things that weren't really there?	_____	_____
5	19	Have you ever gone to anyone for help about your drinking?	_____	_____
5	20	Have you ever been in a hospital because of drinking?	_____	_____
2	21	Have you ever been in a psychiatric hospital or psychiatric unit of a general hospital where drinking was part of the reason for hospitalization?	_____	_____
2	22	Have you ever been seen at a psychiatric or mental health clinic or gone to any doctor, social worker, or counselor for help with an emotional problem where drinking was involved?	_____	_____
2	23	Have you ever been arrested for drunk driving, driving while intoxicated, or driving under the influence of alcoholic beverages? If yes, how many times?	_____	_____
2	24	Have you ever been arrested or taken into custody, even for a few hours, because of drunken behavior of any kind? If yes, how many times?	_____	_____

BRIEF M A S T
SHORT MICHIGAN ALCOHOLISM SCREEN TEST
(M A S T)

1. Do you feel you are a normal drinker? (By normal we mean you drink less than or as much as most other people.)   (No)

2. Does your wife, husband, a parent, or other near relative ever worry or complain about your drinking?   (Yes)

3. Do you ever feel guilty about your drinking?   (Yes)

4. Do friends or relatives think you are a normal drinker?   (No)

5. Are you able to stop drinking when you want to?   (No)

6. Have you ever attended a meeting of Alcoholics Anonymous?   (Yes)

7. Has drinking ever created problems between you and your wife, husband, a parent, or other near relative?   (Yes)

D A S T—DRUG ABUSE SCREENING TEST

1. Have you used drugs other than those required for medical reasons?

2. Have you abused prescription drugs?

3. Do you abuse more than one drug at a time?

*4. Can you get through the week without using drugs (other than those required for medical reasons)?

*5. Are you always able to stop using drugs when you want to?

6. Do you abuse drugs on a continuous basis?

*7. Do you try to limit your drug use to certain situations?

8. Have you had "blackouts" or "flashbacks" as a result of drug use?

9. Do you ever feel bad about your drug use?

10. Does your spouse (or parents) ever complain about your involvement with drugs?

11. Do your friends or relatives know or suspect you abuse drugs?

12. Has drug abuse ever created problems between you and your spouse?

13. Has any family member ever sought help for problems related to your drug use?

14. Have you ever lost friends because of your use of drugs?

15. Have you ever neglected your family or missed work because of your use of drugs?

16. Have you ever been in trouble at work because of drug use?

*Items 4, 5, and 7 are scored in the "no" or false direction.

Module I.3—Overhead #11B

D A S T—DRUG ABUSE SCREENING TEST

17. Have you ever lost a job because of drug abuse?

18. Have you gotten into fights when under the influence of drugs?

19. Have you ever been arrested because of unusual behavior while under the influence of drugs?

20. Have you ever been arrested while driving while under the influence of drugs?

21. Have you engaged in illegal activities in order to obtain drugs?

22. Have you ever been arrested for possession of illegal drugs?

23. Have you ever experienced withdrawal symptoms as a result of heavy drug intake?

24. Have you had medical problems as a result of your drug use (e.g., memory loss, hepatitis, convulsions, bleeding, etc.)?

25. Have you ever been in a hospital for medical problems related to your drug use?

26. Have you ever gone to anyone for help with a drug problem?

27. Have you ever been involved in a treatment program specifically related to drug use?

28. Have you been treated as an out-patient for problems related to drug abuse?

From: **Skinner, H. A. (1982). The drug abuse screening test. *Addictive Behaviors, 7(4)*, 363.**

TRAUMA SCALE SCREENING TOOL

Five questions about history of trauma since 18th birthday:

1. Have you had any fractures or dislocations of your bones or joints?

2. Have you ever been injured in a traffic accident?

3. Have you ever injured your head?

4. Have you ever been in an assault or fight (excluding sports)?

5. Have you ever been injured while drinking?

More than one positive response would indicate a probable drinking problem.

SHORT DRUG AND ALCOHOL HISTORY

A. Alcohol (typical day):

1. How much alcohol do you drink in a day? Size of glass? Ounces?

2. Favorite beverage?

3. Pattern, reasons?

4. Intoxicated? How often?

5. Blackouts?

6. Injured self or others?

7. Drinking interfered with job, friendships, spousal relationship, family relationships?

8. Do you or others worry about your drinking (smoking, caffeine use)?

B. Other Drugs:

1. What *medications* do you take?

2. Types?

3. How often?

4. Pattern, reasons?

5. Medication for sleep, pain?

6. Do you smoke? How many cigarettes, packs daily?

7. How many cups of coffee do you drink daily?

SHORT DRUG AND ALCOHOL HISTORY

C. Brief MSE:

   1. **Consciousness:**

      a. Can client describe current situations, out of the ordinary experiences?

   2. **Orientation:**

      a. Date.

      b. Place.

      c. Daily schedule.

   3. **Attention:**

      a. Concentration.

   4. **Perception:**

      a. Hear or see things?

      b. Smell things that are not there?

   5. **Thought content:**

      a. What sorts of things do you think about a lot?

      b. Problems turning off thoughts?

      c. Fears?

   6. **Thought process:**

      a. Thoughts come fast?

      b. Forgetting: Recent events, past events?

SHORT DRUG AND ALCOHOL HISTORY

7. Self-concept:

   a. What sort of person do you think you are?

   b. Strengths, weaknesses?

   c. Satisfaction with self, liking?

8. Moods:

   a. Feelings of unreality.

   b. Depression.

   c. Feelings against self, others.

   d. Loss, grieving.

   e. Feelings of detachment, alienation.

   f. Anxiety, restlessness, nervousness.

9. Physical complaints related to nerves.

10. Recent life events, reactions to same.

11. Coping strategies.

12. Insight, judgment.

LABORATORY SCREENING

Role of laboratory tests in the diagnosis of alcohol abuse:

1. Few tests available.

2. Tests available are of limited value.

3. Screening questions have higher sensitivity than laboratory tests.

4. Negative laboratory results do not rule out a diagnosis of alcohol abuse/dependence.

Screening questions and history provide the most useful data for diagnosis.

Reprinted with permission from Project Adept, David C. Lewis, M.D., Director. Brown University in Medicine and Center for Alcohol and Addiction Studies.

Module I.3—Overhead #15

LABORATORY VALUES THAT MAY BE ABNORMAL IN ALCOHOLICS

Measurement	Normal Range	Alcoholic Range
Gamma-glutamyl/transferase	Male: 15–85 u/L	Increased
	Female: 5–55 u/L	Increased
Alanine aminotransferase	6–36 u/L	Increased
Aspartate aminotransferase	10–40 u/L	Increased
Alkaline phosphatase	13–39 u/L	Increased
Lactate dehydrogenase	60–120 mg/dL	Increased
Bilirubin (total)	0.3–1.0 mg/dL	Increased
Amylase	4.0–25 u/L	Increased
Uric Acid	3.0–7.0 mg/dL	Increased
Triglyceride	40–150 mg/dL	Increased
Cholesterol	120–220 mg/dL	Increased
Mean corpuscular volume	80–94 u^3	Increased
Prothrombin time	11.02–12.5 sec.	Prolonged
Calcium	8.0–10.5 mg/dL	Decreased
Phosphorus	3.0–4.5 mg/dL	Decreased
Magnesium	1.5–2.0 mEq/L	Decreased
Blood area nitrogen	8–25 mg/dL	Decreased
White blood cell count	4,300–10,000 u/L	Decreased
Platelet count	150,000–300,000/nm	Decreased
Hematocrit	Male: 45–52%	Decreased
	Female: 37–48%	Decreased
Glucose	70–110 mg/dL	Decreased/ Increased

THE SMA-20 AND C.B.C. IN ALCOHOLISM

NORMAL RANGE	High	Low
SGOT	40 I.U.	8 I.U.
SGPT	52 I.U.	0 I.U.
LDH	225 I.U.	100 I.U.
WBC	10.8/cmm	4.7/cmm
ALK PHOS	115 I.U.	30 I.U.
RBC	6.1 cmm / 5.4 cmm	4.7 cmm / 4 cmm
MEAN CORPUSCULAR VOLUME	8.4 cmm	$80.U^3$ / $81.U^3$
PLATELETS		150,000
GGTP	38 U/L	9 U/L
TRI-GLYCERIDES	155 mg/dl	30 mg/dl

Of these ten indicators, three are most indicative of an alcoholism diagnosis: GGTP, MCV, SGOT. When all three are elevated, suspect alcoholism.

BLOOD ALCOHOL LEVEL (BAL/BAC)

Blood Alcohol Level

1. Of limited usefulness because of ethanol's relatively rapid elimination rate.

2. Does not predict patient's overall drinking.

3. An important indicator of tolerance to alcohol if:

    a. BAL > 300 mg/dl recorded at any time.

    b. BAL > 100 mg/dl during routine clinical exam.

    c. BAL > 150 mg/dl without evidence of gross neurological impairment.

Rough Correlation between Blood-Alcohol Level and Behavioral/Motor Impairment

Rising Blood–Alcohol Level*	Expected Effect
20–99	Impaired coordination, euphoria.
100–199	Ataxia, decreased mentation, poor judgment, labile mood.
200–299	Marked ataxia and slurred speech, poor judgment, labile mood, nausea and vomiting.
300–399	Respiratory failure, coma, death.

*mg/100 ml blood (mg % or mg/dl).

From: Schuckit, M. (1979). *Drug and alcohol abuse: A clinical guide to diagnosis and treatment.* New York: Plenum Press.

URINE SCREENING

1. Urine toxicology screens are widely used for detecting substance abuse.

    a. Thin layer chromatography is less sensitive for common drugs of abuse.

    b. Immunoassay procedures are more sensitive.

2. Confirmatory tests are necessary to reduce false positives.

3. False positives may occur with certain foods (e.g., poppy seeds) and medication (e.g., decongestants).

4. Substance use may not be detectable in urine screens.

    a. Some drug use may only be detectable for a short time (as little as 12 hours: cocaine, LSD). Benzodiazepines can last up to 24–48 hours after last dose.

    b. Some drug use is not detectable in urine (inhalants).

DECISION THREE FOR PRIMARY CARE ALCOHOL SCREENING

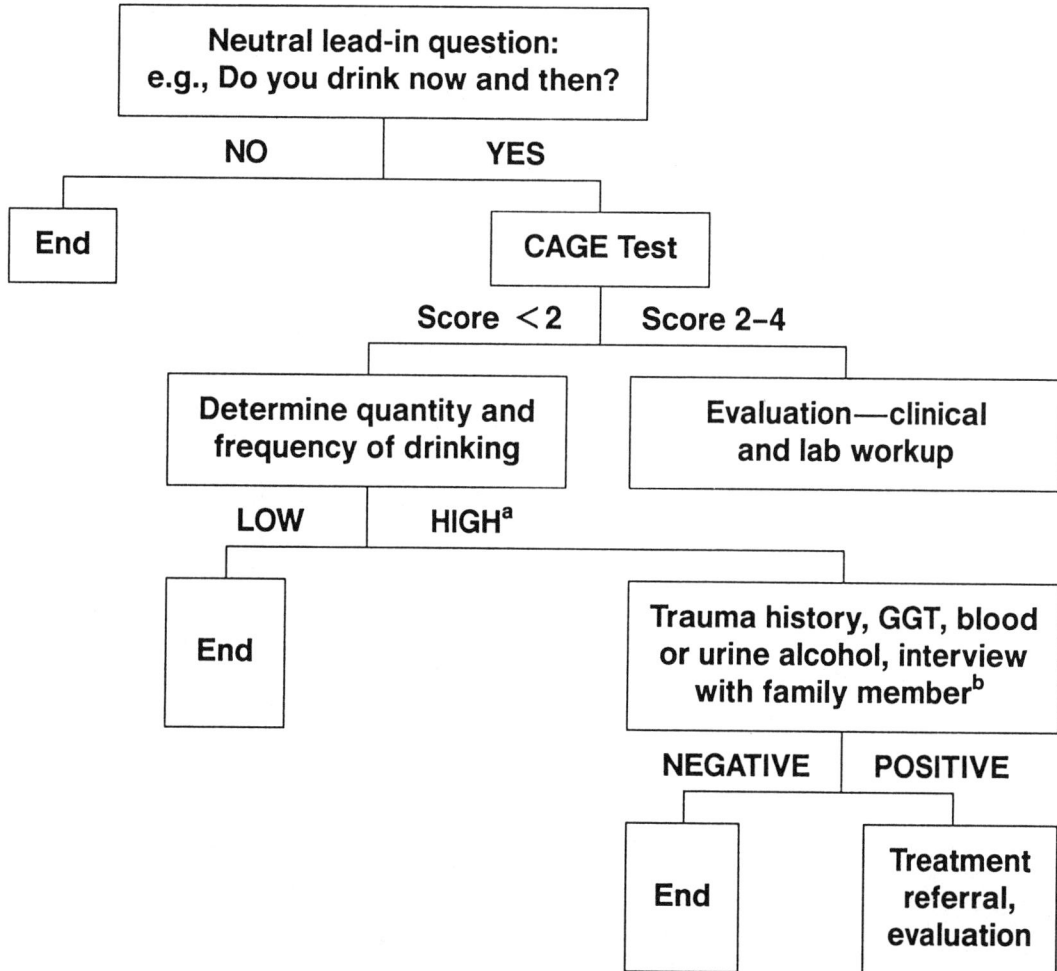

```
              ┌─────────────────────────────────┐
              │   Neutral lead-in question:     │
              │ e.g., Do you drink now and then?│
              └─────────────────────────────────┘
            NO                          YES
      ┌─────────┐                  ┌──────────────┐
      │   End   │                  │  CAGE Test   │
      └─────────┘                  └──────────────┘
                          Score <2           Score 2-4
              ┌─────────────────────────┐  ┌──────────────────────┐
              │ Determine quantity and  │  │  Evaluation—clinical  │
              │  frequency of drinking  │  │    and lab workup     │
              └─────────────────────────┘  └──────────────────────┘
                   LOW         HIGHᵃ
              ┌─────────┐      ┌───────────────────────────────┐
              │         │      │ Trauma history, GGT, blood    │
              │   End   │      │ or urine alcohol, interview   │
              │         │      │ with family memberᵇ           │
              └─────────┘      └───────────────────────────────┘
                              NEGATIVE          POSITIVE
                          ┌─────────┐      ┌──────────────┐
                          │         │      │  Treatment   │
                          │   End   │      │  referral,   │
                          │         │      │  evaluation  │
                          └─────────┘      └──────────────┘
```

SOURCE: Modified from materials produced by NIAAA (1987).

ᵃHigh School consumption is defined as 60 to 80 g of absolute ethanol per day.

ᵇSignificant trauma history would be indicated by a score of two or higher on the five-item trauma scale designed by Israel and colleagues at the Addiction Research Foundation. The questions are asked in the following order: (1) Have you had any fractures or dislocations since you were 18? (2) Have you been injured in a traffic accident? (3) Have you had your head injured? (4) Have you been injured in an assault or fight? (5) Have you been injured after drinking?

SAMPLE REFERRAL FORM

Alcohol and Substance Abuse Intervention Services

INTERVENTION SERVICE PHONE (24 HOUR):

_____

INTERVENTION COORDINATOR NAME:

_____

PHONE:

_____

Referral to Hospital (or Agency) Intervention Service

Patient Name:

_____

Date of Admission:

_____

CRITERIA FOR REFERRAL: (Please check all that apply.)

_____ Evidence of alcohol/drug related problems/dependency.

_____ Patient/family medical history.

_____ Clinical signs of alcohol/drug abuse/dependency elicited upon examination.

Two or more positive responses to the CAGE/Trauma questions:

_____ Have you ever attempted to cut down on your drinking?

_____ Have you ever been annoyed by other people criticizing your drinking?

_____ Have you ever felt guilty about your drinking?

_____ Have you ever taken a morning "eye-opener"?

Since your 18th birthday:

_____   Have you had any fractures or dislocations to your bones or joints?

_____   Have you been injured in a road traffic accident?

_____   Have you injured your head?

_____   Have you been injured in an assault or fight (excluding injuries during sports)?

_____   Have you been injured after drinking?

_____   Hazardous, harmful level of patient's alcohol/drug consumption.

_____   Admission with high BAC and/or Trauma Diagnoses.

_____   Collaborating data, if available

_____

_____

Signature: _____

Date: _____

HANDOUT MASTERS

MODULE I.3 ASSESSMENT OF THE ADULT CLIENT FOR DRUG AND ALCOHOL USE

1. Addictions Nursing Diagnoses (1A, 1B)
2. C A G E Screening Tool
3. Decision Tree for Primary Care Alcohol Screening
4. Screening Tools (C A G E and Trauma Scale)
5. Laboratory Screening: BAL/BAC, Urine Screening (5A, 5B)
6. Laboratory Values That May Be Abnormal in Alcoholics
7. The SMA-20 and C.B.C. in Alcoholism
8. Short Drug and Alcohol History (8A, 8B, 8C)
9. Sample Referral Form

ADDICTIONS NURSING DIAGNOSES

Biological Responses

1. Alteration in nutrition: Less than body requirement.
2. Self-care deficit.
3. Sensory-perceptual alteration.
4. Potential for injury.
5. Sleep pattern disturbance.
6. Potential for infection.
7. Sexual dysfunction.
8. Alteration in comfort: Pain.
9. Altered growth and development: Biological.
10. Activity intolerance.
11. Mobility: Impaired physical.
12. Substance withdrawal.
13. Fluid volume excess.

Cognitive Responses

1. Knowledge deficit related to:
   a. Learning needs.
   b. Agitation.
   c. Cognitive distortion.
2. Alteration in thought processes.
3. Noncompliance.

Module I.3—Handout #1B

ADDICTIONS NURSING DIAGNOSES

Psychosocial Responses

1. Impaired communication.
2. Ineffective individual coping.
3. Alteration in self-concept related to:
   a. Body image.
   b. Self-esteem.
   c. Role performance.
   d. Personal identity.
4. Anxiety.
5. Fear.
6. Social isolation.
7. Dysfunctional family process.
8. Altered parenting.
9. Altered growth and development: Psychosocial.
10. Potential for violence.

Spiritual Responses

1. Spiritual distress.
2. Powerlessness.
3. Hopelessness.
4. Grief.

C A G E SCREENING TOOL

1. **C**—Have you ever felt you ought to *cut down* on your drinking?

2. **A**—Have people *annoyed* you by criticizing your drinking?

3. **G**—Have you ever felt bad or *guilty* about your drinking?

4. **E**—Have you ever had a drink first thing in the morning—an *Eye-Opener*—to steady your nerves or get rid of a hangover?

Module I.3—Handout #3

DECISION THREE
FOR PRIMARY CARE ALCOHOL SCREENING

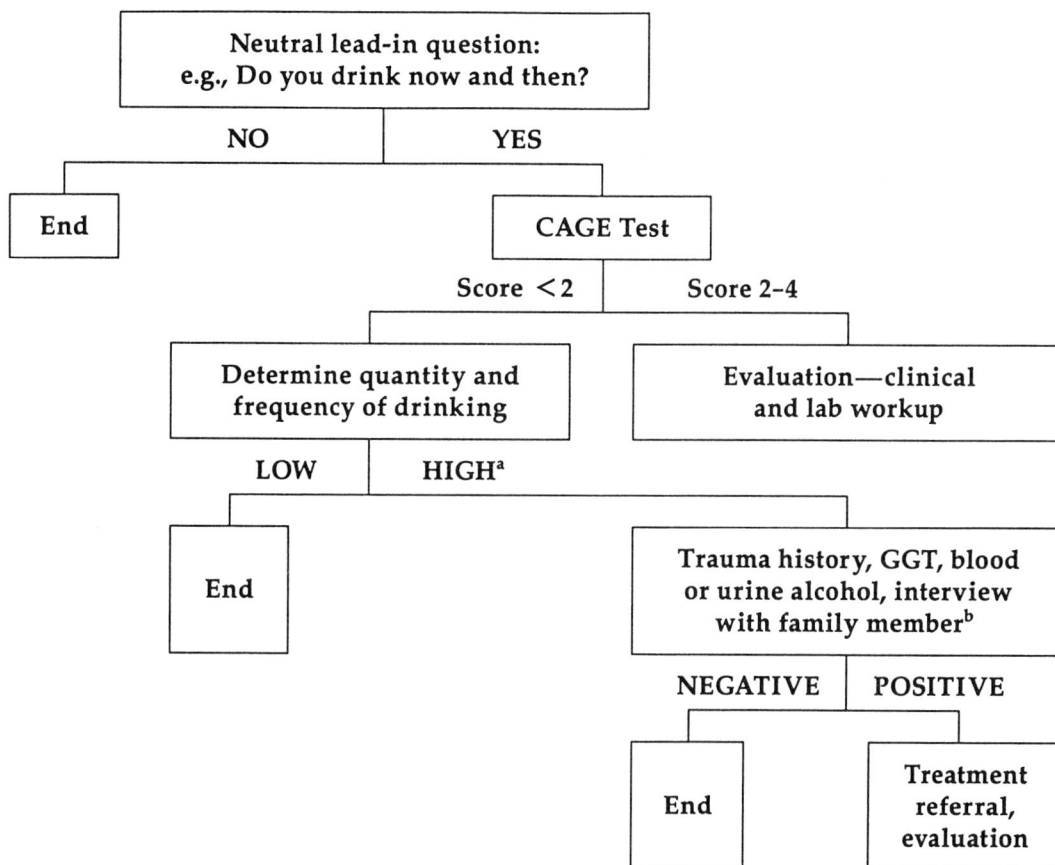

```
                    ┌─────────────────────────────────┐
                    │   Neutral lead-in question:      │
                    │ e.g., Do you drink now and then? │
                    └─────────────────────────────────┘
              NO                              YES
        ┌─────────┐                    ┌──────────────┐
        │   End   │                    │  CAGE Test   │
        └─────────┘                    └──────────────┘
                          Score <2              Score 2-4
              ┌───────────────────────┐   ┌──────────────────────┐
              │ Determine quantity and│   │  Evaluation—clinical  │
              │  frequency of drinking│   │    and lab workup     │
              └───────────────────────┘   └──────────────────────┘
                 LOW          HIGHa
              ┌─────────┐
              │   End   │        ┌──────────────────────────┐
              └─────────┘        │ Trauma history, GGT, blood│
                                 │ or urine alcohol, interview│
                                 │ with family memberb        │
                                 └──────────────────────────┘
                                  NEGATIVE       POSITIVE
                                 ┌─────────┐   ┌────────────┐
                                 │   End   │   │ Treatment  │
                                 │         │   │ referral,  │
                                 └─────────┘   │ evaluation │
                                               └────────────┘
```

SOURCE: Modified from materials produced by NIAAA (1987).

[a]High School consumption is defined as 60 to 80 g of absolute ethanol per day.

[b]Significant trauma history would be indicated by a score of two or higher on the five-item trauma scale designed by Israel and colleagues at the Addiction Research Foundation. The questions are asked in the following order: (1) Have you had any fractures or dislocations since you were 18? (2) Have you been injured in a traffic accident? (3) Have you had your head injured? (4) Have you been injured in an assault or fight? (5) Have you been injured after drinking?

Module I.3—Handout #4

SCREENING TOOLS (C A G E AND TRAUMA SCALE)

C A G E Screening Tool

1. C—Have you ever felt you ought to *cut down* on your drinking?
2. A—Have people *annoyed* you by criticizing your drinking?
3. G—Have you ever felt bad or *guilty* about your drinking?
4. E—Have you ever had a drink first thing in the morning—an *Eye-Opener*—to steady your nerves or get rid of a hangover?

Trauma Scale Screening Tool

Five questions about history of trauma since 18th birthday:

1. Have you had any fractures or dislocations of your bones or joints?
2. Have you ever been injured in a traffic accident?
3. Have you ever injured your head?
4. Have you ever been in an assault or fight (excluding sports)?
5. Have you ever been injured while driving?

More than one positive response would indicate a probable drinking problem.

Module I.3—Handout #5A

LABORATORY SCREENING

Role of Laboratory Tests in the Diagnosis of Alcohol Abuse

1. Few tests available.

2. Tests available are of limited value.

3. Screening questions have higher sensitivity than laboratory tests.

4. Negative laboratory results do not rule out a diagnosis of alcohol abuse/dependence.

Screening questions and history provide the most useful data for diagnosis.

BAL/BAC

Blood-Alcohol Level

1. Of limited usefulness because of ethanol's relatively rapid elimination rate.

2. Does not predict patient's overall drinking.

3. An important indicator of tolerance to alcohol if:

    (1) BAL > 300 mg/dl recorded at any time.

    (2) BAL > 100 mg/dl during routine clinical exam.

    (3) BAL > 150 mg/dl without evidence of gross neurological impairment.

Reprinted with permission from Project Adept, David C. Lewis, M.D., Director. Brown University in Medicine and Center for Alcohol and Addiction Studies.

LABORATORY SCREENING

Rough Correlation between Blood-Alcohol Level and Behavioral/Motor Impairment

Rising Blood-Alcohol Level°	Expected Effect
20–99	Impaired coordination, euphoria.
100–199	Ataxia, decreased mentation, poor judgment, labile mood.
200–299	Marked ataxia and slurred speech, poor judgment, labile mood, nausea and vomiting.
300–399	Respiratory failure, coma, death.

°mg/100 ml blood (mg % or mg/dl).

Urine Screening

1. Urine toxicology screens are widely used for detecting substance abuse.

   a. Thin layer chromatography is less sensitive for common drugs of abuse.

   b. Immunoassay procedures are more sensitive.

2. Confirmatory tests are necessary to reduce false positives.

3. False positives may occur with certain foods (e.g., poppy seeds) and medication (e.g., decongestants).

4. Substance use may not be detectable in urine screens.

   a. Some drug use may only be detectable for a short time (as little as 12 hours: cocaine, alcohol, LSD). Benzodiazepines can last up to 24–48 hours after last dose.

   b. Some drug use is not detectable in urine (inhalants).

From: Schuckit, M. (1979). *Drug and alcohol abuse: A clinical guide to diagnosis and treatment.* New York: Plenum Press.

Module I.3—Handout #6

LABORATORY VALUES THAT MAY BE ABNORMAL IN ALCOHOLICS

Measurement	Normal Range	Alcoholic Range
Gamma-glutamyl/transferase	Male: 15–85 u/L	Increased
	Female: 5–55 u/L	Increased
Alanine aminotransferase	6–36 u/L	Increased
Aspartate aminotransferase	10–40 u/L	Increased
Alkaline phosphatase	13–39 u/L	Increased
Lactate dehydrogenase	60–120 mg/dL	Increased
Bilirubin (total)	0.3–1.0 mg/dL	Increased
Amylase	4.0–25 u/L	Increased
Uric Acid	3.0–7.0 mg/dL	Increased
Triglyceride	40–150 mg/dL	Increased
Cholesterol	120–220 mg/dL	Increased
Mean corpuscular volume	80–94 u^3	Increased
Prothrombin time	11.02–12.5 seconds	Prolonged
Calcium	8.0–10.5 mg/dL	Decreased
Phosphorus	3.0–4.5 mg/dL	Decreased
Magnesium	1.5–2.0 mEq/L	Decreased
Blood area nitrogen	8–25 mg/dL	Decreased
White blood cell count	4,300–10,000 u/L	Decreased
Platelet count	150,000–300,000/nm	Decreased
Hematocrit	Male: 45–52%	Decreased
	Female: 37–48%	Decreased
Glucose	70–110 mg/dL	Decreased/Increased

THE SMA-20 AND C.B.C. IN ALCOHOLISM

NORMAL RANGE	SGOT	SGPT	LDH	WBC	ALK PHOS	RBC	MEAN CORPUSCULAR VOLUME	PLATELETS	GGTP	TRI-GLYCERIDES
(high)	40 I.U.	52 I.U.	225 I.U.	10.8/cmm	115 I.U.	6.1 cmm / 5.4 cmm	8.4 cmm		38 U/L	155 mg/dl
(low)	8 I.U.	0 I.U.	100 I.U.	4.7/cmm	30 I.U.	4.7 cmm / 4 cmm	80.U³ / 81.U³	150,000	9 U/L	30 mg/dl

Of these ten indicators, three are most indicative of an alcoholism diagnosis: GGTP, MCV, SGOT. When all three are elevated, suspect alcoholism.

Module I.3—Handout #8A

SHORT DRUG AND ALCOHOL HISTORY

A. Alcohol (typical day):

    1. How much alcohol do you drink in a day? Size of glass? Ounces?

    2. Favorite beverage?

    3. Pattern, reasons?

    4. Intoxicated? How often?

    5. Blackouts?

    6. Injured self or others?

    7. Drinking interfered with job, friendships, spousal relationship, family relationships?

    8. Do you or others worry about your drinking (smoking, caffeine use)?

B. Other Drugs:

    1. What *medications* do you take?

    2. Types?

    3. How often?

    4. Pattern, reasons?

    5. Medication for sleep, pain?

    6. Do you smoke? How many cigarettes, packs daily?

    7. How many cups of coffee do you drink daily?

SHORT DRUG AND ALCOHOL HISTORY

C. Brief MSE:

   1. Consciousness:

      a. Can client describe current situations, out of the ordinary experiences?

   2. Orientation:

      a. Date.

      b. Place.

      c. Daily schedule.

   3. Attention:

      a. Concentration.

   4. Perception:

      a. Hear or see things?

      b. Smell things that are not there?

   5. Thought content:

      a. What sorts of things do you think about a lot?

      b. Problems turning off thoughts?

      c. Fears?

   6. Thought process:

      a. Thoughts come fast?

      b. Forgetting: Recent events, past events?

   7. Self-concept:

      a. What sort of person do you think you are?

      b. Strengths, weaknesses?

      c. Satisfaction with self, liking?

Module I.3—Handout #8C

SHORT DRUG AND ALCOHOL HISTORY

8. Moods:
    a. Feelings of unreality.
    b. Depression.
    c. Feelings against self, others.
    d. Loss, grieving.
    e. Feelings of detachment, alienation.
    f. Anxiety, restlessness, nervousness.
9. Physical complaints related to nerves.
10. Recent life events, reactions to same.
11. Coping strategies.
12. Insight, judgment.

SAMPLE REFERRAL FORM

Alcohol and Substance Abuse Intervention Services

INTERVENTION SERVICE PHONE (24 HOUR):

_____

INTERVENTION COORDINATOR NAME:

_____

PHONE:

_____

Referral to Hospital (or Agency) Intervention Service

Patient Name:

_____

Date of Admission:

_____

CRITERIA FOR REFERRAL (Please check all that apply.):

_____ Evidence of alcohol/drug related problems/dependency.

_____ Patient/family medical history.

_____ Clinical signs of alcohol/drug abuse/dependency elicited upon examination.

Two or more positive responses to the CAGE/Trauma questions:

_____ Have you ever attempted to cut down on your drinking?

_____ Have you ever been annoyed by other people criticizing your drinking?

_____ Have you ever felt guilty about your drinking?

_____ Have you ever taken a morning "eye-opener"?

Since your 18th birthday:

_____   Have you had any fractures or dislocations to your bones or joints?

_____   Have you been injured in a road traffic accident?

_____   Have you injured your head?

_____   Have you been injured in an assault or fight (excluding injuries during sports)?

_____   Have you been injured after drinking?

_____   Hazardous, harmful level of patient's alcohol/drug consumption.

_____   Admission with high BAC and/or Trauma Diagnoses.

_____   Collaborating data, if available:

_____

_____

Signature: _____

Date: _____

RECOMMENDED TEACHING STRATEGIES AND SAMPLE ASSIGNMENTS

RECOMMENDED TEACHING STRATEGIES

- Role-playing using simulated client situations
- Dyadic exercises in history-taking with peers or relatives
- Media presentations on history-taking
- Lecture
- Videotaping of history-taking
- Use of case studies to formulate diagnoses

SAMPLE ASSIGNMENTS

Role-Play Teaching Format

1. Role-play a client assessment for substance abuse using one of the assessment tools (MAST, DAST, CAGE).

2. Discussion group regarding comfort, biases, feelings when assessing clients for substance use/abuse.

TEST QUESTIONS AND ANSWERS

TEST QUESTIONS

Instructions: Questions 1–13. Below are a number of case vignettes. Answer the questions following each vignette with the letter indicating the correct choice.

A friend accompanies Mr. Peter Willard to the substance abuse unit of the hospital, where he is to be admitted for detoxification from alcohol.

1. While obtaining a nursing history, the nurse questions Mr. Willard about the amount of alcohol he consumes daily. The nurse can expect that Mr. Willard will most probably answer the question by:

   a. exaggerating the amount.

   b. underestimating the amount.

   c. indicating he does not know the amount.

   d. stating he can't remember.

2. The most important reason for investigating the amount of alcohol Mr. Willard has consumed during the 24–48 hours before admission is to help determine:

   a. how far the disease has progressed.

   b. the degree of severity of withdrawal.

   c. whether the patient will experience delirium tremens.

   d. whether the patient should be considered an alcoholic.

3. The nurse who could probably relate most effectively with Mr. Willard is one who has an attitude of:

   a. morality.

   b. optimism.

   c. acceptance.

   d. indulgence.

4. Mr. Willard could not remember the events of the past weekend, although he had receipts in his pockets from several shops where he made purchases on Saturday. This problem is illustrative of a condition known as:

   a. blackout.

   b. a hangover.

c. a dry drunk syndrome.

d. an alcoholic hallucinosis.

5. After a day of abstinence, Mr. Willard has coarse tremors of the hands, which make it hard for him to feed himself. He asks the nurse how long it will be before his "shakes" go away. On which of the following statements should the nurse base her response?

   a. The tremors can only be relieved by a further intake of alcohol.

   b. The tremors usually disappear after about two days of abstinence.

   c. The tremors may persist for several days or even longer after alcohol intake has stopped.

   d. The tremors are a permanent condition due to irreversible central nervous system damage.

Mrs. Gina Baxter, a 44-year-old homemaker, enters the hospital for treatment of cirrhosis of the liver. She is accompanied by her husband.

6. Most of the information about Mrs. Baxter has come from her husband, who says his wife sees no connection between her liver disorder and her alcohol intake. He reports that she believes she drinks very little and that her family is making something out of nothing. Which of the following defense mechanisms is the patient using?

   a. Denial.

   b. Displacement.

   c. Rationalization.

   d. Reaction formation.

7. Besides her cirrhosis, Mrs. Baxter suffers from numbness, itching, and pain in her extremities and is prone to foot drop. This disorder of the nervous system is termed:

   a. neuralgia.

   b. Bell's palsy.

   c. neurasthenia.

   d. peripheral neuritis.

8. Mrs. Baxter has neurological damage. A precautionary measure is for the nurse to be especially careful when giving nursing care that includes:

   a. cleansing the patient's skin.

   b. massaging the patient's feet.

   c. turning the patient from side to side.

   d. applying heat to the patient's lower legs.

Ms. Alice Choate, 22, is brought in her parents' limousine from a cold-water flat, where she has been living with several other drug addicts, to the emergency room of a psychiatric hospital. Ms. Choate is a known heroin user.

9. In the past, Ms. Choate occasionally used cocaine. For which of the following telltale signs should the nurse look to help detect whether the patient has recently abused this drug?

   a. Red, excoriated nostrils.

   b. Clear, constricted pupils.

   c. White patchy areas on the tongue.

   d. Lumpy abscesses in intramuscular areas.

10. Ms. Choate starts methadone therapy. If Ms. Choate experiences acute toxicity from the methadone, the nurse is most likely to note that the patient displays signs of:

    a. fever.

    b. colitis.

    c. renal shutdown.

    d. respiratory depression.

Ms. Lola Albert, a 36-year-old mother of two children, is brought by ambulance to the emergency room of the hospital after taking an overdose of barbiturates. A male friend arrives a short time later, carrying some of her personal belongings.

11. Ms. Albert went into shock at home and is semi-comatose on admission. If death occurs shortly, the cause of death would most likely be:

    a. kidney failure.

    b. cardiac standstill.

    c. internal hemorrhaging.

    d. respiratory depression.

12. Before her hospitalization, Ms. Albert needed increasingly larger doses of barbiturates to achieve the same euphoric effect she initially realized from their use. From this information, the nurse should plan care while taking into account that Ms. Albert is most probably suffering from a drug:

    a. tolerance.

    b. addiction.

    c. habituation.

    d. dependence.

13. By which of the following symptoms could Ms. Albert probably have been identified as a chronic user of barbiturates in the days before her hospitalization?

    a. Drooling, fainting, and illusions.

    b. Sluggishness, ataxia, and irritability.

    c. Diaphoresis, twitching, and sneezing.

    d. Suspiciousness, tachycardia, and edema.

Module I.3

Instructions: Select the one best answer to the question from the choices given.

14. Which of the following substances is associated with abuse only—that is, physiological dependence is not an established outcome?

    a. Alcohol.

    b. Barbiturates.

    c. Amphetamines.

    d. Cocaine.

15. Which of the following symptoms should the nurse expect to encounter in a client going through alcohol withdrawal?

    a. Slurred speech, ataxia.

    b. Coarse tremors of the hand, general malaise, anxiety.

    c. Hallucinations and seizures.

    d. Cirrhosis of the liver.

16. The main feature of amphetamine withdrawal is:

    a. agitation.

    b. increased heart rate and respirations.

    c. nausea and vomiting.

    d. depressed mood.

17. The initial effect of cocaine on the user is a:

    a. feeling of increased self-confidence and well-being.

    b. clouded sensorium.

    c. heightened sexual drive.

    d. calming drowsiness.

18. Which approach by the nurse to a drug-dependent client would be most useful in an initial interview?

    a. What do you drink?

    b. Which drug do you prefer if you can get it?

    c. Do you use booze, shoot up, or snort?

    d. Do the people around you approve of your self-destructive habits?

19. The message the treatment team gives to the drug-dependent client when breaking through the client's defenses is that:

    a. there is never a valid reason to use the substances of abuse and dependency.

    b. under extreme stress, the client may be forced to use drugs from which he has withdrawn.

    c. the client has been sick and is, therefore, excused for behavior while under the influence of drugs.

    d. the client has hurt himself and others by his drug-dependent behavior.

ANSWER KEY

1. b
2. b
3. c
4. a
5. c
6. a
7. d
8. d
9. a
10. d
11. d
12. a
13. b
14. d
15. b
16. d
17. a
18. b
19. a

BIBLIOGRAPHY

MODULE I.3 ASSESSMENT OF THE ADULT CLIENT FOR DRUG AND ALCOHOL USE

American Nurses' Association, Drug and Alcohol Nursing Association, & National Nurses Society on Addiction. (1987). *The care of clients with addictions: Dimensions of nursing practice.* Kansas City, MO: Author.

American Nurses' Association, & National Nurses Society on Addictions. (1988). *Standards of addictions nursing practice with selected diagnoses and criteria.* Kansas City, MO: Author.

American Psychiatric Association. (1987). *DSM-IIIR.* Washington, DC: Author.

Babb, D., & Jenkins, B. (1990). Action stat!: Alcohol withdrawal syndrome. *Nursing, 20*(10), 33.

Barnes, H. N., Aronson, M. D., & DelBanco, T. L. (1987). *Alcoholism: A guide for the primary care physician.* New York: Springer-Verlag.

Bates, B. (1983). *A guide to physical examination* (3rd ed.). Philadelphia: Lippincott.

Brodsley, L. (1982). Avoiding a crisis: The assessment. *American Journal of Nursing, 82*(12), 1865–1871.

Brown, S. A., Christiansen, B. A., & Goldman, M. S. (1987). Alcohol expectancy questionnaire: An instrument for assessment and adult alcohol expectancies. *Journal of Studies on Alcohol, 48*(5), 483–491.

Burgess, A. (1990). *Psychiatric nursing* (5th ed.). Norwalk: Appleton & Lange.

Cohen, S., & Gallant, D. M. (1981). Diagnosis of drug and alcohol abuse. *Medical Monograph Series, 1*(Serial No. 6).

Cohn, L. (1982). The hidden diagnosis. *American Journal of Nursing, 82,* 1862–1864.

Dubiee, D. (1990). Action stat! Cocaine overdose. *Nursing, 20*(3), 33.

Ewing, J. A. (1978). Recognizing, confronting, and helping the alcoholic. *American Family Physician, 16*(5), 107–114.

Gallant, D. (1987). *Alcoholism: A guide to diagnostic intervention and treatment.* New York: W. W. Norton & Co.

Grimes, J., & Burns, E. (1989). *Health assessment in nursing practice.* Boston: Jones & Bartlett Publishers, Inc.

Haber, J., Priu-Hoskins, P., McMahon, A. L. & Sideleau, B. (1991). *Comprehensive psychiatric nursing* (3rd ed.). New York: McGraw-Hill.

Newton, M., Wulf, B. G., Lindeman, M., & Volcek, M. K. (1986). When the nurse suspects drug abuse. *Plastic Surgery Nursing, 6*(3), 113–115.

Phipps, W., Long, B., & Woods, N. (1987). *Medical-surgical nursing concepts and clinical practice* (3rd ed.). St. Louis, MO: C. V. Mosby Co.

Podrosky, D. L., & Sexton, D. L. (1988). Nurses' reaction to difficult patients. *Images, 26,* 16–20.

Potter, P., & Perry, A. (1989). *Fundamentals of nursing concepts, process, and practice* (2nd ed.). St. Louis, MO: C. V. Mosby.

Povenmire, K., & House, M. A. (1990). Recognizing the cocaine addict. *Nursing, 20*(5), 46–48.

Schuckit, M. (1979). *Drug and alcohol abuse: A clinical guide to diagnosis and treatment.* New York: Plenum Press.

Thompson, J., McFarland, G., Hirsh, J., Tucker, S., & Bowers, A. (1989). *Mosby's manual of clinical nursing* (2nd ed.). St. Louis, MO: C. V. Mosby Co.

Zahourek, R. (1986). Identification of the alcoholic in the acute care setting. *Critical Care Quarterly, 8*(4), 1–10.

MODULE I.4
PHARMACOLOGY

Elizabeth A. Duthie, MA, RN
Janet S. D'Arcangelo, MA, RN, C

Madeline A. Naegle, PhD, RN, FAAN
Project Director
Janet S. D'Arcangelo, MA, RN, C
Project Coordinator

Project SAEN
SUBSTANCE ABUSE
EDUCATION IN NURSING

CONTENT OUTLINE

I.   Introduction

    A. Pharmacotherapeutics Related to Substance Abuse

    B. Issues Relevant to Nursing

II. Common Terms Related to Abuse/Dependency

    A. Habituation

    B. Misuse

    C. Abuse

    D. Dependence

    E. Tolerance

    F. Addiction

    G. Dual Addiction

    H. Mixed Addiction

III. Routes of Administration

IV. Over-the-Counter Drugs

V.   Alcohol

VI. Prescription Drugs

    A. Central Nervous System Depressants

        1. Barbiturates

        2. Non-barbiturate sedatives

        3. Anti-anxiety agents

    B. Central Nervous System Stimulants

        1. Amphetamines

        2. Anorexiants (Anorectics)

    C. Narcotics and Other Controlled Substances

Module I.4

VII. Street and Socially Misused Drugs

    A. CNS Stimulants

    B. Narcotics

    C. Hallucinogens

    D. Volatile Inhalants

    E. Marijuana, Hashish, "Weed," "Hash"

    F. Nicotine

    G. Caffeine

    H. Anabolic Steroids

CONTENTS

I. INTRODUCTION

A. Pharmacotherapeutics Related to Substance Abuse

1. The 1960s brought new hope for psychiatric patients with the introduction of psychotropic medications. Patients who had been previously considered untreatable were now responding to therapy and able to move back into society. The American public was introduced to the concept that there are legitimate reasons for using medications to deal with emotional problems.

   This concept was enhanced further by the introduction of Valium. It became one of several drugs that would be perceived by the medical profession and the general public as having many benefits with no serious side effects. It would be many years before the addictive properties of Valium were recognized and an acknowledgment was made that it was not a harmless drug.

   The 1960s brought attitudinal changes toward medications and drugs that have contributed to the drug-related problems of the 1980s and 1990s. These attitudinal changes are exemplified by a recent admission interview with a 23-year-old female being admitted for elective surgery. When she was asked if she had any history of drug use for medical or recreational purposes, she replied "nothing more serious than coke." It is a common misconception that recreational drug use is not a problem. This is reflected in an escalated abuse of prescription drugs and street drugs.

2. More people die annually from prescription drugs obtained legally but used improperly than from all illegal substances combined (Gold, 1988).

3. Almost 25 million people have tried cocaine (Gold, 1988). This means that one out of 10 Americans has experimented with cocaine.

4. Crack has brought substance abuse to lower socioeconomic groups and is easily used (smoked).

5. Substance abuse spans all geographic regions, ethnic groups and social classes. Substance abuse is a widespread problem and an inevitable reality for nursing practitioners in the 1990s.

B. Issues Relevant to Nursing

1. As competent health care providers, nurses need to know how to assess and recognize the manifestations accompanying substance abuse. An individual's substance abuse alters every aspect of life functions: physical, psychological and interpersonal.

   Identifying that a substance abuse problem exists is frequently a difficult process. This process extends from the emergency room with a comatose patient suspected of having overdosed, to a classroom with an adolescent who is experiencing behavioral problems potentially related to substance abuse.

   Acknowledgment and self-assessment of one's own drug use contribute to a comprehensive understanding of these issues.

2. This module will provide the practitioner with a sound theoretical knowledge of the physical manifestation of drugs, thus allowing the practitioner to identify

an actual or potential problem and the need for intervention. It examines drugs at a physiological level to assist practitioners in recognizing the symptoms a client may manifest when under the influence of drugs.

3. Each drug is presented according to symptoms of acute intoxication, overdose and withdrawal, with accompanying treatment modalities introduced. The drugs are examined from medical, nursing and lay perspectives. This includes teaching street names for various drugs so that communication with clients may be enhanced.

4. Polysubstance abuse has become much more common than an isolated or single abuse pattern. Common drug combinations and interactions are discussed in this module.

II. COMMON TERMS RELATED TO ABUSE/DEPENDENCY

A. Habituation

1. Pattern of repeated drug use in absence of actual physical need for the drug.
2. No desire for increased use.
3. No withdrawal manifestations.

B. Misuse

1. Used for purposes other than those for which they are intended.
2. Common among people, especially the elderly, who self-medicate for a variety of reasons.

C. Abuse

1. Drug use patterns outside the limits acceptable by society which impact negatively on psychological, physiological, and social functioning.
2. A concept that is, in part, culturally defined.
3. May be combined with misuse.

D. Dependence

1. Reliance on a drug to a degree in which abstinence will cause an impairment in function.
2. Psychological dependence is characterized by a compulsive need to experience pleasurable response from the drug.
3. Physical dependence is an altered physiological state resulting from prolonged drug use; regular use is necessary to prevent withdrawal.

E. Tolerance

1. Decreased effect of a drug resulting from repeated exposure.
2. It is also possible to develop cross-tolerance to other drugs in the same category.

F. Addiction

1. Compulsive drug use for both physical and psychological reasons.

G. Dual Addiction

1. Simultaneous dependence on substances that have similar effects, such as alcohol and other CNS depressants (e.g., benzodiazepine, Valium).

H. Mixed Addiction

1. Dependence on more than one substance, not necessarily similar in effect, such as alcohol and cocaine.

III. ROUTES OF ADMINISTRATION

A. By Mouth (PO). Tablet or liquid

1. Examples: Codeine, Noctec, Alcohol.

B. Smoked

1. Examples: Marijuana, Crack.

C. Inhaled

1. Examples: Benzene, Nitrous Oxide, PCP.

D. Intravenous (IV)

1. Examples: Heroin, Cocaine.

E. Intradermal (Skin-popping)

1. Example: Heroin.

IV. OVER-THE-COUNTER DRUGS

A. Most Commonly Abused Relative to Appetite or Weight Control

B. Misuse

1. Example: Ex-Lax.

C. Self-Medication

1. Example: Dexatrim.

V. ALCOHOL—A MAJOR CNS DEPRESSANT

A. Signs of Alcohol Intoxication

1. Euphoria.
2. Altered judgment.
3. Impaired motor coordination (falls with multiple bruises).
4. Inability to concentrate.
5. Memory loss (alcoholic blackout).

6. Profound respiratory and cardiovascular depression.

7. Coma.

B. Problems Associated with Chronic Alcohol Use

1. GI disturbances (GI bleeds).

2. Liver damage (palmar erythema).

3. Pancreatitis.

4. Neuronal damage (peripheral tremors, neuropathy).

5. Cardiac impairment.

6. Malnutrition (anorexia).

7. Psychotic disturbances.

8. Blood dyscrasias and anemias.

C. Signs of Alcohol Withdrawal

1. Tremors.

2. GI disturbances.

3. Anxiety.

4. Insomnia.

5. Confusion.

6. Weakness.

7. Delusions.

D. Delirium Tremens (DTs)

1. Fever.

2. Tachycardia.

3. Tremors.

4. Profuse diaphoresis.

5. Agitation.

6. Disorientation.

7. Hallucinations (visual, tactile).

8. Convulsions.

E. Treatment of Acute Alcohol Withdrawal

1. Hydration.

2. Sedation (paraldehyde).

3. Anticonvulsants (Valium).

4. Vitamin B6 injections.

5. Antacids.

6. Referral to supportive social agencies (e.g., A.A.).

F. Potential for Addiction: HIGH

VI. PRESCRIPTION DRUGS

A. Central Nervous System Depressants

1. Barbiturates.

   a. Examples: Seconal (secobarbital), Red Devils, Nembutal (pentobarbital), Yellow Jackets.

   b. Barbiturate intoxication.

      (1) Slurred speech.

      (2) Disorientation.

      (3) Impaired motor coordination.

      (4) Poor judgment.

      (5) Confusion.

      (6) Emotional instability.

   c. Barbiturate overdose.

      (1) Decreased respirations.

      (2) Rapid and weak pulse.

      (3) Cyanosis.

      (4) Mydriasis.

      (5) Coma.

      (6) Respiratory paralysis.

   d. Barbiturate withdrawal reactions.

      (1) Anxiety.

      (2) Weakness.

      (3) Anorexia.

      (4) Insomnia.

      (5) Tremors.

      (6) Confusion and disorientation.

      (7) Delirium.

      (8) Hallucinations.

      (9) Convulsions.

  e. Treatment of barbiturate overdose and withdrawal is symptomatic.

  f. Potential for Addiction: HIGH.

2. Non-barbiturate sedatives.

  a. Example: Methaqualone, quaaludes, ludes.

  b. Non-barbiturate sedative overdose reactions.

      (1) Convulsions.

      (2) Rigidity.

      (3) Coma.

  c. Non-barbiturate sedative withdrawal reactions.

      (1) Nausea.

      (2) Headache.

      (3) Cramping.

      (4) Toxic psychosis.

      (5) Severe convulsions.

      (6) Insomnia.

  d. Treatment of non-barbiturate withdrawal is supportive.

  e. Potential for Addiction: HIGH.

3. Anti-anxiety agents.

  a. Example: Valium (Diazepam), a Benzodiazepine.

  b. Anti-anxiety agent withdrawal reactions.

      (1) Cramping.

      (2) Sweating.

      (3) Agitation.

      (4) Disorientation.

      (5) Confusion.

      (6) Tremors.

      (7) Depression.

      (8) Auditory/visual hallucinations.

      (9) Paranoia.

  c. Valium must be withdrawn gradually.

  d. Potential for Addiction: HIGH.

Pharmacology

B. CNS Stimulants

1. Amphetamines: Uppers, speed, bennies.

   a. Examples:

      (1) Dextroamphetamine (Dexedrine), Dexies.

      (2) Amphetamine sulfate (Amphetamine), Beans.

      (3) Methamphetamine.

   b. General characteristics.

      (1) Suppress fatigue.

      (2) Increase alertness.

      (3) Enhance psychomotor performance.

      (4) Induce a temporary state of well-being.

      (5) Frequently administered IV.

      (6) Instantaneous euphoria or orgasmic-like reaction.

      (7) After a period of several days, person becomes exhausted, lapsing into long periods of sleep and depression ("crash").

   c. Stimulant overdose reactions.

      (1) Insomnia.

      (2) Increased BP, AR, palpitations.

      (3) Excitation.

      (4) Convulsions.

      (5) Hyperreflexia.

      (6) Hostility.

      (7) Impulsiveness.

      (8) Hallucinations.

      (9) Confusion.

      (10) Paranoid ideation.

      (11) Death.

   d. Stimulant withdrawal reactions.

      (1) Fatigue.

      (2) Muscle pain.

      (3) Lethargy.

      (4) Depression.

259

    e. Treatment of stimulant overdose.

        (1) Quiet environment.

        (2) Support of vital functions.

        (3) Valium (diazepam) for sedation.

        (4) Urinary acidifiers increase drug excretion.

    f. Potential for Addiction: HIGH.

2. Anorexiants (Anorectics).

    a. Examples: Benzophetamine, Phendimetrazine.

    b. General characteristics:

        (1) Indirect acting sympathomimetics.

        (2) Same spectrum of pharmacological and toxicological actions as amphetamines.

        (3) Less potential for habituation than amphetamines.

        (4) Fewer cardiovascular, CNS and gastrointestinal side effects when used in appropriate dose range.

        (5) Chronic ingestion produces many of the symptoms of prolonged amphetamine use.

            (a) Insomnia.

            (b) Tachycardia.

            (c) Elevated blood pressure.

            (d) Anxiety and restlessness.

        (6) Potential for Addiction: UNCLEAR.

3. Cocaine: This CNS stimulant is not a prescription drug. It is discussed with Street and Socially Misused Drugs.

C. Narcotics and Other Controlled Substances

1. Types.

    a. Opiates.

        (1) Morphine.

        (2) Codeine.

    b. Semi-synthetic.

        (1) Hydromorphone (Dilaudid).

        (2) Heroin (this narcotic has no current accepted medical uses and is discussed with Street and Socially Misused Drugs).

    c. Synthetic.

        (1) Methadone.

        (2) Meperidine.

2. Narcotic overdose reactions.

    a. Depressed level of consciousness, obtunded to comatose.

    b. Depressed respirations leading to apnea and respiratory arrest.

    c. Pulmonary edema, aspiration pneumonia or atelectases.

    d. Bradycardia, marked hypotension and shock.

    e. Gastrointestinal atony.

3. Narcotic withdrawal reactions.

    a. Withdrawal is characterized by rebound excitability in those organs whose functions were previously depressed.

    b. Physiological manifestations.

        (1) Stomach cramps, nausea, vomiting, diarrhea.

        (2) Diaphoresis.

        (3) Hypertension.

        (4) Backaches, muscle aches.

        (5) Lacrimation, rhinorrhea, gooseflesh, yawning.

        (6) Mydriasis.

    c. Psychological manifestations include:

        (1) Anxiety, irritability and restlessness.

        (2) In severe withdrawal, paranoia, violence, fear, depersonalization.

4. Initial treatment of narcotic reactions.

    a. Is similar to that for other depressants: Symptomatic.

    b. Assessment of baseline vital signs.

    c. Support of vital functions.

    d. Evaluation of mental/emotional state.

5. Potential for Addiction: HIGH.

VII. STREET AND SOCIALLY MISUSED DRUGS

A. CNS Stimulants: Examples: Cocaine, Crack

1. Cocaine is a natural product extracted from leaves of the coca plant. It may be smoked by inhaling fumes of heated cocaine. This is known as "free-basing." Cocaine may also be snorted by inhaling via nasal passages. Cocaine heated to the liquid state may be injected intravenously. Crack is a crystallized form of cocaine. It is melted in a water pipe and smoked.

2. Immediate reaction to the use of cocaine/crack is an intense euphoria achieved in less than 10 seconds; this reaction lasts 10–15 minutes.

3. Immediate physiological effects of cocaine/crack use:

    a. Tachycardia.

    b. Increased blood pressure.

4. Overdose of cocaine/crack use (may be immediate since there is little quality control in the street drug culture).

    a. Arrhythmias.

    b. Tremors.

    c. Convulsions.

    d. Respiratory failure.

    e. Cardiovascular collapse.

    f. Death.

5. Psychological effects of cocaine/crack.

    a. Overwhelming psychological dependence rapidly develops.

    b. Euphoria.

    c. Depression.

    d. Verbosity.

    e. Inability to concentrate.

    f. Insomnia, sleep disorders.

    g. Altered sexual drive.

    h. Reduced sense of humor.

    i. Antisocial behavior.

    j. Hallucinations, visual disturbances.

    k. Compulsive behavior.

6. Treatment of cocaine/crack overdose.

    a. Supportive.

    b. Resuscitative measures are frequently unsuccessful, resulting in death.

7. Potential for Addiction: HIGH.

B. Narcotics

1. Example: Heroin, "H."

2. Usual mode of administration is IV.

3. Immediate responses.

    a. Sensation of exquisite pleasure, "orgasmic rush."

    b. Euphoria.

    c. Relaxation.

    d. Feeling of detachment.

    e. Indifference to anxiety or pain.

4. Heroin overdose reactions.

    a. Stupor.

    b. Pinpoint pupils.

    c. Cold, clammy skin.

    d. Respiratory depression.

    e. Hypotension.

    f. Bradycardia.

    g. Coma, death.

5. Treatment of heroin overdose.

    a. Narcan (naloxone)—must be used cautiously. Precipitous withdrawal from heroin may result in death.

    b. Respiratory support (ventilator).

    c. Vasopressors.

6. Heroin withdrawal reactions.

    a. Yawning.

    b. Perspiration.

    c. Restlessness.

    d. Anorexia.

    e. Irritability.

    f. Stomach cramps.

    g. Diarrhea.

    h. Fever, chills.

    i. Tremors, jerking motions.

    j. Tachycardia.

    k. Hypertension.

    l. Noncardiogenic pulmonary edema.

7. Treatment of heroin withdrawal: Substitute methadone.

8. Potential for Addiction: HIGH.

C. Hallucinogens

1. Examples.

    a. LSD.

    b. Mescaline.

    c. MDMA ("XTC").

    d. PCP—often classified by itself, has greater risk of pathophysiological manifestations.

2. General characteristic of use of these drugs is a profound distortion of reality.

3. Physiological responses to hallucinogens.

    a. Confusion, delirium.

    b. Amnesia.

    c. Distortion of time, place, distance.

    d. Delusions, hallucinations.

    e. Impaired judgment.

    f. Severe depression.

4. Psychic alterations reported as "pleasant."

    a. Euphoria.

    b. Elation.

    c. Vivid color imagery.

    d. Synthesiasis: Hearing colors, seeing sounds.

5. Psychic alterations described as "bad trips."

    a. Anxiety.

    b. Panic.

    c. Severe depression.

    d. Suicidal tendencies.

6. Flashbacks of "bad trips" may occur up to 5 years after drug use and are precipitated by stress, anxiety, or use of psychotropic drugs (e.g., marijuana).

7. Treatment of "bad trips."

    a. Supportive, non-threatening environment.

    b. Maintain reassuring verbal contact ("talking down").

    c. Mild sedatives (benzodiazepines).

8. Treatment of PCP "bad trips."

    a. Sedatives.

    b. Urinary acidifiers.

c. Isolate patient: Decrease stimulation. Verbal contact may precipitate acute psychotic and involuntary muscle reactions.

9. Potential for Addiction: PSYCHOLOGICAL DEPENDENCE ONLY.

D. Volatile Inhalants

1. Examples.
   a. Toluene (glues).
   b. Gasoline.
   c. Fluorocarbons (aerosols).
   d. Nitrous oxide (anesthetic).
   e. Nitrites (amyl, isobutyl commonly used as heart stimulant medications), "poppers."
2. General effects of use of inhalants.
   a. CNS excitation.
   b. Exhilaration.
   c. Dizziness.
   d. Unconsciousness.
   e. Auditory, visual hallucinations.
   f. Drowsiness.
   g. Hypotension.
   h. Stupor.
   i. Coma.
   j. Heightened sexual response due to profound vasodilation.
3. Pathophysiological conditions associated with common inhalants.
   a. Toluene: Renal tubular acidosis.
   b. Gasoline: Chemical pneumonitis.
   c. Fluorocarbons: Sensitize myocardium to catecholamines; arrhythmias.
   d. Nitrous oxide: Peripheral neuropathy.
   e. Nitrites: Methemoglobinemia—the presence of methemoglobin in the blood, causing cyanosis due to the inability of red cells to release oxygen.
4. Treatment of overdose of inhalants.
   a. Oxygen.
   b. Respiratory support.
   c. Avoid vasopressors, as these may induce life-threatening arrhythmias.
5. Potential for Addiction: PSYCHOLOGICAL DEPENDENCE ONLY.

E. Marijuana, Hashish, "Weed," "Hash"

1. General effects.

    a. Sense of relaxation and well-being.

    b. Euphoria.

    c. Altered sensory perception.

    d. Impaired psychomotor function.

    e. Decreased attention span.

    f. Compromised driving ability.

    g. Disorientation.

    h. Disorganized thought processes.

2. Effects of prolonged use.

    a. Pulmonary toxicity.

    b. Impaired immune response.

    c. Personality and behavioral changes.

3. "Reverse tolerance": Smaller amount of drug elicits desired psychic effects.

4. Potential for Addiction: MODERATE.

F. Nicotine

1. Nicotine is found in tobacco in a 1–2% concentration.

2. Nicotine is rapidly absorbed by the lungs, producing a mild central stimulatory effect.

3. Physiological effects.

    a. Decreased skeletal muscle tone.

    b. Reduced appetite.

    c. Vasoconstriction.

4. Nicotine withdrawal symptoms.

    a. Nausea.

    b. Diarrhea.

    c. Increased appetite.

    d. Headache.

    e. Drowsiness.

    f. Insomnia.

    g. Irritability.

    h. Poor concentration.

5. Prolonged abstinence.

   a. Decrease in blood pressure.

   b. Decrease in heart rate.

   c. Increase in peripheral blood flow.

   d. Reduction in respiratory difficulties.

   e. Weight gain.

6. Risk factors associated with cigarette smoking.

   a. Cancer of the lung and bladder.

   b. Coronary artery disease.

   c. Emphysema.

7. Potential for Addiction: PSYCHOLOGICAL DEPENDENCE.

G. Caffeine

1. Physiological effects.

   a. CNS and cardiac stimulant.

   b. Relaxes smooth muscles in blood vessels and bronchi.

   c. Diuresis occurs because of increased renal blood flow.

   d. Gastric acid secretion increased and appetite suppressed.

   e. Euphoria and/or increased feeling of energy.

   f. Constricts cerebral blood vessels (used in headache remedies).

2. Caffeinism.

   a. A syndrome caused by excessive caffeine intake.

   b. Characteristics.

      (1) Marked anxiety.

      (2) Affective symptoms.

      (3) Psychophysiological complaints.

3. Symptoms of caffeine toxicity.

   a. Central Nervous System.

      (1) Jitteriness.

      (2) Restlessness.

      (3) Nervousness.

      (4) Excitement.

    b. Cardiovascular.

       (1) Flushed face.

       (2) Palpitations.

       (3) Diuresis.

    c. Gastrointestinal.

       (1) Nausea.

       (2) Gastric irritation, pain.

4. Caffeine withdrawal symptoms.

    a. Headache.

    b. Irritability.

    c. Tremulousness.

5. Common sources of caffeine.

    a. Brewed coffee (60–180 mg./5 oz.).

    b. Colas (34–58 mg./12 oz.).

    c. Brewed tea (20–90 mg./5 oz.).

    d. Cocoa (2–20 mg./5 oz.).

6. Potential for Addiction: MODERATE.

H. Anabolic Steroids

1. General information.

    a. Anabolic steroids are compounds derived from testosterone or prepared synthetically.

    b. Medical uses of anabolic steroids are in the treatment of specific anemias and among the many modalities in some cancer therapies.

2. Common perceptions of effects of anabolic steroids.

    a. Increased skeletal muscle mass.

    b. Enhanced physical performance of skeletal muscles.

    c. Increased body weight.

    d. Improved athletic abilities.

3. Abused primarily by athletes and young males for their effects on muscle mass.

4. There is no conclusive evidence to support that the perceived advantages are medically accurate.

5. Potential adverse consequences.

    a. Masculinization and virilization (desired effect for abusers).

    b. Personality disorders and aggressiveness.

    c. Testicular atrophy.

    d. Oligospermia and erectile dysfunction.

    e. Fatal hemorrhagic liver disease.

6. Potential for Addiction: PSYCHOLOGICAL DEPENDENCE ONLY.

MODULE I.4
PHARMACOLOGY

INSTRUCTOR'S GUIDE

Elizabeth A. Duthie, MA, RN

Madeline A. Naegle, PhD, RN, FAAN
Project Director
Janet S. D'Arcangelo, MA, RN, C
Project Coordinator

Project SAEN
SUBSTANCE ABUSE
EDUCATION IN NURSING

CONTENTS

MODULE DESCRIPTION

This module describes the physiological and behavioral effects of commonly abused drugs. Drug misuse, abuse, and dependence will be defined as related to drug interaction, drugs in combination, and behavioral and physiological changes. The addictive and toxic potential of classes of drugs will be emphasized. Clients' learning processes and health needs in relation to drugs are addressed.

TIME FRAME

3 hours

PLACEMENT

Basic Sciences are prerequisites for this module.

LEARNER OBJECTIVES

Upon successful completion of this module, the learner will:

1. List common drugs of abuse by generic, trade, and street names.
2. Describe pharmacological properties of classes of commonly abused drugs.
3. Describe the behavioral effects of commonly abused drugs.
4. Define terms commonly used in relation to drugs of abuse.
5. Describe the assessment process for the client under the influence of a drug.
6. Describe effects of drug abuse/dependence which require nursing intervention.
7. Describe the interactional effect of the abuse of multiple drugs.
8. Describe interventions utilized for clients in toxic drug states.

RECOMMENDED READINGS

GENERAL READINGS

Malseed, R. (1985). Drug dependence and addiction. In R. Malseed, *Pharmacology: Drug therapy and nursing considerations*. Philadelphia: J. B. Lippincott.

Matthewson, M. (Ed.) (1989). *Pharmacotherapeutics* (2nd ed.). Philadelphia: F. A. Davis.

FACULTY READINGS

Busto, V. (1986). Patterns of benzodiazepine abuse and dependence. *British Journal of Addictions, 81*(1), 87–94.

Cushman, P. (1986). Sedative drug interactions of clinical importance. *Recent Developments in Alcohol, 4*, 61–83.

Gawin, F. H., & Ellingwood, E. H. (1988). Cocaine and other stimulants: Action, abuse and treatment. *New England Journal of Medicine, 318*, 1173–1182.

Goldstein, D. B. (Ed.) (1983). *The pharmacology of alcohol*. New York: Oxford University Press.

Sullivan, J. B., et al. (1979). Management of tricyclic antidepressant toxicity. *Topics in Emergency Medicine, 1*(3), 65–71.

Zerwecki, J., & Gordon, D. (Eds.) (1989). *The nursing clinics of North America*. Philadelphia: W. B. Saunders.

STUDENT READINGS

Gold, M. S. (1988). *The facts about drugs and alcohol*. Washington, DC: Psychiatric Institute of America.

Hahn, A. B., Oestereich, S. J. K., & Borkin, R. (1986). *Pharmacology in nursing*. St. Louis: C. V. Mosby.

Naegle, M. (1989). Utilizing the nursing process with the client who abuses drugs and alcohol. In M. Matthewson (Ed.), *Pharmacotherapeutics* (2nd ed.). Philadelphia: F. A. Davis.

Vourakis, C., & Bennett, G. (1979). Angel dust: Not heaven sent. *American Journal of Nursing, 79*, 649–652.

RECOMMENDED AUDIOVISUAL
AND
OTHER RESOURCES

AUDIOVISUAL RESOURCES

1. Psychoactive Drugs

Using information from the San Francisco Drug Detoxification and Rehabilitation Project, this film surveys the effects of psychoactive drugs on the nine systems of the human body, demonstrating how each system functions, and how a drug intended for one body system can throw another into disequilibrium. The five categories of psychoactive drugs covered are: sedative hypnotics (Valium), opioids and opiates (heroin), stimulants (amphetamines), psychedelics (LSD, marijuana), and alcohol. **Available from New York State Council on Alcoholism and other Drug Addiction, Inc., 155 Washington Avenue, Third Floor, Albany, New York 12210. Phone: (518) 436-1077.**

2. Living with Antabuse Therapy

This thought-provoking videotape dramatizes one family's reactions to the father's involvement in Antabuse therapy. It presents detailed information about Antabuse therapy and promotes discussion about how it affects the patient and his family. 18 minutes. **Available from the Health Sciences Consortium, 201 Silver Cedar Court, Chapel Hill, North Carolina 27514. Phone: (919) 942-8731. VHS #R861-VI-048, purchase ($195).**

Module I.4

OVERHEAD MASTERS

MODULE I.4 PHARMACOLOGY

1. Substance Abuse Terms
2. Routes of Administration
3. Pharmacokinetics of Drugs of Abuse
4. Index of Physiological Addictive Power
5. Types of Drugs—Prescribed and Unprescribed
6. Alcohol (6A, 6B, 6C, 6D, 6E)
7. Central Nervous System Depressants (7A, 7B, 7C, 7D, 7E, 7F)
8. Central Nervous System Stimulants (8A, 8B, 8C, 8D)
9. Narcotics—Opiates
10. Cocaine, Crack (10A, 10B, 10C, 10D)
11. Narcotics—Heroin (11A, 11B, 11C, 11D)
12. Psychotomimetics (Hallucinogens) (12A, 12B, 12C)
13. Volatile Inhalants (Amyl Nitrites) (13A, 13B)
14. Marijuana, Hashish (14A, 14B)
15. Nicotine (15A, 15B)
16. Caffeine (16A, 16B)
17. Anabolic Steroids (17A, 17B)

SUBSTANCE ABUSE TERMS

1. *Habituation:* Pattern of repeated drug use in the absence of an actual physical need for the drug. There is no desire for increased use. There are no withdrawal manifestations.

2. *Misuse:* Used for purposes other than those for which they are intended. Common among people, especially the elderly, who self-medicate for a variety of reasons.

3. *Abuse:* Drug use patterns outside the limits acceptable by society and which impact negatively on psychological, physiological, and social functioning of an individual. It is a concept that is, in part, culturally defined. Drug abuse may be combined with misuse.

4. *Dependence:* Reliance on a drug to a degree in which the absence will cause an impairment in function.

   a. *Psychological dependence* is characterized by a compulsive need to experience pleasurable response from the drug.

   b. *Physical dependence* is an altered physiological state resulting from prolonged drug use; regular use is necessary to prevent withdrawal.

5. *Tolerance:* Decreased effect of a drug resulting from repeated exposure. It is also possible to develop cross-tolerance to other drugs in the same category.

6. *Addiction:* Compulsive drug use for both physical and psychological reasons.

7. *Dual Addiction:* Simultaneous dependence on substances that have similar effects, such as alcohol and other CNS depressants (e.g., the benzodiazepine, Valium).

8. *Mixed Addiction:* Dependence on more than one substance, not necessarily similar in effect, such as alcohol and cocaine.

ROUTES OF ADMINISTRATION

1. **By mouth (PO). Tablet or liquid.**

   Examples: Codeine, Noctec, Alcohol.

2. **Smoked.**

   Examples: Marijuana, Crack.

3. **Inhaled.**

   Examples: Benzene, Nitrous Oxide, PCP (Angel Dust).

4. **Parenteral: IM, IV, SC.**

   Examples: Morphine, Heroin.

5. **Intradermal (Skin-popping).**

   Example: Heroin.

PHARMACOKINETICS OF DRUGS OF ABUSE

Ingested Orally

SUBSTANCE NAME	ONSET	PEAK	DURATION
Alcohol (10–12 oz. beer on an empty stomach)	5–10 min.	30–40 min.	1 hr.
Anorectic (Benzophetamine)	30–60 min.	1–2 hr.	4–6 hr.
Anxiolytic (Valium)	30–60 min.	1–2 hr.	3–4 hr.
Barbiturate (Seconal)	5–15 min.	15–30 min.	3–5 hr.
Caffeine (Coffee)	10–15 min.	30–60 min.	6–8 hr.
Narcotic (Percodan)	10–15 min.	30–60 min.	4–5 hr.

INDEX OF PHYSIOLOGICAL ADDICTIVE POWER

HIGH

Crack

Cocaine

Heroin

Morphine

Demerol

Barbiturates

Amphetamines

Alcohol

Marijuana

Minor Tranquilizers

Codeine

Sedative Hypnotics

Bromides

Nicotine

LOW   Caffeine

Module I.4—Overhead #5

TYPES OF DRUGS—PRESCRIBED AND UNPRESCRIBED

1. CNS Depressants
2. CNS Stimulants
3. Narcotics
4. Psychotomimetics
5. Inhalants
6. Marijuana, Hashish
7. Nicotine
8. Caffeine
9. Anabolic Steroids

Module I.4—Overhead #6A

ALCOHOL

A. **Signs of Alcohol Intoxication:**
1. Euphoria.
2. Altered judgment.
3. Impaired motor coordination (falls with multiple bruises).
4. Inability to concentrate.
5. Memory loss (alcoholic blackout).
6. Profound respiratory and cardiovascular depression.
7. Coma.

ALCOHOL

B. **Problems Associated with Chronic Alcohol Abuse:**

1. GI disturbances (GI bleeds).

2. Liver damage (palmar erythema).

3. Pancreatitis.

4. Neuronal damage (peripheral tremors, neuropathies).

5. Cardiac impairment.

6. Malnutrition (anorexia).

7. Psychotic disturbances.

ALCOHOL

C. Alcohol Withdrawal:
1. Tremors.
2. GI disturbances.
3. Anxiety.
4. Insomnia.
5. Confusion.
6. Weakness.
7. Delusions.

ALCOHOL

D. Delirium Tremens (DTs):
    1. Fever.
    2. Tachycardia.
    3. Tremors.
    4. Profuse diaphoresis.
    5. Agitation.
    6. Disorientation.
    7. Hallucinations (visual, tactile).
    8. Convulsions.

ALCOHOL

E. Treatment of Acute Alcohol Withdrawal (Symptomatic):

1. Hydration.

2. Sedation (paraldehyde).

3. Anticonvulsants (Valium).

4. Vitamin B6 injections.

5. Antacids.

6. Referral to supportive social agencies (e.g., A.A.).

CENTRAL NERVOUS SYSTEM DEPRESSANTS—BARBITURATES

A. Barbiturate Intoxication:

1. Slurred speech.

2. Disorientation.

3. Impaired motor coordination.

4. Poor judgment.

5. Confusion.

6. Emotional instability.

CENTRAL NERVOUS SYSTEM DEPRESSANTS—BARBITURATES

B. Barbiturate Overdose:

1. Decreased respirations.

2. Rapid and weak pulse.

3. Cyanosis.

4. Mydriasis.

5. Coma.

6. Respiratory paralysis.

CENTRAL NERVOUS SYSTEM DEPRESSANTS—BARBITURATES

C. Barbiturate Withdrawal Reactions:

1. Anxiety.

2. Weakness.

3. Confusion and disorientation.

4. Anorexia.

5. Insomnia.

6. Tremors.

7. Delirium and hallucinations.

8. Convulsions.

Treatment of Barbiturate Overdose and Withdrawal Is Symptomatic.

CENTRAL NERVOUS SYSTEM DEPRESSANTS—NON-BARBITURATE SEDATIVES

A. Drug of Choice: Methaqualone (Quaaludes).

B. Principal Effect Desired: As a "downer."

C. Non-Barbiturate Sedative Overdose:

1. Convulsions.

2. Rigidity.

3. Coma.

CENTRAL NERVOUS SYSTEM DEPRESSANTS—NON-BARBITURATE SEDATIVES

D. Non-Barbiturate Sedative Withdrawal:

1. Nausea.

2. Headache.

3. Insomnia.

4. Cramping.

5. Toxic psychosis.

6. Severe convulsions.

Treatment of Non-Barbiturate Sedative Overdose and Withdrawal Is Supportive.

CENTRAL NERVOUS SYSTEM DEPRESSANTS—ANTI-ANXIETY AGENTS

A. Example: Valium (diazepam).

B. Anti-Anxiety Agent Withdrawal Reactions:

1. Cramping.

2. Sweating.

3. Tremors.

4. Agitation.

5. Depression.

6. Paranoia.

7. Auditory/Visual hallucinations.

8. Confusion.

9. Disorientation.

Gradual Drug Withdrawal Is Used in the Treatment of Anti-anxiety Agent Abuse.

CENTRAL NERVOUS SYSTEM STIMULANTS—AMPHETAMINES ("UPPERS")

A. General Characteristics:

1. Suppress fatigue.

2. Increase alertness.

3. Enhance psychomotor performance.

4. Induce a temporary state of well-being.

B. Methamphetamine ("Speed"):

1. Administered IV.

2. Instantaneous euphoria or orgasmic-like reaction.

3. "Crash" (after a period of several days, person becomes exhausted, lapsing into long periods of sleep and depression).

CENTRAL NERVOUS SYSTEM STIMULANTS—AMPHETAMINES ("UPPERS")

C. CNS Stimulant Overdose:

1. Insomnia.

2. Increased BP.

3. Increased AR, palpitations.

4. Excitation.

5. Hyperreflexivity.

6. Impulsiveness.

7. Hostility.

8. Confusion.

9. Paranoid ideation.

10. Hallucinations.

11. Convulsions.

12. Death.

CENTRAL NERVOUS SYSTEM STIMULANTS—AMPHETAMINES ("UPPERS")

D. CNS Stimulant Withdrawal:

   1. Fatigue.

   2. Muscle pain.

   3. Lethargy.

   4. Depression.

E. Treatment of CNS Stimulant Overdose:

   1. Quiet environment.

   2. Support of vital functions.

   3. Valium (diazepam) for sedation.

   4. Urinary acidifiers markedly increase amphetamine excretion.

CENTRAL NERVOUS SYSTEM STIMULANTS—ANOREXIANTS (ANORECTICS)

A. Examples: Benzophetamine, phendimetrazine.

B. General Characteristics:

1. Indirect acting sympathomimetics.

2. Same spectrum of pharmacological and toxicological actions as amphetamines.

3. Less potential for habituation than amphetamines.

4. Fewer cardiovascular, CNS and gastrointestinal side effects when used in the appropriate dose range.

5. Chronic ingestion produces many of the symptoms of prolonged amphetamine use:

   a. Insomnia.

   b. Tachycardia.

   c. Elevated blood pressure.

   d. Anxiety and restlessness.

Module I.4—Overhead #9

NARCOTICS—OPIATES

A. Common Prescribed Narcotics (by Generic and Common Trade Names):
1. Codeine.
2. Hydromorphone (Dilaudid).
3. Morphine (Duramorph).
4. Meperidine (Demerol).
5. Methadone (Dolophine).
6. Levophanol (Levo-Dromoran).
7. Oxycodone (Percodan).
8. Pentazocine (Talwin).
9. Propoxyphene (Darvon).

B. Desired Effect: Pain relief.

NARCOTICS—COCAINE

A. General Information:

1. Cocaine is a natural product extracted from the leaves of the coca plant.

2. Cocaine may be smoked, sniffed or injected:

   a. Smoking: Known as "free-basing," inhaling fumes of heated cocaine.

   b. Snorting: Sniffing, inhaling via the nasal passages.

   c. Injection: IV administration of cocaine heated to liquid state.

3. Crack is a hardened form of cocaine smoked in a water pipe.

4. Crack produces an intense euphoria in less than 10 seconds, lasting 10–15 minutes.

NARCOTICS—COCAINE

B. **Physiological Effects of Cocaine Use (May Be Immediate):**

1. Tachycardia.

2. Increased BP.

3. Respiratory failure.

4. Cardiovascular collapse.

5. Death.

NARCOTICS—COCAINE

C. Psychological Effects of Cocaine Use:

1. Rapid development of overwhelming psychological dependence.

2. Euphoria.

3. Verbosity.

4. Inability to concentrate.

5. Compulsive behavior.

6. Insomnia/sleep disorders.

7. Depression.

8. Altered sex drive.

9. Reduced sense of humor.

10. Antisocial behavior.

11. Hallucinations or visual disturbances.

NARCOTICS—COCAINE

D. Cocaine Overdose:

1. Arrhythmias.

2. Tremors.

3. Convulsions.

4. Respiratory failure.

5. Cardiovascular collapse.

6. Death.

Treatment of Cocaine Overdose Is Supportive.
Resuscitative Measures Are Frequently Unsuccessful, Resulting in Death.

NARCOTICS—HEROIN

A. General Characteristics:

1. Heroin is a semi-synthetic narcotic which has no current accepted medical uses. It is considered to be a street/socially misused drug.

2. Heroin is used intravenously (IV).

B. Effect Desired by IV Heroin User:

1. Sensation of exquisite pleasure ("orgasmic rush").

C. Immediate Responses to IV Heroin Use:

1. Euphoria.

2. Relaxation.

3. Feeling of detachment.

4. Indifference to anxiety or pain.

5. Increased risk of HIV/AIDS.

NARCOTICS—HEROIN

D. Complications of Chronic IV Heroin Use:

    1. Malnutrition.

    2. Poor hygiene.

    3. Infections from unsterile needles.

    4. Vasculitis.

    5. Hepatitis.

    6. Endocarditis.

NARCOTICS—HEROIN

E. Overdose of IV Heroin:

1. Hypotension.

2. Bradycardia.

3. Respiratory depression.

4. Stupor.

5. Pinpoint pupils.

6. Cold, clammy skin.

7. Coma.

8. Death.

F. Treatment of IV Heroin Overdose:

1. Narcan (naloxone).

2. Respiratory support.

3. Vasopressors.

CAUTION: Use Narcan Cautiously to Avoid Precipitous Withdrawal,
Which May Result in Death.

NARCOTICS—HEROIN

G. IV Heroin Withdrawal:

   1. Yawning.

   2. Irritability.

   3. Tremors.

   4. Perspiration.

   5. Stomach cramps.

   6. Jerking motions.

   7. Restlessness.

   8. Diarrhea.

   9. Tachycardia.

   10. Anorexia.

   11. Fever, chills.

   12. Hypertension.

   13. Noncardiogenic pulmonary edema.

Treatment of IV Heroin Withdrawal Is to Substitute Methadone.

PSYCHOTOMIMETICS (HALLUCINOGENS)

A. Examples:

    1. LSD.

    2. Mescaline.

    3. Phencyclidine ("PCP"), though usually classified by itself.

B. General Effects of Hallucinogens:

    1. A profound distortion of reality.

    2. Experience of drug effects known as a "trip" or "tripping."

C. Physiological Responses from Hallucinogen Ingestion:

    1. Distortion of time, place, distance.

    2. Impaired judgment.

    3. Severe depression.

    4. Amnesia.

    5. Confusion, delirium.

    6. Delusions, hallucinations.

PSYCHOTOMIMETICS (HALLUCINOGENS)

D. Psychic Alterations Reported as "Pleasant":

1. Euphoria.

2. Elation.

3. Vivid color imagery.

4. Synthesthiasis:

   a.   Hearing colors.

   b.   Seeing sounds.

E. Characteristics of "Bad Trips":

1. Anxiety.

2. Panic.

3. Severe depression.

4. Suicidal tendencies.

5. Flashbacks of "bad trips" may occur up to 5 years after drug use and are precipitated by stress, anxiety or use of psychotropic drugs (e.g., marijuana).

PSYCHOTOMIMETICS (HALLUCINOGENS)

F. Treatment of "Bad Trips":

   1. Supportive, non-threatening environment.

   2. Reassuring verbal contact ("talking down").

   3. Mild sedatives (benzodiazepines).

G. Additional Considerations in Treatment of "Bad Trips" Precipitated by PCP Use:

   1. Sedatives.

   2. Urinary acidifiers.

   3. Isolation of patient: Verbal contact may precipitate acute psychotic and involuntary muscle reactions.

VOLATILE INHALANTS (AMYL NITRITES)

A. Effects of Inhalants:

    1. CNS excitation.

    2. Exhilaration.

    3. Auditory or visual hallucinations.

    4. Hypotension.

    5. Dizziness.

    6. Drowsiness.

    7. Stupor.

    8. Delirium.

    9. Coma.

    10. Unconsciousness.

    11. Profound vasodilation contributes to heightened sexual response.

VOLATILE INHALANTS (AMYL NITRITES)

     B. Treatment of Overdose of Inhalants:

         1. Oxygen.

         2. Respiratory support.

         3. Avoid vasopressors, as these may induce life-threatening arrhythmias.

MARIJUANA

A. Effects of Marijuana Use:
1. Sense of relaxation and well-being.
2. Euphoria.
3. Decreased attention span.
4. Impaired psychomotor function.
5. Altered sensory perception.
6. Compromised driving ability.
7. Disorientation.
8. Disorganized thought processes.

MARIJUANA

B. Effects of Prolonged Use of Marijuana:
1. Pulmonary toxicity.
2. Impaired immune response.
3. Personality and behavioral changes.
C. "Reverse Tolerance" Phenomenon: Smaller amount of drug elicits the desired effects.

Marijuana Is Addictive

NICOTINE

A. General Information:

    1. Rapidly absorbed by lungs, producing mild stimulatory effect.

    2. Found in tobacco in a 1%–2% concentration.

B. Risk Factors Associated with Cigarette Smoking:

    1. Lung cancer.

    2. Bladder cancer.

    3. Coronary artery disease.

    4. Emphysema.

C. Physiological Effects of Nicotine Ingestion:

    1. Decreased skeletal muscle tone.

    2. Reduced appetite.

    3. Vasoconstriction.

NICOTINE

D. Symptoms of Nicotine Withdrawal:

1. Irritability.

2. Insomnia.

3. Nausea.

4. Diarrhea.

5. Headache.

6. Increased appetite.

7. Poor concentration.

8. Drowsiness.

E. Effects of Prolonged Abstinence from Nicotine:

1. Blood pressure decreases.

2. Heart rate decreases.

3. Peripheral blood flow increases.

4. Respiratory difficulties are reduced.

5. Weight gain.

CAFFEINE

A. Physiological Effects of Caffeine:

1. CNS and cardiac stimulant.

2. Relaxes smooth muscle in the blood vessels and bronchi.

3. Diuresis occurs because of increased renal blood flow.

4. Gastric acid increased and appetite suppressed.

5. Euphoria and/or increased feeling of energy.

6. Constricts cerebral blood vessels (used in headache remedies).

B. Caffeinism: A syndrome caused by excessive caffeine intake, characterized by:

1. Marked anxiety.

2. Affective symptoms.

3. Psychophysiological complaints.

C. Common Sources of Caffeine:

1. Brewed coffee (60–180 mg./5 oz.).

2. Colas (34–58 mg./12 oz.).

3. Brewed tea (20–90 mg./5 oz.).

4. Cocoa (2–20 mg./5 oz.).

CAFFEINE

D. Caffeine Toxicity:

   1. Central Nervous System:

      a. Jitteriness.

      b. Restlessness.

      c. Nervousness.

      d. Excitement.

   2. Cardiovascular:

      a. Flushed face.

      b. Palpitations.

      c. Diuresis.

   3. Gastrointestinal:

      a. Nausea.

      b. Gastric irritation, pain.

E. Caffeine Tolerance and Dependence May Develop.

F. Caffeine Withdrawal Symptoms:

   1. Headache.

   2. Irritability.

   3. Tremulousness.

ANABOLIC STEROIDS

A. Abused Primarily by Athletes and Young Males for Their Effects on Muscle Mass.

B. Abused Because of the Following Perceptions:

   1. Increased skeletal muscle mass.

   2. Enhanced physical performance of skeletal muscles.

   3. Increased body weight.

   4. Improved athletic abilities.

There Is No Conclusive Evidence to Support That These Perceived Advantages Are Medically Accurate.

ANABOLIC STEROIDS

B. Potential Adverse Consequences:

1. Masculinization and virilization (desired effect for abusers).

2. Personality disorders and aggressiveness.

3. Testicular atrophy.

4. Oligospermia and erectile dysfunction.

5. Fatal hemorrhagic liver disease.

Anabolic Steroids Are Non-Addicting But Psychic Dependence May Occur.

HANDOUT MASTERS

MODULE I.4 PHARMACOLOGY

1. Substance Abuse Facts
2. Substance Abuse Terms
3. Types of Drugs and Street Names (3A, 3B)
4. Classes of Abused Drugs and Their Actions (4A, 4B, 4C)
5. What Could Happen If You Drink While Taking Any of These Drugs (5A, 5B, 5C)
6. Medications Containing Alcohol (6A, 6B)

Module I.4—Handout #1

SUBSTANCE ABUSE FACTS

1. Almost 25 million people have tried cocaine in the U.S.—this means one out of 10 Americans.

2. 5.8 million people use cocaine per month.

3. The American drug of choice is still marijuana, with 18 million people using it per month.

4. Sixty percent (60%) of people between the ages of 18 and 35 have tried an illegal drug.

5. Thirty percent (30%) of people between the ages of 12 and 17 have used an illegal drug at least once.

6. More people die annually from prescription drugs obtained legally, but used improperly, than from all illegal substances combined.

7. Drunk drivers account for 60% of all traffic deaths each year.

8. Crack has brought substance abuse in epidemic proportions to lower socioeconomic groups because it is cheap, easily obtained and easily used (by smoking).

9. The age of the typical abuser continues to drop annually.

10. Substance abuse spans all geographic regions, ethnic groups, and social classes.

11. Statistics indicate earlier first use of drugs—dropping below junior high school levels into pre-teen age groups.

12. The most frequently abused drugs by adolescents are: alcohol, marijuana, tobacco, illegal prescription stimulants, and cocaine.

13. Adolescents who smoke or drink are far more likely to abuse illegal drugs.

14. Kids are more likely to use drugs in combinations and sooner than adults.

15. Teenagers are far more vulnerable to developmental problems, and even brain damage, because their body systems are not fully developed.

Module I.4—Handout #2

SUBSTANCE ABUSE TERMS

1. *Habituation:* Pattern of repeated drug use in the absence of an actual physical need for the drug. There is no desire for increased use. There are no withdrawal manifestations.

2. *Misuse:* Used for purposes other than those for which they are intended. Common among people, especially the elderly, who self-medicate for a variety of reasons.

3. *Abuse:* Drug use patterns outside the limits acceptable by society and which impact negatively on psychological, physiological, and social functioning of an individual. It is a concept that is, in part, culturally defined. Drug abuse may be combined with misuse.

4. *Dependence:* Reliance on a drug to a degree in which the absence will cause an impairment in function.

   a. *Psychological dependence* is characterized by a compulsive need to experience pleasurable response from the drug.

   b. *Physical dependence* is an altered physiological state resulting from prolonged drug use; regular use is necessary to prevent withdrawal.

5. *Tolerance:* Decreased effect of a drug resulting from repeated exposure. It is also possible to develop cross-tolerance to other drugs in the same category.

6. *Addiction:* Compulsive drug use for both physical and psychological reasons.

7. *Dual Addiction:* Simultaneous dependence on substances that have similar effects, such as alcohol and other CNS depressants (e.g., the benzodiazepine, Valium).

8. *Mixed Addiction:* Dependence on more than one substance, not necessarily similar in effect, such as alcohol and cocaine.

TYPES OF DRUGS AND COMMON STREET NAMES (A)

CNS Depressants:

Alcohol	Booze, white lightning
Barbiturates:	Goofballs, dolls, downers
Seconal (Secobarbital)	Red Devils, Seccy
Nembutal (Pentobarbital)	Yellow Jackets, Nembies
Non-Barbiturates:	
Methaqualone (Quaaludes)	Ludes
Anti-Anxiety Agents:	
Valium (Diazepam)	Tranqs
Librium	Roaches

CNS Stimulants:

Amphetamines:	Bennies, Uppers, Pep Pills
Dexedrine (Dextroamphetamine)	Dexies
Amphetamine sulfate (Amphetamine)	Beans
Methamphetamines	Speed
Cocaine, Crack	Coke, Snow, Flake
Cocaine and Heroin	Speedball
Anorectics	

Module I.4—Handout #3B

TYPES OF DRUGS AND COMMON STREET NAMES (B)

Narcotics:

    Opiates:

Morphine	M, Microdots
Codeine	Terp (cough syrup)

    Semi-synthetic:

Hydromorphone (Dilaudid)	
Heroin	H, Horse, Junk, Shit, Skag, Smack

    Synthetic:

Methadone	Dollies
Meperidine (Demerol)	

Psychotomimetics (Hallucinogens):

LSD	Acid, Blue Dots
Mescaline	Mescal
MDMA (XTC)	Ecstasy
Phencyclidine (PCP)	Angel Dust, Goon, Shermans, Superjoint, Whack

Volatile Inhalants:

Amyl Nitrites	Poppers
Toluene, Gasoline	
Fluorocarbons	
Nitrous Oxide	

Cannabinoids:

Marijuana	Acapulco Gold, Grass, Hay, Hemp, Joint, Mary Jane, Pot, Reefer, Roach
Hashish	Bang, Hash, Sweet Lucy

Nicotine

Caffeine

Steroids

Module I.4—Handout #4A

CLASSES OF ABUSED DRUGS AND THEIR ACTIONS

General Type of Drug	Drug Effects	Drug Name	Site of Action	Length of Effect	Potential for Addiction
CNS DEPRESSANTS					
1. Sedative hypnotics	Drowsiness/sedation/sleep, escape/loss of inhibition, reduction of aggressive and sexual drives, emotional instability, poor judgment.	Barbiturates: Seconal, Nembutal, Amytal, Tuinal, Barbiturate-like (Quaaludes) Benzodiazepines, Minor tranquilizers (Librium, Valium).	CNS (ascending reticular activating system). Taken orally and ingested.	Usual onset: 30–45 min. Usual duration: 4–5 hr.	HIGH: Tolerance and life-threatening withdrawal occur. Cross-tolerance to all CNS depressants occurs.
2. Alcohol	Relaxation, sedation, release of inhibition. Objective signs: Incoordination, nausea, ataxia, vomiting, impaired cognitive function, slurred speech.	Beverage alcohol: beer, wine, liquor.	Taken orally. CNS Respiratory system.	Usual onset: 20 min.–1 hr. Dose-related.	HIGH: Tolerance and life-threatening withdrawal occur.
CNS STIMULANTS					
3. Stimulants	Euphoria/grandiosity, energy, excitation, relief of fatigue, depression, wakefulness, suppression of appetite, aggressive feelings, paranoia, reproductive dysfunction in women. Objective signs: Sweating, dilated pupils, weight loss, vital signs elevated, tremors, seizures.	Amphetamine, (Methamphetamine, Dexedrine), Cocaine, Crack (free base), Caffeine.	CNS (Synapses).	Usual duration: 2–6 hr. Rapid onset; Brief duration: Up to 30 min.	HIGH: Tolerance and withdrawal occur. HIGH: Tolerance and withdrawal occur.

Module I.4—Handout #4B

CLASSES OF ABUSED DRUGS AND THEIR ACTIONS

General Type of Drug	Drug Effects	Drug Name	Site of Action	Length of Effect	Potential for Addiction
NARCOTICS					
4. Opioids (narcotics, synthetic narcotics)	Analgesia, euphoria, escape, reduction in sexual and aggressive drives, sedation, sleepiness. Objective signs: Hypertension, respiratory depression, constipation, impaired intellectual function.	Codeine, Morphine, Heroin, Dilaudid, Methadone, Demerol.	Bind in receptor sites, CNS, GI tract. Taken orally and injected, inhaled.	Usual onset: 20–30 min. Usual duration: 4–8 hr.	HIGH: Tolerance and withdrawal occur.
HALLUCINOGENS					
5. Psychedelic drugs	Euphoria, altered perceptions, somatic effects (dizziness, tremors, weakness, nausea), psychotic-like symptoms, flashbacks. Objective signs: Dilated pupils, emotional swings, suspiciousness, paranoia, bizarre behavior, increased BP.	LSD, Psilocybin, Mescaline, MDA (Ecstasy), DOM, DMT.	CNS (modify neurotransmitters). Taken orally.	Usual onset: 30–40 min. Usual duration: 8–12 hr. Mescaline: 12–14 hr. LSD: 10–12 hr.	Psychological dependence only.
6. Phencyclidines	Detachment from surroundings, decreased sensory awareness, illusions of superhuman strength, acute intoxication. Objective signs: Flushing, fever, sweating, coma, agitation, incoherent, speech, aggression.	PCP (Angel Dust).	CNS. Inhaled.	Rapid onset: 2–3 min., up to 45 min. Prolonged effects.	Psychological only.

Module I.4—Handout #4C

CLASSES OF ABUSED DRUGS AND THEIR ACTIONS

General Type of Drug	Drug Effects	Drug Name	Site of Action	Length of Effect	Potential for Addiction
INHALANTS					
7. Inhalants	Euphoria, giddiness, headache, fatigue. Objective signs: Increase in vital signs, damage to kidneys, and liver, disorientation.	Benzene (paint thinner, cleaning fluid, glue), Nitrites, Freons, Nitrous Oxide.	Cardiac effects, CNS, Inhaled.	Rapid absorption.	Psychological only.
CANNABINOIDS					
8. Cannabinoids	Failure in judgment/ memory, mild intoxication, euphoria, relaxation, sexual arousal, panic states and psychosis in high doses.	Marijuana, Hashish (THC, Cannabis saliva).	CNS, Cardiovascular system, Smoked.	Admin./dose dependent. Usual onset: 20–30 min. Usual duration. 3–7 hr. Objective signs: Reddened eyes; heart rate to 140/bpm; pulse, respirations, BP increase.	MODERATE: Psychological dependence and long-term effects occur.

From: Naegle, M.A. (1989). *Psychiatric mental health nursing: A client-centered approach.* Philadelphia: J. B. Lippincott.

Module I.4—Handout #5A

WHAT COULD HAPPEN IF YOU DRINK
WHILE TAKING ANY OF THESE DRUGS?

The chart below lists classes of drugs which have been reported to interact with alcohol. It must be emphasized that this only represents the smallest part of the whole alcohol-drug interaction picture. It is not meant to replace the advice of your doctor or pharmacist.

ANALGESICS, NARCOTIC

(Demoral, Darvon, Dilaudid, etc.)

When used alone, both alcohol and narcotic drugs cause a reduction in the function of the central nervous system. When used together, this effect is even greater, and may lead to loss of effective breathing function (respiratory arrest). Death may occur.

ANALGESICS, NON-NARCOTIC

(Aspirin, APC, Pabalate, etc.)

Even when used alone, some non-prescription pain relievers can cause bleeding in the stomach and intestines. Alcohol also irritates the stomach and can aggravate the bleeding, especially in ulcer patients.

ANTIALCOHOL PREPARATIONS

(Antabuse, Calcium Carbamide)

Use of alcohol with medications prescribed to help alcoholic patients keep from drinking results in nausea, vomiting, headaches, high blood pressure, and possible erratic heartbeat. Can result in death.

ANTICOAGULANTS

(Panwarfin, Dicumarol, Sintrom, etc.)

Alcohol can increase the ability of these drugs to stop blood clotting, which in turn can lead to life-threatening or fatal hemorrhages.

ANTICONVULSANTS

(Dilatin, Diphenyl, EKKO, etc.)

Drinking may lessen the ability of the drug to stop convulsions in a person.

ANTIDEPRESSANTS

(Tofranil, Pertofrane, Triavil, etc.)

Alcohol may cause an additional reduction in central nervous system functioning and lessen a person's ability to operate normally. Certain wines like Chianti may cause a high blood pressure crisis.

Module I.4—Handout #5B

WHAT COULD HAPPEN IF YOU DRINK
WHILE TAKING ANY OF THESE DRUGS?

ANTIDIABETIC AGENTS/HYPOGLYCEMICS

(Insulin, Diabenese, Orinase, etc.)

Because of the possible severe reaction to combining alcohol and insulin or the oral antidiabetic agents, and because alcohol interacts unpredictably with them, patients taking any of these medications should avoid alcohol.

ANTIHISTAMINES

(Most cold remedies, Actifed, Coricidin, etc.)

Taking alcohol with this class of drugs increases their calming effect and a person can feel quite drowsy, making driving and other activities that require alertness more hazardous.

ANTIHYPERTENSIVE AGENTS

(Serpasil, Aldomet, Esidrix, etc.)

Alcohol may increase the blood pressure lowering capability of some of these drugs, causing dizziness when a person gets up. Some agents will also cause a reduction in the function of the central nervous system.

ANTIBIOTICS

(Flagyl, Chloromycetin, Seromycis, etc.)

In combination with alcohol, some may cause nausea, vomiting, and headache, and possibly convulsions, especially those taken for urinary tract infections.

CENTRAL NERVOUS SYSTEM STIMULANTS

(Most diet pills, Dexedrine, Caffeine, Ritalin)

Because the stimulant effect of this class of drugs may reverse the depressant effect of the alcohol on the central nervous system, these drugs can give a false sense of security. They do *not* help intoxicated persons gain control of their movements.

DIURETICS

(Diuril, Lasix, Hydromox, etc.)

Combining alcohol with diuretics may cause reduction in blood pressure, possibly resulting in dizziness.

Module I.4—Handout #5C

WHAT COULD HAPPEN IF YOU DRINK
WHILE TAKING ANY OF THESE DRUGS?

PSYCHOTROPICS

(Tindal, Mellaril, Thorazine, etc.)

Alcohol and the major tranquilizers cause additional depression to the central nervous system function, which can result in severe impairment of voluntary movements such as walking or using the hands. The combination can also cause a loss of effective breathing function and can be fatal.

SEDATIVE HYPNOTICS

(Doriden, Quaalude, Nembutal, etc.)

Alcohol in combination further reduces the function of the central nervous system, sometimes to the point of coma or loss of effective breathing (respiratory arrest). This combination can be fatal.

SLEEP MEDICINES

It is likely that non-prescription sleeping medicines, to the degree that they are effective, will lead to the same kind of central nervous system depression when combined with alcohol as the minor tranquilizers. (See below.)

TRANQUILIZERS—MINOR

(Miltown, Valium, Librium, etc.)

Tranquilizers in combination with alcohol will cause reduced functioning of the central nervous system, especially during the first weeks of drug use. This results in decreased alertness and judgment, and can also lead to household and automotive accidents.

VITAMINS

Continuous drinking can keep vitamins from entering the blood stream. However, this situation stops when a person stops drinking.

From: National Council on Alcoholism, Northern Jersey Area, Inc., 60 South Fullerton Avenue, Room 211, Montclair, New Jersey 07042.

MEDICATIONS CONTAINING ALCOHOL*

Drug	Percentage of Alcohol	Drug	Percentage of Alcohol
Actol Expectorant	12.5	Dramamine Liquid	5.0
Alurate Elixir	20.0	Elixophyllin	20.0
Ambenyl Expectorant	5.0	Elixophyllin-KI	10.0
Aromatic Elixir	22.0	Ephedrine Sulfate Syrup	
Asbron Elixir	15.0	U.S.P.	3.0
Atarax Syrup	0.5	Ephedrine Sulfate Syrup-Not	
Bactrim Suspension	0.3	U.S.P.	12.0
Tr. Belladonna	67.0	Feosol Elixir	5.0
Benadryl Elixir	14.0	Fer-In-Sol Syrup	5.0
Bentyl-Pb Syrup	19.0	Fer-In-Sol Drops	0.2
Benyiin Expectorant	5.0	Geriplex-FS	18.0
Brondecon Elixir	20.0	Gevrabon	18.0
Bronkolixir	19.0	Hycotuss Expectorant & Syrup	10.0
Butibel Elixir	7.0	Hydryllin Compound	5.0
Calcidrine Syrup	6.0	Iberet Liquid	1.0
Cas Evac	18.0	Ipecac Syrup	2.0
Aromatic Cascara Sagrada	18.0	Isuprel Comp. Elixir	19.0
Cerose & Cerose DM Expect	2.5	Kaochlor	5.0
Cheracol & Cheracol D	3.0	Kaon	5.0
Chlor-Trimeton Syrup	7.0	Kay-Ciel Elixir	4.0
Choledyl Elixir	2.0	Lanoxin Elixir Pediatric	10.0
Citra Forte Syrup	2.0	Lomotil Liquid	1.0
Cologel Liquid	5.0	Luffyllin-GG	1.0
Conar Expectorant	5.0	Marax Syrup	5.0
Coryban D	7.5	Mediatric Liquid	1.0
Decadron Elixir	5.0	Mellaril Concentrate	3.0
Demazin Syrup	7.5	Minocin Syrup	5.0
Dexedrine Elixir	1.0	Modane Liquid	5.0
Dilantin Suspension	0.6	Mol Iron Liquid	4.0
Dilaudid Cough Syrup	5.0	Nembutal Elixir	1.0
Dimacol Liquid	4.0	Nico-Metrazol Elixir	1.0
Dimetane Elixir	3.0	Novahistine DH	5.0
Dimetane Expectorant	3.5	Novahistine DMX	1.0
Dimetane Expectorant-DC	3.5	Novahistine Expectorant	7.5
Dimetapp Elixir	2.3	Novahistine Elixir	5.0
Donnagel	3.8	Nyquil Cough Syrup	2.0
Donnagel PG	5.0	Organidin Elixir	23.0
Donnatal Elixir	2.0	Ornacol Liquid	8.0
Doxinate Liquid	5.0	Tincture Paregoric	4.0

*Space does not permit listing all products containing alcohol. Consult a pharmacist for information about other products.

Module I.4—Handout #6B

MEDICATIONS CONTAINING ALCOHOL*

Drug	Percentage of Alcohol	Drug	Percentage of Alcohol
Parelixir	18.0	Rondec-DM	0.6
Parepectolin	0.69	Roniacol Elixir	8.0
Periactin Syrup	5.0	Serpasil Elixir	1.0
Pertussin 8 Hour Syrup	9.5	Tedral Elixir	1.0
Phenergan Expectorant Plain	7.0	Temaril Syrup	5.7
Phenergan Expectorant with Codeine	7.0	Terpin Hydrate Elixir	4.0
Phenergan Expectorant VC, Plain	7.0	Terpin Hydrate Elixir with Codeine	4.0
Phenergan Expectorant VC, with Codeine	7.0	Theolixir	2.0
		Theo Organidin Elixir	1.0
Phenergan Expectorant Pediatric	7.0	Triaminic Expectorant	5.0
Phenergan Syrup Fortis		Triaminic Expectorant D.H	5.0
(25 mg)	1.5	Tussar-2 Syrup	5.0
Phenobarbital Elixir	14.0	Tussar SF Syrup	1.0
Polaramine Expectorant	7.2	Tussend	6.0
P.B.Z. Exp. with Codeine and		Tussi-Organidin	1.0
Ephedrine	6.0	Tuss-Ornade	7.5
P.B.Z. Exp. with Ephedrine	6.0	Tylenol Drops	7.0
Propadrine Elixir	16.0	Tylenol Elixir	7.0
Quibron Elixir	15.0	Tylenol with Codeine Elixir	7.0
Robitussin	3.5	Ulo-Syrup	6.65
Robitussin-AC	3.5	Valadol Liquid	9.0
Robitussin-CF	1.4	Vicks Formula 44	10.0
Robitussin-DM	1.4	Vita Metrazol Elixir	15.0
Robitussin-PE	1.4	Potassium Chloride Sol	
		(Standard)	10.0
		(A no alcohol solution can be requested)	

---

*Space does not permit listing all products containing alcohol. Consult a pharmacist for information about other products.

From: Berger, J., et al. (1979, February 28). Medications containing alcohol. *Patient Care, 13*(4), 103.

Note:

1. Mouthwashes—Scope, Listerine, Cepacol, Colgate 100, Micrin all have approximately 15–25%.

2. All elixirs contain some alcohol.

3. The following antitussives do not contain alcohol:

   Hycodan Syrup   Orthoxicol Syrup

   Hycomine Syrup   Actifed C Expectorant

   Triaminicol Syrup   Omni-Tuss

   Tussionex Suspension   Ipsatol Syrup

4. Other nonalcoholic liquids:

   Chloraseptic mouthwash/gargle   Sudafed Syrup

   Liquiprin (acetaminophen)   Quadrinal Susp.

   Alupent Syrup   Actifed Syrup

   Noctec Syrup   Triaminic Syrup

   Vistaril Susp.   Naldecon Syrup

   Antacids   Nydrazid Syrup

   Kaopectate and Pargel, etc.

RECOMMENDED TEACHING STRATEGIES AND SAMPLE ASSIGNMENTS

RECOMMENDED TEACHING STRATEGIES

- Lecture
- Discussion
- Media

SAMPLE ASSIGNMENTS

1. Assignment of students to clinical setting designed for treatment of substance abuse.

2. Cite nursing considerations necessary before and during administration of benzodiazepines.

3. Ask students to be ready to identify significant drug interactions possible with barbiturates, paying attention to both most likely interactants and resulting interactions.

4. Take time to review carefully possible side effects and adverse reactions to amphetamines. Ask: Why are amphetamines contraindicated in hypertension or cardiovascular diseases?

5. Assign students to develop client education teaching plan for amphetamines, anorexiants and analeptics.

From: McKenry, L., & Salerno, E. (1989). *Mosby's pharmacology in nursing: Instructor's manual and test bank.* Philadelphia: C. V. Mosby.

TEST QUESTIONS AND ANSWERS

TEST QUESTIONS

1. Match the drug name (combination) with the street name:

   a. _____ amyl nitrite   1. speed ball

   b. _____ methaqualone (quaaludes)   2. poppers

   c. _____ amphetamine/opiate combination   3. angel dust

   d. _____ barbiturates (secobarbital)   4. ludes

   e. _____ phencyclidine (PCP)   5. red devils

2. Alcoholics are prone to the development of cross-tolerance with barbiturates. The implications of this in treating an alcoholic with barbiturates suggest that one should:

   a. decrease the barbiturate dose.

   b. increase the barbiturate dose.

   c. avoid the use of barbiturates.

   d. maintain normal doses until a toxicity develops.

3. Mary Henry is a 28-year-old mother of three who enters the emergency room with a fractured arm. She states that she fell three days ago but did not think it was serious. Your assessment results in the following findings. Which symptom does not classify as a possible indicator of alcoholism?

   a. Palmar erythema.

   b. Multiple bruises.

   c. Paranoia.

   d. Fine hand tremors.

4. James Robbins enters the emergency room with delirium, Cheyne-Stokes respirations, rapid pulse, and severe anxiety. Because he is delirious he is unable to tell you what drugs he took. The signs suggest which of the following substances?

   a. Heroin.

   b. Free based cocaine.

   c. Phencyclidine (PCP).

   d. Methaqualone (quaaludes).

5. Narcan (naloxone) is used in the treatment of acute heroin overdose. One of the dangers in using Narcan is:

   a. precipitating acute withdrawal symptoms.

   b. aggravating cardiac arrhythmias.

   c. inducing profound hypotension.

   d. exacerbating agitated, paranoid behavior.

6. Undesirable reactions ("bad trips") are a significant problem associated with phencyclidines (PCP). Select the treatment modality which should *not* be employed in treating acute overdose:

   a. Sedatives to control agitation.

   b. Urinary acidifiers to facilitate excretion.

   c. Isolation to minimize stimuli.

   d. Frequent verbal contact to provide support.

7. Select the physiological changes which accompany cannabis saliva (marijuana) use:

   a. Running nose, anorexia, papillary constriction.

   b. Elevated heart rate, conjunctival congestion, enhanced appetite.

   c. Impaired speech, loss of coordination, and elevated blood pressure.

   d. Euphoric sensation ("rush"), nausea, and feeling of detachment.

8. Volatile nitrites (e.g., amyl nitrite) have increased in popular use because heightened sensations of orgasm may occur during sexual intercourse. Select the physiological action which explains this phenomenon:

   a. Profound vasodilation.

   b. Reflex bradycardia.

   c. Mild hypertension.

   d. Cutaneous flushing.

9. Acute amphetamine withdrawal is characterized by:

   a. paranoia, hostility, agitation, and tremors.

   b. convulsions, tachycardia, and profound emotional withdrawal.

   c. confusion, psychosis, amnesia, and visual hallucinations.

   d. fatigue, muscle pain, lethargy, and depression.

10. Ellen Trammers is a 16-year-old who enters the emergency room in acute pulmonary edema. She has "track marks" indicating I.V. drug abuse. Which substance is most likely to be the precipitating agent?

    a. Heroin.

    b. Crack.

    c. Phencyclidines (PCP).

    d. Free based cocaine.

Module I.4

ANSWER KEY

1. a-2
   b-4
   c-1
   d-5
   e-3
2. b
3. c
4. b
5. a
6. d
7. b
8. a
9. d
10. c

BIBLIOGRAPHY

MODULE I.4 PHARMACOLOGY

Ahmad, G. (1987). Abuse of Phencyclidine (PCP): A laboratory experience. *Journal of Clinical Toxicology, 25*(4), 341–346.

Berkowitz, B. A. (1976). Relationship of pharmacokinetics to pharmacological activity: Morphine, methadone, naloxone. *Clinical Pharmacokinetics,1*(3), 219–230.

Berger, J., Clark, T., Cruse, J. et al. (1979). Medications containing alcohol. *Patient Care, 13*(4).

Boning, J. (1985). Benzodiazepine dependence: Clinical neuro-biological aspects. *Advances in Biochemical Psychopharmacology, 40,* 185–192.

Buffum, J. (1982). Pharmacosexology: The effects of drugs on sexual function. *Journal of Psychoactive Drugs, 14*(1–2), 5–44.

Busto, V. (1986). Patterns of benzodiazepine abuse and dependence. *British Journal of Addictions, 81*(1), 87–94.

Cushman, P. (1986). Sedative drug interactions of clinical importance. *Recent Developments in Alcohol, 4,* 61–83.

Duncan, D. J., & Shaw, E. B. (1985). Anabolic steroids: Implications for the nurse practitioner. *Nurse Practitioner, 10*(12), 13–15.

Freund, G. (1984). Biomedical causes of alcohol abuse. *Alcohol, 1*(2), 129–131.

Gawin, F. H., & Ellingwood, E. H. (1988). Cocaine and other stimulants: Action, abuse and treatment. *New England Journal of Medicine, 318,* 1173–1182.

Gold, M. S. (1988). *The facts about drugs and alcohol* (3rd ed., rev.). Washington, DC: Bantam, Psychiatric Institute of America Press.

Goldstein, D. B. (Ed.) (1983). *The pharmacology of alcohol.* New York: Oxford University Press.

Hahn, A. B., Oestereich, S. J. K., & Borkin, R. (1986). *Pharmacology in nursing.* St. Louis: C. V. Mosby.

Ho, A. K. S., Chen, R. C. A., & Morrison, J. M. (1977). Opiate ethanol interaction studies. In K. Blum (Ed.), *Alcohol and opiates* (pp. 89–202). New York: Academic Press.

Malseed, R. (1985). Drug dependence and addiction. In R. Malseed (Ed.), *Pharmacology: Drug therapy and nursing considerations.* Philadelphia: J. B. Lippincott.

Matthewson, M. (Ed.). (1989). *Pharmacotherapeutics* (2nd ed.). Philadelphia: F. A. Davis.

McKenry, L., & Salerno, E. (1989). *Mosby's pharmacology in nursing: Instructor's manual and test bank*. Philadelphia: C. V. Mosby.

Naegle, M. A. (1989). Utilizing the nursing process with the client who abuses drug and alcohol. In M. Matthewson (Ed.), *Pharmacotherapeutics* (2nd ed.). Philadelphia: F. A. Davis.

Peterson, R. G., & Rumack, B. H. (1977). Treating acute acetaminophen poisoning with acetylcysteine. *Journal of American Medical Association, 237*, 2406–2407.

Shlafer, M., & Marieb, E. (1989). *The nurses' pharmacology and drug therapy*. Menlo Park, CA: Addison-Wesley.

Smith, D. (1984). Benzodiazepine dependence potential: Current studies and trends. *Journal of Substance Abuse Treatment, 1*(3), 163–167.

Spiker, D. G. (1975). Tricyclic antidepressant overdose: Clinical presentation and plasma levels. *Clinical Pharmacologic Therapy, 18*(5), 539–546.

Spitz, H., & Rosecan, J. (Eds.) (1987). *Cocaine abuse: New directions in treatment and research*. New York: Brunner/Mazel.

Sullivan, J. B., et al. (1979). Management of tricyclic antidepressant toxicity. *Topics in Emergency Medicine, 1*(3), 65–71.

Teped, H. (1985). Biochemical basis of alcoholism: Statements and hypotheses of present research. *Alcohol, 2*(6), 711–788.

Vourakis, C., & Bennett, G. (1979). Angel dust: Not heaven sent. *American Journal of Nursing, 79*, 649–652.

Wesson, D., & Smith, D. (1977). *Barbiturates: Their uses, misuse and abuse*. New York: American Science Press.

West, R. J., & Russell, M. A. (1985). Dependence on nicotine chewing gum. *Journal of the American Medical Association, 256*, 3214–3215.

Zerwecki, J., & Gordon, D. (Eds.) (1989). *The nursing clinics of North America*. Philadelphia: W. B. Saunders.

MODULE I.5
DYSFUNCTIONAL PATTERNS
IN FAMILIES WITH DRUG AND
ALCOHOL PROBLEMS

Kem Louie, PhD, RN, CS

Madeline A. Naegle, PhD, RN, FAAN
Project Director
Janet S. D'Arcangelo, MA, RN, C
Project Coordinator

Project SAEN
SUBSTANCE ABUSE
EDUCATION IN NURSING

CONTENT OUTLINE

I. Drug and Alcohol Use in Families

    A. Populations at Risk

    B. Patterns of Alcohol and Other Drug Use

II. Familial History and Genetic Factors Related to Risk for Drug and Alcohol Problems

    A. Research on Family and Genetic Predisposition

    B. Utilizing the Genogram in Understanding Family History

    C. Role Modeling and Social Learning Theory

    D. The Family History Model of Alcoholism

    E. The "Shame Bound" Family Model

    F. The Dysfunctional Family Model

    G. Family History of Drug and Alcohol Dependence, Psychiatric Illness

III. Patterns of Family and Childhood Disturbances Associated with Family Drug Use

    A. Deviations From Normal Development of Children With Fetal Alcohol Syndrome and Fetal Alcohol Effects

    B. Children with AIDS

    C. Developmental Disturbance in Children of Addicted Parents

    D. Adaptive Roles and Coping Strategies

    E. Physical and Sexual Abuse

    F. Domestic Violence

IV. Alterations in Family Process Related to Drug Use

    A. Overview of Family Roles and Communication Patterns

V. Nursing Interventions with the Drug Using Family

A. Must Be Sensitive to Cultural and Ethnic Differences in Values and Health Practices

B. Health Teaching

C. Screening and Early Identification

D. Referral

E. Evaluation of Interventions

I. DRUG AND ALCOHOL USE IN FAMILIES

A. Populations at Risk

1. The prevalence of alcoholism and other drug addictions in American society place families and their members at risk for the development of highly dysfunctional patterns, a variety of dependencies and emotional illness. Abuse or dependence on alcohol or other drugs by a family member results in distortions of traditional patterns of family interaction related to role structure, communication, completion of developmental tasks and other patterns which impede smooth family functioning.

2. Drug using patterns occur in a social context and may also serve to sustain family dynamics and contribute to family unity through symptomatic behavior (Bernal, Rodriguez, Diamond, 1990).

3. An estimated 18 million American adults have a serious drinking problem or are alcoholic. Another 5.5 million probably need treatment for drug dependence (Institute of Medicine, 1990). An estimated 6.6 million children under the age of 18 live in homes with at least one alcoholic parent (Russell, 1984); the number of children living with other drug dependent parents is unknown.

4. In addition to dysfunctional interactional patterns, cultural, economic and trans-generational patterns influence the outcomes of drug use on children.

B. Patterns of Alcohol and Other Drug Use

1. Of individuals over the age of 12 residing in American household, 85% have used alcohol at least once. This same population has a 37% use of illicit drugs.

2. Adolescent drug use is a frequently identified "family" problem.

   a. Drinking usually begins in adolescence and by age 18, about 90% have used alcohol.

      (1) By age 13, approximately 30% of boys and 22% of girls drink alcohol.

      (2) By age 18, 92% of boys and 73% of girls drink alcohol.

   b. In 1988, 24.7% of individuals ages 12–17 had used illicit drugs 1990).

      (1) Marijuana use is highest among individuals in the 18–25 year-old group.

   c. Peer group behavior and drug use by parents are the most influential factors in adolescent drug use (See Module 1.6).

3. Patterns of drug use vary by geographic region, gender, age, socioeconomic group, race, and ethnicity.

   a. Fathers more frequently have problems with alcohol and other drugs than do mothers.

   b. Family traditions and rituals influence the acceptance of drug use and values developed in relation to drug use.

   c. Changes in the family system where drugs are used can be viewed as attempts to adapt.

d. Patterns of drug use, such as drug related behaviors, frequency of intoxication and the extent to which drug use limits economic resources, influence the impact of alcohol and drug-related problems on the family.

II. FAMILIAL HISTORY AND GENETIC FACTORS RELATED TO RISKS FOR ALCOHOL AND DRUG PROBLEMS

A. Research on familial and genetic predisposition suggests that certain factors may predispose individuals to alcohol and other drug problems. Since alcoholism appears repeatedly from generation to generation, questions of environmental versus constitutional variables continue:

1. Studies of adopted children of alcoholics conducted in Sweden, Denmark and the United States and Finland indicate that children of alcoholics had a high rate of alcoholism even when raised by adoptive parents rather than their alcoholic biologic parents (Bohman, 1978; Bohman, Sigvardsson & Cloniger, 1981; Cadoret & Gath, 1978; Cadoret, Cain & Grove, 1980; Bohman, Sigvardsson & Cloniger, 1981; Goodwin, 1971; Goodwin, Schulsinger, Hermanson, Guze & Winokur, 1973, 1975).

2. Biological marker studies have also been implemented; subjects are studied prior to extensive exposure to alcohol with the hope of identifying indicators of alcoholism. Findings are inconsistent.

3. Biochemical deficiencies which may be inherited have also been linked to alcohol and other drug use. Reductions in serotonin (Boismare, et al., 1987), endorphins (Barret, Bourhis, Buffet, Danel and Debru, 1987) have been suggested in some studies, and Dole and Nyswander (1976) suggest that endorphin deficiencies in heroin addicts are compensated for with methadone.

4. Other physiologic factors related to alcoholism include variation in alcohol dehydrogenase (ADH) and aldehyde dehydrogenase (ALDH), and monoamine oxidase (MAO) levels (Kinney, J. (1991). *Clinical Manual of Substance Abuse* St. Louis, MO: Mosby–Yearbook.)

B. Utilizing the Genogram in Understanding Family History

1. The "genogram" is similar to a family tree, but it describes information not only on family members' relationships to one another, but over three generations. Information includes: gender, births, birth order, death, date and cause of death, marital status, and health problems.

   a. Formats for constructing genograms vary from simple to complex. A sample is in the study guide. Standard symbols are used to connote gender, death, and relationship linkages. The historian can add symbols to represent events or character traits of interest.

   b. The genogram is well-utilized in the history taking and family assessment or in early treatment, and is most valuable when all family members participate in its formulation.

C. Role Modeling and Social Learning Theory

1. The excessive use of alcohol and other drugs provides a model for family members which is frequently passed from generation to generation.

2. When drinking or drug using becomes the central organizing principle for the family system, behaviors are learned which function to maintain a homeostasis of the system.

3. Learned patterns of behavior include rigid family roles, and roles which enable the continuation of the dysfunctional drug taking behavior, such as "enabling."

4. Attitudes about the acceptability of drug using as a coping mechanism may develop in family members.

5. Positive reinforcement may be learned through role modeling whereby children experience positive effects of drug use, then increase usage, ultimately, using to fend off withdrawal symptoms.

D. The Family History Model of Alcoholism (Steinglass, 1980)

1. Alcohol use becomes the central organizing principle for the daily life of the family system. Families cycle through two different and predictable interactional states, one associated with sobriety and one associated by intoxication.

2. Patterns of family development in the alcoholic family consist of a series of progressive stages which can be observed and differentiated from non-alcoholic family developmental phases.

E. The "Shame Bound" Family Model (Fossum and Mason, 1986)

1. Families where one or more members are addicted to compulsive behaviors, including substance abuse, exhibit patterns of shame.

2. A shame-bound family is one with a self-sustaining, multi-generational system of interaction among individuals loyal to a set of rules demanding control, perfectionism, blame and denial.

3. The pattern of shame serves to inhibit or defeat healthy growth and development, including the attainment of intimacy, a defined separate identity, and the perpetuation of shame within subsequent family relationships and family systems.

F. The Dysfunctional Family Model (Bowen, 1978)

1. Bowen described dysfunctional families as characterized by an "undifferentiated family ego mass" where the family system is emotionally connected by tensions and anxieties.

2. Families are "undifferentiated" when none of the members can function independently from the whole. Family members are "differentiated" by degree; low differentiation of family members leads to anxiety, fears of acting alone,

low self-esteem and a poorly defined sense of a separate self. People tend to choose marital partners who are similar to them in level of differentiation.

3. "Triangulation" occurs in families when a two-member emotional subsystem, i.e., husband and wife, relieve tension by shifting the focus from their relationship by incorporating a third person, or possibly a substance.

4. Interactional processes within the family system and its "subsystems" create patterns, including triangulating, which become fixed over time and are learned from one generation to the next.

G. Family History of Drug and/or Alcohol Dependence, Psychiatric Illness

1. Families with members who are alcohol and/or drug dependent show a higher rate of psychiatric disturbance than families in the general population.

2. The presence of "dual diagnosis" or "co-morbidity" increases the complexity of assessment and treatment of the family.

3. Co-existing psychiatric disturbances include schizophrenia, manic-depressive illness, and personality disorders.

4. Co-existing disorders exacerbate one another, although they may be of separate etiologies.

5. The dually diagnosed individual is frequently a poly-substance abuser. (Carey, 1989).

6. Alcoholism itself is a "traumatic" experience and may cause psychopathology in the abuser (Bean-Bayog, 1988).

III. PATTERNS OF FAMILY AND CHILDHOOD DISTURBANCES ASSOCIATED WITH FAMILY DRUG USE

A. Deviations from Normal Development in Children with Fetal Alcohol Syndrome and Fetal Alcohol Effects (See Module II.1)

1. Children with these disturbances require assistance with psychomotor and learning tasks.

2. Families require assistance in accessing appropriate social and health services.

B. Children with AIDS

1. The human immunodeficiency virus is most frequently transmitted to infants by mothers who are intravenous drug users or partners of intravenous drug users.

2. Rates of transmission of HIV are rising most rapidly among women and intravenous drug users of color.

3. Children born to seropositive mothers may be seropositive at birth or convert within the first 18 months to 10 years of life.

4. These children may manifest congenital problems and disorders associated with premature labor and delivery or be asymptomatic for many months after birth.

5. The multiple problems experienced by these children require ongoing involvement with health care providers.

6. Extensive periods of illness and premature deaths of children and parents pose complex social, ethical and health care problems.

C. Developmental Disturbance in Children of Alcohol and Drug Abusers

1. Research studies on children in this population have focused primarily on children of alcoholics. Findings suggest that a variety of differences exist between children of alcoholics and children of non-alcoholics; research limitations, including inadequate numbers of studies, prohibit generalizations about all children who grow up with alcoholic parents and children in families where parents are addicted to other drugs and dually addicted.

2. Children of alcoholic parents appear to be at risk for cognitive, emotional and behavioral problems.

   a. They often have academic problems such as poor grades and failure to complete schooling (Miller & Jang, 1977).

   b. Psychological disorders in children include higher levels of anxiety and depression, and general stress (Schuckit & Chiles, 1978; Moos & Billings, 1982; Anderson & Quast, 1983).

   c. Children of alcoholics appear to be at risk for delinquency and truancy, and conduct disorders (West & Prinz, 1987; Rimmer, 1982).

   d. Additional psychological stresses for children are associated with the consequences of drug use, such as separation and divorce, incarceration of a parent, parental psychological disturbance, and unstable parent-child relationships.

   e. Clinical observations of children of cocaine (crack) using mothers suggest problems in parental attachment, learning lags, and impaired social and psychomotor skills.

   f. Developmental problems experienced as a result of parental alcoholism appear to contribute to adolescent suicide (Meyer and Phillips, 1990).

3. Parental drug and alcohol use does not appear to negatively affect development in all children. In one study, 41% of children of alcoholics developed problems (Werner, 1985).

   a. Emotional stress in children appears to lessen when parents stop drinking.

   b. Research suggests that children of parents with other disturbances, i.e., schizophrenia, exhibit similar problems to children of drug using parents (Garmezy, 1974).

   c. These children experience problems disengaging from the family system and establishing independence (Harbin & Mazian, 1975).

   d. Repetition of learned, interactional, self-defeating patterns in later relationships is a common pattern.

D. Physical and Sexual Abuse

1. Alcohol dependence is a factor in more than one third of reported child abuse cases.

2. Women recovering from alcohol and other drug abuse report high incidences of physical and sexual abuse (Menicucci & Wermuth, 1989).

3. Parental alcohol dependence is linked with physical and sexual abuse and incest (Boyer, 1989).

E. Domestic Violence

1. Alcohol is reported as a factor in 40% of all family court problems and 56% of all fights or assaults in U.S. homes (Covington, 1986).

2. Statistics link domestic violence with the abuse of alcohol in 50–90% of cases studied (Lerner, 1986).

IV. ALTERATIONS IN FAMILY PROCESS RELATED TO DRUG USE

A. Overview of Family Roles and Communication Patterns

1. Communication patterns in families where alcoholism or drug dependence exist are dysfunctional and characterized by:

   a. Unclear, mixed, or conflicting messages.

   b. Avoidance of confrontation direct eye contract.

   c. Inconsistent messages about feelings.

   d. Secret keeping.

   e. Speaking for others.

   f. Inhibitions of emotional expression.

2. Lower levels of cohesion.

3. Lower levels of intellectual orientation.

4. Decreased capacity for independent functioning.

5. Boundaries between parents and children become fluid and ill defined.

6. Emotional nurturance and basic care taking is inconsistent and may result in deprivation.

7. Family members share a collectively low self-concept fostered by powerlessness to change the addicted member's behavior. There is a preoccupation with:

   a. Projection of problems outward: blame.

   b. Attempts to control others' behavior.

   c. Shame.

8. Family roles are altered.

   a. Role reversal between parent and child may occur. The child becomes "parentified" taking on responsibilities for the adult or acting as a surrogate parent.

   b. Spouses assume complementary but unbalanced roles such as "over-functioning" and "under-functioning."

   c. Rigid role structures may develop:

      1. The addicted person may assume a "victim" role to cope with feelings of shame, guilt, fear, and pain.

      2. Children assume consistent role behaviors which help define identity and contribute to homeostasis in an unstable system.

V. NURSING INTERVENTIONS WITH THE DRUG USING FAMILY

A. Must Be Sensitive to Cultural and Ethnic Differences in Values and Health Practices

B. Health Teaching: The Nurse Provides Counseling and Health Teaching About:

1. Drug use, abuse, addiction, and recovery.
2. Health maintenance.
3. Stress management.
4. Problem solving and coping skills.
5. Relapse prevention.
6. Participation in aftercare/rehabilitation.
7. Roles of self-help programs.

C. The Nurse Participates in Screening and Identification of Alcohol/Drug Related Problems and Individuals at Risk

1. Obtains a drug history.

   a. Prior experience with drug use (inclusive of alcohol).

   b. Age of onset of substance abuse.

   c. Positive family history.

   d. Types of drugs used.

   e. Amount of drug used.

   f. Frequency of drug use.

   g. Frequency of intoxication and consequences.

2. Performs a nursing assessment.

   a. Conducts history and physical to assess health status.

   b. Identifies accompanying health compromising behaviors.

3. Develops a nursing care/treatment plan.

   Screening for Substance Use (RAFFT) for Adolescents:

   a. Do you drink or use drugs to RELAX, feel better about yourself, or to fit in?

   b. Do you ever drink alcohol or use drugs when you are ALONE?

   c. Do you or any of your closest FRIENDS drink or use drugs?

   d. Does a close FAMILY member have a problem with alcohol or drug use?

   e. Have you ever gotten into TROUBLE from drink or drug use (e.g., skipping school, bad grades, or trouble with the law or parents)? (Kinney, 1991).

D. Referral

1. Substance abuse specific: Self-help groups.

   a. Twelve Step Programs.

      (1) Alcoholics Anonymous.

      (2) Al-Anon.

      (3) Ala-Teen.

      (4) Ala-Tot.

      (5) Cocaine Anonymous.

      (6) Narcotics Anonymous.

      (7) Adult Children of Alcoholics.

         (a) Women for Sobriety.

         (b) S.O.S.

         (c) SOAR.

2. Community services.

   a. Public housing accessibility.

   b. Welfare, food stamps, WIC program.

   c. Mental health centers.

   d. Emergency shelters or housing resources.

   e. Subsidized child care.

   f. Child guidance center.

E. Evaluation of Interventions

1. Frequently identified nursing diagnoses.

   a. Altered growth and development.

   b. Altered family process.

   c. Altered health maintenance.

   d. Altered parenting.

   e. Disturbance of self-concept.

   f. Ineffective individual coping.

   g. Ineffective family coping.

   h. Parental self-esteem disturbance.

   i. Potential for injuries.

2. Evaluation of intervention.

   a. Parents demonstrate appropriate use of resources to deal with stress.

   b. Parents cope adaptively with stress, using new behaviors that enhance personal and family growth.

   c. Parents demonstrate positive parent-child interaction and are able to effectively discipline children without anger or violence.

   d. Parents have a realistic perception of the child's abilities.

   e. Parents' expectations of the child's skills and behaviors are age appropriate.

   f. Parents express pleasure and pride in parental role performance.

   g. Family members demonstrate satisfactory role performance and an ability to modify roles.

   h. Family members demonstrate equal concern for each other without favor or blame directed to a specific member.

   i. Child's development is within normal parameters.

   j. Child and parent demonstrate adaptive changes in their interactions.

   k. Child's behavior is age appropriate and child demonstrates self-confidence.

   l. Parents demonstrate support and affirmation of child's abilities.

   m. Parents establish and use a positive support system (Mott, 1990).

MODULE I.5
DYSFUNCTIONAL PATTERNS
IN FAMILIES WITH DRUG AND
ALCOHOL PROBLEMS

INSTRUCTOR'S GUIDE

Kem Louie, PhD, RN

Madeline A. Naegle, PhD, RN, FAAN
Project Director
Janet S. D'Arcangelo, MA, RN, C
Project Coordinator

Project SAEN
SUBSTANCE ABUSE
EDUCATION IN NURSING

CONTENTS

MODULE DESCRIPTION

This module is designed to facilitate the student's understanding of the impact of drug and alcohol use on child development and family process. Family assessment for the identification of parenting problems, dysfunctional family roles, and dysfunctional communication patterns will be reviewed in the context of child development. Studies will integrate nursing principles into health teaching and interventions which reflect an understanding of dysfunctional patterns manifested in relation to family drug use.

TIME FRAME

3 hours

PLACEMENT

Family Development, Parent-Child Nursing, Maternity Nursing, Community Health

LEARNER OBJECTIVES

Upon successful completion of the module, the learner will:

1. List familial and genetic factors which place individuals at risk for the development of drug and alcohol problems.

2. Describe common drug and alcohol use patterns in families.

3. Describe behavioral signs frequently observed in children of drug dependent parents.

4. Describe roles developed by family members in response to drug use.

5. Identify drug-related communication patterns in families where drug use is common.

6. Demonstrate knowledge of key components of drug education in the health teaching of school age children by families and care providers.

7. Demonstrate strategies for effective health teaching with families about the risks and problems of drug use.

RECOMMENDED READINGS

FACULTY READINGS

Anderson, E. E., & Quast, W. (1983). Young children in alcoholic families: A mental health needs assessment and intervention/prevention strategy. *Journal of Primary Prevention, 3,* 174–187.

Bowen, M. (1974). Alcoholism as viewed through family systems theory and family psychotherapy. In F. A. Seixas, R., Cadoret, S., Eggleston, (Eds.) *The Person with Alcoholism* (pp. 115–122). New York: New York Academy of Sciences.

Cadoret, R. J., & Gath, A. (1978). Inheritance of alcoholism in adoptees. *British Journal of Psychiatry, 132,* 252–258.

Friensen, V. I. (1983). The family in the etiology of alcoholism: Toward a balance perspective (Advances in) *Alcohol and Substance Abuse, 2*(40), 77–86.

Kaufman, E. (Ed.) (1983). *Power to Change: Family Case Studies in the Treatment of Alcoholism.* New York: Gardner.

Miller, D. & Jang, M. (1977). Children of alcoholics: A longitudinal study. *Social Work Research and Abstracts, 13,* 23–29.

Werner, E. E. (1985). Resilient offspring of alcoholics: A longitudinal study from birth to age 18. *Journal of Studies on Alcohol. 47,* (1), 34–40.

STUDENT READINGS

Blechman, E. (1982). Conventional wisdom about familial contributions to substance abuse. *American Journal of Drug and Alcohol Abuse, 9*(1), 35–54.

Chychula, N. (1984). Screening for substance abuse in primary care settings. *Nurse Practitioner, 9,* 15–24.

Fisk, N. B. (1986). Alcoholism: Ineffective family coping. *American Journal of Nursing, 896*(5), 586–587.

Kiehne, A. M. (1988). Children in the addicted family: An overview. *Holistic Nursing Practice, 2*(4), 14–19.

Rowe, J. (1989). Nursing assessment of children of alcoholics, *Journal of Pediatric Nursing, 4*(4), 248–254.

RECOMMENDED AUDIOVISUAL
AND
OTHER RESOURCES

AUDIOVISUAL RESOURCES

1. **Crisis Intervention: Families Under Stress**

   Identifies needs of families whose members are acutely ill. Available from American Journal of Nursing Company. Twenty-eight minutes. Videocassette and Study Guide. Rental, ($60), sale ($275.00). American Journal of Nursing Company Educational Services Division, 555 West 57th Street, New York, NY, 10019-2961. (800) 223-2282.

2. **Child Abuse**

   Emphasizes an understanding of the origins of child abuse and focuses on prevention, detection, and management. Available from American Journal of Nursing Company. Videocassette rental ($60) and sale ($275.00). American Journal of Nursing Company Educational Services Division, 555 West 57th Street, New York, NY, 10019-2961. (800) 223-2282.

3. **Soft is the Heart of a Child**

   A dramatic rendering of a classic alcoholic family system in which mother and children are affected by father's alcoholism. Available from Hazelden Educational Materials. Thirty minutes. Film rental ($70), purchase ($375.00). Videocassette rental ($50), purchase ($250). Hazelden Educational Materials, 15251 Pleasant Valley Road, Box 176, Center City, MN 55012-0176. (800) 328-9000.

4. **A Child's View**

   In simple, understandable terms, Dr. Black explains alcoholism and drug abuse with pictures and stories gathered from youngsters in therapy groups where a parent was completing treatment for alcoholism. Geared specifically for young children living in alcoholic homes, this video presents alcoholism as seen through a child's eyes. It is the perfect visual companion to the presenter's book,

My Dad Loves Me, My Dad Has a Disease. 45 minutes. Available from Hazelden. Hazelden Educational Materials, 15251 Pleasant Valley Road, Box 176, Center City, MN 55012-0176. (800) 328-9000.

5. **Alcohol and the Family: The Breaking Point**

This film develops awareness that the families of alcoholics are as much in need of professional help as the alcoholics themselves. The film depicts the destructive behavioral patterns of the families and friends of two alcoholics. It shows that when family members seek help for themselves, recognizing that rescue of the alcoholic is beyond their overtaxed emotional resources, the change in their own behaviors becomes a stimulus for change in the alcoholic's behavior. 29 minutes. **Available from AIMS Media #9797 rental ($75) or purchase ($395). Aims Media, Inc., 6901 Woodley Avenue, Van Nuys, CA, 91406-4878. (800) 267-2467.**

6. **Alcohol, Children, And The Family**

The destructive effects of alcoholism on families, with special focus on children, are examined in this program. Dr. Timmen L. Cermak provides a solid background for examination of the harm done to children in chemically dependent families. After reviewing the developmental needs of children that are met in healthy families where one or both of the parents are alcoholic. Children of alcoholics must deal with the loss of a safe environment, loss of communication, distortion of roles, loss of continuity, and loss of privacy. Dr. Cermak discusses the problem of co-dependency and shows how non-alcoholic family members contribute to the lack of health in the family. Infants, toddlers, children, and adolescents have very different needs. The effects of dysfunction at each stage of development are described in detail. By the Hospital Satellite Network. 20 minutes. **Available from AIMS Media, Inc., 6901 Woodley Avenue, Van Nuys, CA, 91406-4878. (800) 267-2467.**

7. **Another Chance**

A view of the intensely personal process of a woman who unravels the complex story of generations of dependent family behavior through counseling and experiential therapy sessions. By Sharon Wegscheider-Cruse. 32 minutes. **Available from Hazelden. Hazelden Educational Materials, 15251 Pleasant Valley Road, Box 176, Center City, MN 55012-0176. (800) 328-9000.**

8. **Children Of Denial**

Children of alcoholics are affected by their parent's alcoholism and/or other drug dependency. Dr. Claudia Black, in a warm and sensitive style, examines what happens to these children and offers some answers to the problems. She discusses the three basic tenets which rule the lives of many children of alcoholics: "Don't talk;" "Don't trust;" "Don't feel." 28 minutes. **Available from Hazelden. Hazelden Educational Materials, 15251 Pleasant Valley Road, Box 176, Center City, NM 55012-0176. (800) 328-9000.**

9. Choice Making

Drawing upon her long-term work in the field of chemical dependency, Sharon Wegscheider-Cruse, the author of Another Chance, describes how a person can transcend family trauma by making sometimes hard but necessary choices. 30 minutes. Available from Hazelden. Hazelden Educational Materials, 15251 Pleasant Valley Road, Box 176, Center City, MN 55012-0176. (800) 328-9000.

10. The Family Trap

Explaining that addiction destroys not only the addict but the family as well, this film offers a revealing look into the survival roles that are adopted by the family members of a dependent person. By Sharon Wegscheider-Cruse. 30 minutes. Available from Hazelden. Hazelden Educational Materials, 15251 Pleasant Valley Road, Box 176, Center City, MN 55012-0176. (800) 328-9000.

11. Lots Of Kids Like Us

This film tells the story of two children as they try to cope with their father's alcoholism. The children are burdened by intense feelings of guilt and are often exposed to physical and emotional abuse as they remain silent in order to keep the "family secret." The film is direct and supportive as it offers viewers the messages, "You're not alone" and "It's not your fault." 28 minutes. Available from NYSCA. New York State Council on Alcoholism, Film Library, 155 Washington Avenue, Albany, New York 12210. Phone (518) 432-8281 or (800) 252-2557.

OVERHEAD MASTERS

MODULE I.5 DYSFUNCTIONAL PATTERNS IN FAMILIES WITH DRUG AND ALCOHOL PROBLEMS

1. Factors Influencing the Impact of Parental Alcoholism on Children
2. Factors Influencing the Origins and Continuance of Long Term Family Drug Abuse
3. Nursing Interventions with Drug Abusing Families

Module I.5—Overhead #1

FACTORS INFLUENCING THE IMPACT OF PARENTAL ALCOHOLISM ON CHILDREN

Child's Age at Onset of Parent Alcoholism

Ethnicity

Religion

Social Class

Family Sex Roles

Cultural Variations

Family Structure

From: Nardi, P. (1981). Children of alcoholics: A role theoretical perspective. *The Journal of Social Psychology, 115,* 237–245.

Module I.5—Overhead #2

FACTORS INFLUENCING THE ORIGINS AND CONTINUANCE OF LONG-TERM FAMILY DRUG ABUSE

Cultural Variations

Social Class Differences

Individual and Family Life Cycle Development

Gender

From: Menicucci & Wermuth (1989). Expanding the family systems approach: Cultural, class, developmental and gender influences in drug abuse, *Journal of Family Therapy, 12* (2), 129–192.

Module I.5—Overhead #3

NURSING INTERVENTIONS WITH DRUG ABUSING FAMILIES

Health Teaching
Counseling on Drug Use, Abuse, and Addiction
Referral to Appropriate Treatment Facilities and Community Agencies
Advocacy for Patients and Families

HANDOUT MASTERS

MODULE I.5 DYSFUNCTIONAL PATTERNS IN FAMILIES WITH DRUG AND ALCOHOL PROBLEMS

     1. Genogram—Principles

     2. Sample Genogram

GENOGRAM—PRINCIPLES

Formats for constructing genograms vary from fairly simple to extremely complex. The basic symbols are:

□ = Male   ○ = Female

⊠ ⊗ = Died. Write year, age, and cause of death next to symbol.

m = Married. Insert year and place.

⫲ = Divorced

= = Close bond between two family members

〰 = Conflict between two family members

A, D, E = Alcohol, drug, or eating disorder. Place letter on top of the symbol for that person.

PA, SA = Physical or sexual abuse. Place the letters on top of the symbol for that person.

Module I.5—Handout #2

SAMPLE GENOGRAM

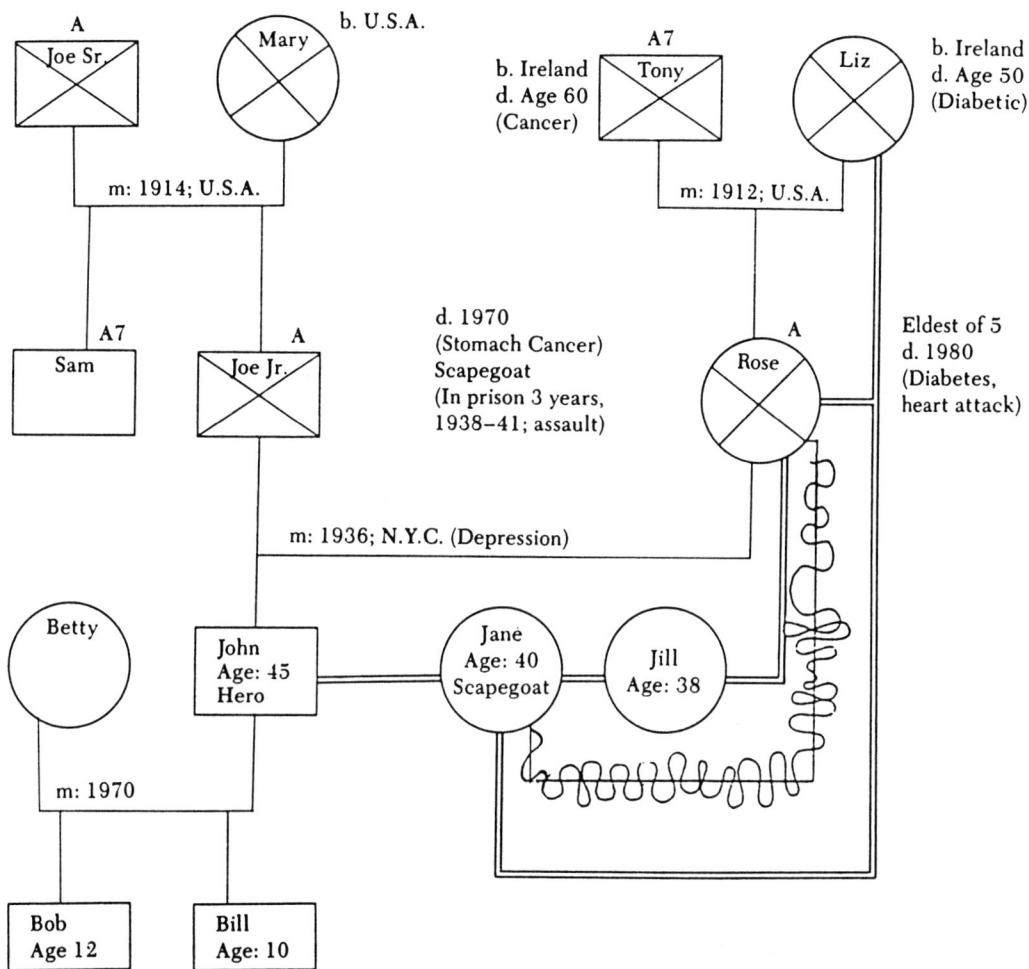

A

Joe Sr.

b. U.S.A.

Mary

m: 1914; U.S.A.

A7

Sam

A

Joe Jr.

d. 1970
(Stomach Cancer)
Scapegoat
(In prison 3 years,
1938–41; assault)

A7

Tony

b. Ireland
d. Age 60
(Cancer)

Liz

b. Ireland
d. Age 50
(Diabetic)

m: 1912; U.S.A.

A

Rose

Eldest of 5
d. 1980
(Diabetes,
heart attack)

m: 1936; N.Y.C. (Depression)

Betty

John
Age: 45
Hero

Jane
Age: 40
Scapegoat

Jill
Age: 38

m: 1970

Bob
Age 12

Bill
Age: 10

Reprinted with permission from Marlin, E. (1987). Harper & Row. New York: 1987.

RECOMMENDED TEACHING STRATEGIES AND SAMPLE ASSIGNMENTS

RECOMMENDED TEACHING STRATEGIES

- Attendance at Family Self-Help Programs (Adult Children of Alcoholics, Al-Anon)
- Family interviews
- Home visits
- Role playing
- Use of genogram

TEST QUESTIONS AND ANSWERS

TEST QUESTIONS

1. The single most important factor which places family members at risk for drug abuse is:

   a.   accessibility of drugs.

   b.   alcohol or drug abuse problem relatives.

   c.   truant behavior by children.

   d.   peer group drug use.

2. Roles adopted by children in families with an alcoholic parent represent:

   a.   task assignment.

   b.   efforts to achieve stability.

   c.   ways of coping with feelings.

   d.   manipulative behaviors.

3. Developmental impairment in children of alcohol/drug users include:

   a.   impaired psychomotor skills.

   b.   sensory deprivation.

   c.   sociopathic personalities.

   d.   congenital syphilis.

4. Children in families where alcohol and drugs are used often learn which of the following coping strategies?

   a.   projection of blame onto others.

   b.   sublimation of social anxiety.

   c.   avoidance of all drug use.

   d.   over investment in religion.

5. Drug use occurs in a social context. In assessing the family, the health care provider should:

   a.   obtain documentation of ethnic background.

   b.   recognize personal ethnic and class bias.

c. expect that families will deny family illnesses.

d. limit data gathering to the drug history.

6. Drug use patterns may be sustained by family dynamics because:

a. family traditions sanction drug use.

b. family members feel loyal in support of one another.

c. family members believe that drug users deserve to suffer the consequences.

d. the behavior is not viewed as deviant.

7. Later problems which result from rigid family roles include:

a. inability to modify behavior to accommodate relationships.

b. inability to be gainfully employed.

c. inability to relate to siblings.

d. lack of communication with parents.

8. Communication is distorted in families where a member is frequently intoxicated because:

a. drugs inhibit verbal expression.

b. emotional messages are inconsistent and conflicting.

c. no one speaks during periods when the drug user is intoxicated.

9. Children of alcohol and drug dependent parents show varying responses to parental addiction because:

a. denial restricts their acknowledgement of the problem.

b. the non-addicted parent attempts to compensate for the problem.

c. characteristics of the family system temper the response.

d. they are "survivors."

10. Incest and sexual abuse are frequently associated with drug abuse because:

a. children seek to please the addicted parent.

b. boundaries within the family are blurred.

c. drug dependent parents cannot express affection.

d. such families are in constant states of chaos.

ANSWER KEY

1. b
2. b
3. a
4. a
5. b
6. b
7. a
8. b
9. b
10. b

BIBLIOGRAPHY

MODULE I.5 DYSFUNCTIONAL PATTERNS IN FAMILIES WITH DRUG AND ALCOHOL PROBLEMS

Ablon, J. (1983). Family behavior in alcoholism. In B. Tabakoff, P. Sutker, & C. Randall. (Eds.), *Medical and social aspects of alcohol abuse* (pp. 139–160). New York: Plenum Press.

ANA (1988). *Standards of addictions nursing practice with selected diagnoses and criteria.* Kansas City: Author.

Anderson, E. E., & Quast, W. (1983). Young children in alcoholic families: A mental health needs assessment and intervention/prevention strategy. *Journal of Primary Prevention, 3,* 174–187.

Barret, L., Bourhis, F., Buffet, H., Danel, V. & Debru, J. L. (1987). Determination of B-endorphin in alcoholic patients in acute stages of intoxication: Relation with Naloxone therapy. *Drug and Alcohol Dependence, 19,* 71–78.

Bean-Bayog, M. (1988). Alcoholism as a cause of psychopathology. *Hospital and Community Psychiatry, 39*(4), 352–354.

Bernal, G., Rodriguez, C., & Diamond, G. (1990). Contextual therapy: Brief treatments of an addict and spouse. *Family Process, 29,* 59–71.

Bingham, H., & Bargain, T. (1985). Children of alcoholic families. *Journal of Psychosocial Nursing, 23*(12), 13–15.

Blechman, E. (1982). Conventional wisdom about familial contributions to substance abuse. *American Journal of Drug and Alcohol Abuse, 9*(1), 35–54.

Bohman, M. (1978). Some genetic aspects of alcoholism and criminating. A population of adoptees. *Archives of General Psychiatry, 35,* 269–276.

Bohman, M., Sigvardsson, S., & Cloriger, C. R. (1981). Maternal inheritance of alcohol abuse: Cross fostering analysis of adopted women. *Archives of General Psychiatry, 38,* 965–969.

Boismare, F., Lhuintre, J. O., Daoust, M., Moore, N., Sallgant, C., & Hillemand, B. (1987). Platelet affinity for serotonpin is increased in alcoholics and former alcoholics: A biological marker for dependence? *Alcohol and Alcoholism, 22,* 155–159.

Bowen, M. (1974). Alcoholism as viewed through family systems theory and family psychotherapy. In F. A. Seixas, R. Cadoret, S. Eggleston, (Eds.). *The Person With Alcoholism* (pp. 115–122). New York: New York Academy of Sciences.

Bowen, M. (1978). *Family therapy in clinical practice.* New York: Jason Aronson.

Boyer, P. A. (1989). A guide to theory of families with a chemically dependent parent. *Psychotherapy, 26* (1), 88–95.

Cadoret, R. J., Cain, C. A., & Gove, W. M. (1980). Development of alcoholism in adoptees raised apart from alcoholic biologic relatives. *Archives of General Psychiatry, 37,* 561–563.

Cadoret, R. J., & Gath, A. (1978). Inheritance of alcoholism in adoptees. *British Journal of Psychiatry, 132,* 252–258.

Carey, K. (1989). Emerging treatment guidelines for mentally ill chemical abuses. *Hospital and Community Psychiatry, 40*(4), 341–342.

Chychula, N. (1984). Screening for substance abuse in primary care settings. *Nurse Practitioners, 9,* 15–24.

Covington, S. S. (1986). Physical, emotional and sexual abuse. *Focus, 3,* 10–11, 37, 42–44.

Cotroneo, M. (1976). Addiction, alienation and parenting. *Nursing Clinics of North America, 11*(3), 517–26.

Dole, V. P., & Nyswander, M. (1976). Methadone maintenance treatment: A ten year perspective. *Journal of the American Medical Association, 235,* 2117–2119.

Elkin, M. (1984). *Families under the influence.* New York: W.W. Norton.

Elles, M. (1986). Interventions with alcoholics and their families. *Nursing Clinics of North America, 21*(3), 493–504.

Fisk, N. B. (1986). Alcoholism: Ineffective family coping. *American Journal of Nursing, 896*(5), 586–587.

Friensen, V. I. (1983). The family in the etiology and treatment of drug abuse: Toward a balanced perspective. *Advances in Alcohol and Substance Abuse, 2*(4), 77–86.

Fossum, M., & Mason, M. (1986). *Facing shame: Families in recovery.* New York: W.W. Norton.

Foster, R. L., Hunsberger, M. M., & Anderson, J. J. (1989). *Family centered nursing care of children,* Philadelphia: W.B. Saunders Co.

Garmezy, N. (1974). Children at risk: The search for antecedents of schizophrenia. Part II: Ongoing research programs, issues, and intervention. *Schizophrenia Bulletin, 9,* 55–125.

Glynn, T. J. (1984). Adolescent drug use & family environment: A review. *Journal of Drug Issues, 14,* 271–298.

Goodwin, D. W. (1971). Is alcoholism hereditary? A review and critique. *Archives of General Psychiatry, 25,* 545–549.

Goodwin, D. W., Schulsinger, F., Hermansen, L., Guze, S. B., & Winokur, G. (1975). Alcoholism and the hyperactive child syndrome. *Journal of Nervous and Mental Disease, 160,* 349–353.

Goodwin, D. W., Schulsinger, F., Hermansen, L., Guze, S. B., & Winokur, G. (1973). Alcohol problems in adoptees raised apart from alcoholic biologic parents. *Archives of General Psychiatry, 28,* 238–242.

Harbin, H. T., & Mazian, H. M. (1975). The families of drug abusers: A literature review. *Family Process, 14,* 411–431.

Hofling, C. K., & Lewis, J. (1980). *The Family: Evaluational Treatment*. New York: Brunner/Mazel.

Institute of Medicine (September 19, 1990). News from the Institute of Medicine. Washington, D.C.: National Academy of Sciences.

Kaufman, E. (Ed.) (1983). *Power to change: Family case studies in the treatment of alcoholism*. New York: Gardner.

Kiehne, A. M. (1988). Children in the addicted family: An overview. *Holistic Nursing Practice, 2*(4), 14–19.

Kinney, J. (1991). *Clinical manual of substance abuse*, St. Louis: Mosby.

Lawson, G., Peterson, J. S. & Lawson, A. (1983). *Alcoholism and the family: A guide to treatment and prevention*. Rockville, MD: Aspen.

Lerner, R. (1986). Children in family treatment: Are they still forgotten? *Focus, 3*, 6–7, 45.

Menicucci, L., & Wermuth, L. (1989, Summer). Expanding the family systems approach: Cultural, class, developmental and gender influences in drug abuse. *American Journal of Family Therapy, 12*, (2), 129–192.

Meyer, D., & Phillips, W. (1990). No safe place: Parental alcoholism and adolescent suicides *American Journal of Psychotherapy, XLIV*(4), 552–562.

Miller, D., & Jang, M. (1977). Children of alcoholics: A 20-year longitudinal study. *Social Work Research & Abstracts, 3*, 23–29.

Moos, R. H., & Billings, A. G. (1982). Children of alcoholics during the recovery process: Alcoholic and matched control families, *Addictive Behaviors, 7*, 155–163.

Mott, J., Sr., & Sperhac, A. M. (1990). *Nursing care of children and families*, 2nd edition. Redwood City, CA: Addison-Wesley.

Nardi, P. M. (1984). Children of alcoholics: A role-theoretical perspective. *The Journal of Social Psychology, 115*, 237–245.

Orford, J., & Harwin, J. (Eds.) *Alcohol and the family*. New York: St. Martin's Press, 1982.

Perez, J. F. (1986). *Coping with the alcoholic family*. Indiana: Accelerated Development, Inc.

Regan, D. C., Erlich, S., & Finnegan, L. (1987). Infants of drug addicts: At risk for child abuse, neglect, and placement in foster care. *Neurotoxicology and Teratology, 9*(4), 315–319.

Rimmer, J. (1982). The children of alcoholics: An exploratory study. *Children and youth review, 4*, 365–373.

Rowe, J. (1989). Nursing assessment of children of alcoholics. *Journal of Pediatric Nursing, 4*(4), 248–254.

Russel, M., Henderson, C., & Blume, S. B. (1984). Children of alcoholics: A review of the literature. New York: Children of Alcoholics Foundation.

Schuckit, M., & Chiles, J. A. (1978). Family history as a diagnostic aid in two samples of adolescents. *Journal of Nervous and Mental Disease, 66*(3), 165–176.

Schuckit, M., & Goodwin, D. W. (1972). A study of alcoholism in half siblings. *American Journal of Psychiatry, 128*(9), 1132–36.

Steinglass, P. (1980). A life history model of the alcoholic family. *Family Process, 19*(3), 211–225.

Steinglass, P. (1981). The alcoholic family at home. *Archives of General Psychiatry, 38,* 578–584.

Steinglass, P., Bennett, L., Wolin, S. & Reiss, D. (1987). *The alcoholic family.* New York: Basic Books.

Werner, E. E. (1985). Resilient offspring of alcoholics: A longitudinal study from birth to age 18. *Journal of Studies on Alcohol, 47*(1), 34–40.

Wegscheider, S. (1981). *Another chance: Hope & health for the alcoholic family,* Science & Believer.

West, M. O., & Prinz, R. J. (1987). Parental alcoholism and childhood psychopathology. *Psychological Bulletin, 102, 2,* 204–218.

MODULE I.6
THE ADOLESCENT WHO USES DRUGS AND ALCOHOL

Madeline A. Naegle, PhD, RN, FAAN

Madeline A. Naegle, PhD, RN, FAAN
Project Director
Janet S. D'Arcangelo, MA, RN, C
Project Coordinator

Project SAEN
SUBSTANCE ABUSE
EDUCATION IN NURSING

CONTENT OUTLINE

D. Social Factors

    1. Peer Influence

    2. Drug Using Social Contexts

    3. Societal Influences

E. Psychological Factors and Related Behaviors

    1. Coping Mechanisms

    2. Motivational Factors

    3. Psychopathology

    4. Behaviors Suggesting Use

III. Assessment of Factors Specific to the Drug Using Adolescent

A. Experimentation and Risk Taking

B. The Heavy Drinker

C. Developmental and Health Needs

D. The Sero-Positive Adolescent

E. The Pregnant Adolescent

IV. Nursing Intervention

A. The Nurse as Care Provider

    1. Identification and Screening

    2. Health Teaching

    3. Community Resources

    4. Early Intervention and Referral

    5. Inpatient Treatment

B. The Nurse as Health Educator

    1. Formal Educational Programs

    2. The Community

    3. The School

CONTENTS

I. PATTERNS OF ADOLESCENT DRUG USE

A. Prevalence of Drinking

1. After nicotine, alcohol is the drug most widely used by adolescents.

   a. Of high school seniors, 4.2% are daily drinkers (Johnston, O'Malley & Bachman, 1988).

   b. Heavy drinking occurs disproportionately among male adolescents.

   c. In recent years, female adolescents are drinking in numbers approaching those of their male peers.

   d. In 1983, there were an estimated 3.3 million problem drinkers among youth in the 14 to 17 age group.

   e. Alcohol consumption by adolescents has remained relatively stable since 1980 at a level of 92% of adolescents having used the drugs.

B. Prevalence of Use of Drugs Other Than Alcohol

1. Street drugs.

   a. The use of cocaine and crack among adolescents has maintained a steady level in recent years, while other illicit drug use has declined (Johnston, O'Malley, & Bachman, 1988).

   b. Of the 12- to 17-year-olds, 16% report some illicit drug use in the first year of high school (National Institute of Drug Abuse 1990); however, Kandel reported a 1989 reduction by half in adolescents reporting use of an illicit drug (Kandel, 1989).

   c. Of the adolescents surveyed in particular studies, 5–15% report daily marijuana use.

   d. Marijuana is the most widely used illicit drug (47% used); cocaine/crack is second.

   e. Sedatives, hypnotics, and tranquilizers were used by a small percentage (3–6%) of high-school seniors in 1988 (Johnston, O'Malley, & Bachman, 1988).

2. Abused and misused prescription drugs.

   a. Data on the prevalence of steroid use by adolescent males and females are not available, clinical data suggest that it is widespread among competitive high school athletes.

3. Nicotine.

   a. Longitudinal studies suggest that 24% of adolescents aged 16–18 smoked cigarettes; males smoke less frequently (21%) than females, who have increased percentage of use over recent years (27%). (Pirie, Murray, & Luepter, 1988).

Module I.6

C. Patterns of Drug Use in Adolescents

1. Gender variations.

   a. Males use alcohol and illicit drugs at a disproportionately higher rate than females; males are more frequently daily users of marijuana (Kandel, 1989).

   b. Adolescent females are drinking in numbers approaching their male peers.

   c. A higher percentage of female adolescents now smoke cigarettes (27%) than do male adolescents (21%).

   d. Drinking behaviors of adolescent girls correlate most closely with habits of their best friends; males most closely pattern their fathers.

   e. Twice as many males as females reported marijuana use in 1990 (NIDA, 1990).

   f. Female adolescents are more likely to use and abuse prescription drugs and stimulants.

2. Age.

   a. Initation of youth into drinking and drug use occurs at younger ages than ever before.

   b. Of the 12- to 17-year-old youths, 25.9% reported drinking alcohol in 1990 at age 12 (NIDA, 1990).

   c. Drug use increases with age.

   d. Drug use appears to progress from "soft" drugs like alcohol and marijuana to heroin or other drugs. These introductory substances are referred to as "gateway" drugs (Kandel, 1982).

3. Race.

   a. In racial ethnic groups, blacks are more likely to abstain from alcohol; the heaviest rates of alcohol use occur among Native Americans and Oriental ethnic groups.

   b. Cocaine use is highest among Hispanics (1.9%), with blacks (1.7%) and whites (0.6%) using with less prevalence (NIDA, 1990).

   c. In illicit drug use, Alaskan native youth appear more likely to have used an illicit substance, followed by white, black and Hispanic youth. Orientals appear to have shown the least likelihood of illicit drug abuse (Radosevic, Lanza-Kaduce, Akers, & Krohn, 1980).

4. Variables.

   a. Illicit drug use by youth varies by geographic region; it is highest in the West (25%), compared to the Northeast, North Central and South (20%).

   b. Widespread use of inhalants is common in the Southwest among economically disadvantaged youth.

   c. The use of phencyclidine (PCP) appears to vary by geographic region, with highest rates in large cities (Johnston, O'Malley, & Bachman, 1988).

     d. The use of heroin and PCP appears concentrated at the lower end of the socio-economic scale (Johnston, O'Malley & Bachman, 1988).

  5. Socioeconomic variables.

     a. Drug use by adolescents occurs in all socioeconomic groups, but may vary with the accessibility of drug by cost and type.

     b. Drug use as a pattern emerges from the interaction of multiple factors.

     c. The profile of the adolescent who drinks most frequently and intensely is that of the white, higher SES, urban or rural mode with a weak family orientation (Martin & Pritchard, 1991).

     d. Inhalants, particularly glue, gasoline, and toluene are used frequently by economically disadvantaged youth (Oetting, Edwards, & Beauvais, 1988).

II. FACTORS INFLUENCING USE

A. Adolescents at Risk

  1. Adolescents who begin early use of drugs, particularly alcohol, frequently embark upon a drug using hierarchy characterized by progression to stronger drugs and more frequent use (Kandel, 1975). "Gateway drugs," those that precede heavier use, are alcohol and marijuana.

  2. Adolescents with histories of alcohol abuse were four times as likely to have major depressive disorders; this was especially true for females (Deykin, Levy, & Wells, 1987).

  3. Adolescents with major psychiatric disorders may self-medicate with alcohol and illicit drugs, thereby complicating the symptomatology and identification of substance abuse problems.

  4. Risks for drug dependence appear to increase for adolescents from broken homes, homes where family income is higher than for others, where the father's education level is low (Kandel, 1989).

  5. High risk groups: "gateway" drug users, the economically disadvantaged and children of substance abusers.

  6. Physical and sexual abuse increase risks (Schiff, Caviola, & Harrison, 1989).

B. Attitudinal Factors

  1. Attitudes about drug use.

     a. Attitudes that support the use of alcohol and experimentation with other drugs as "normal" are common among adolescents and young adults.

     b. Adolescents with tolerant attitudes toward drugs are more likely to use than adolescents with negative attitudes (Johnston, 1985).

     c. Positive or negative attitudes toward drug use are outcomes of socializing processes by parents and peer groups.

2. Alienation and affiliation.

   a. The relationship between political and/or social alienation and drug use seems unclear and subject to changes in social trends.

   b. Drug use may represent alienation from parental values.

3. Developmental patterns.

   a. The need to establish an identity and values separate from those of parents is a developmental task that may relate to choices about drug use.

   b. The sense of well-being and invulnerability common to adolescence interferes with assessment of drug-taking risks.

   c. Choice of a vocation and skill development related to future goals is compromised by drug use.

   d. Social skill acquisition is compromised by drug use.

C. Family Factors

1. Family history.

   a. History of alcohol and/or other drug dependencies in parents, siblings or others.

   b. Family history of depression in female relatives of women who use, and sociopathic personality disorders in relatives of male users (Meyer, 1986).

2. Parental values about drug use and patterns of drug use are major shaping factors in adolescent drug-user behaviors.

3. Quality of parent-child relationships.

   a. Common problems in families of drug-using adolescents include:

      (1) Role rigidity.

      (2) Generational boundary breakdown.

      (3) Communication problems.

      (4) Marital tension.

      (5) Differences in goals and values (Potter-Efron & Potter, 1986).

   b. Absence of parental involvement correlates positively with drug use.

   c. Higher percentages of nonusers report close parent-child relationships (Harford & Grant, 1987).

4. The relationship between religious values and drug use by adolescents is unclear, although firm religious beliefs appear to inhibit drinking or drug use (Rohrbaugh & Jessor, 1975).

D. Social Factors

1. Peer influence.

   a. With parental influence, peer influence is considered the most significant variable in adolescent drinking and drug use (Brooks, Nomura, & Cohen, 1989).

b. Patterns of use of family and peers are considered the best predictors of frequency of and attitudes toward use.

2. Drug-using social contexts.

   a. Adolescents most frequently drink and use drugs with same-age peers.

   b. Perceived pressure from peers and fear of disapproval are often given as reasons for use (Radosevic, et al, 1980).

3. Societal influences.

   a. Societal demands for drugs make drug use and drug dealing profitable.

   b. Widespread availability of drugs makes them accessible to young people with limited resources.

   c. A well-defined drug subculture supports drug use in normative patterns.

   d. A social environment that views risk taking as desirable.

E. Psychological Factors and Related Behaviors

Studies suggest reasons for alcohol and other drug use in adolescents.

1. In a study of 12- to 17-year-olds, users identified alcohol as something to alter mood and resolve conflict, as well as to "cope" with personal problems.

2. Motives for the use of marijuana and other drugs appear to relate to:

   a. Tension reduction, relief of boredom, and depression.

   b. Expanded awareness, increased insight.

   c. Drug effect, feeling mellow, getting along better with friends.

   d. Experimentation and sensation-seeking (Segal, 1983).

3. Adolescents using drugs are described as having more psychological symptoms than nonusers, including:

   a. Depression.

   b. Feelings of inadequacy.

   c. Frustration.

   d. Feelings of helplessness.

   e. Immaturity.

   f. Self-alienation.

   g. Poor object relations.

   h. Suicidal gestures and behaviors (Pallikkathayil & Tweed, 1983).

4. Behavior patterns suggesting drug and alcohol abuse include:

   a. Changes in school performance and failing grades.

   b. Absenteeism from school or work.

   c. Withdrawal from social activities.

   d. Signs of chronic or acute depression.

   e. Recurrent accidents or fights.

   f. Involvement with the law—such as drunk and disorderly conduct, vandalism, Drinking While Intoxicated violations.

   g. Unexplained expenditures and petty theft.

   h. Preoccupation with social activities centered on drug or alcohol use.

   i. Repeated overt intoxications.

   j. Decreased interaction with family members and peers (modified from Jones, 1985).

III. ASSESSMENT OF FACTORS SPECIFIC TO THE DRUG USING ADOLESCENT

A. Experimentation and Risk Taking

1. Adolescent drug users risk parental discovery and reaction, community disapproval, adverse effects on school work and possible discipline, and negative impacts on health.

2. Adolescents who are more accepting of risk taking in general are more likely to engage in substance abuse (Keyser-Smith & Stoil, 1987).

3. Identification of risk taking behaviors in adolescents is useful in shaping education about, and management of, drug using behaviors.

B. Heavy Drinking

1. Heavy-drinking adolescents constitute about 5% of the adolescent population.

2. Identification and early intervention should be tailored to adolescent needs.

3. Ala-Teen is an appropriate complement to treating the adolescent.

4. Family treatment is the optimal complement to treating the adolescent.

5. Student assistance programs (SAP) provide a structure for early intervention.

C. Developmental and Health Needs

Modifications in classifications and nursing diagnosis reflect developmental and health needs of the adolescent (ANA, 1988).

D. The Sero-Positive Adolescent

1. Assessment should include.

   a. Testing and counseling, confidentiality issues.

   b. Comprehensive health history, including a sexual history.

    c. Review of sexual practices, including gender and number of partners, use of condoms, contraceptive methods, usual sexual activities, high risk encounters and activities,—i.e., involvement with prostitution and sex in exchange for drugs, history of sexual abuse and/or incest.

    d. Comprehensive drug use history.

        (1) Sources of drugs.

        (2) Paraphernalia and needle sharing.

        (3) Safer sex practices.

    e. Knowledge of health risks.

        (1) Implications of drug use—i.e. direct impact of alcohol and marijuana on the immune system.

        (2) Knowledge of HIV.

        (3) Knowledge of familial history and implications of drug use.

E. The Pregnant Adolescent

  1. Assessment should be comprehensive, with special attention to.

    a. Drug use history including nicotine use.

    b. Sexual practices.

    c. High-risk sexual activity.

    d. Understanding of fetal effects of alcohol and other drugs.

    e. Assessment of support systems to deter drug use.

    f. Contacts and service connections in the HCDS.

IV. NURSING INTERVENTION

A. The Nurse as Care Provider

  1. Identification and screening should be conducted in all settings in which adolescents receive nursing care.

    a. Identification is contingent upon observation of deviations from normal individual and family patterns.

    b. Informal history taking on individual and family drug use is appropriate to all general nursing roles.

    c. All nursing assessments should include questions on alcohol, illicit, over-the-counter and prescription-drug use, as well as nicotine and caffeine use.

    d. All nursing assessments should explore the interfaces between drug use and high-risk sexual practices as well as sexual contact with members of high-risk groups.

    e. The problem oriented screening instrument for teenagers (POSIT) is a helpful resource (Appendix).

2. Health teaching of adolescents.

    a. Description of pathologic patterns of alcohol and drug use.

    b. Description of non-drug related alternative modes of coping with psychological stress.

    c. Impact of alcohol and drug use for growth and optimal health.

    d. Information on drug effects.

        (1) Regular use.

        (2) Behavioral manifestation of drug effects.

        (3) Factors that place the adolescent at risk for drug dependence.

3. Community resources should be known to the nurse and utilized in student teaching including.

    a. Al-Anon, Ala-Teen, self-help groups.

    b. Students Against Drunk Driving (SADD).

    c. Mothers Against Drunk Drivers (MADD).

    d. Support of non-alcoholic recreational activities.

    e. Community agencies focused on alcohol and drug problems, i.e., Council on Alcoholism.

    f. Support of Student Assistance Programs (SAP).

4. Early intervention/referral is a part of nursing's early intervention.

    a. The nurse refers students and families for evaluation by advanced practitioners of addiction nursing.

    b. The nurse refers, as appropriate, to specialized treatment centers.

    c. The nurse coordinates resources of agencies and providers to assist students and families.

5. Inpatient treatment requires nursing care.

    a. Inpatient treatment is indicated for:

        (1) Adolescents who are severely physically dependent.

        (2) Patients/clients who do not qualify or who have failed in outpatient treatment.

        (3) Intravenous drug abusers and individuals who free base.

        (4) Dually diagnosed adolescents.

        (5) Adolescents needing isolation from their environment.

    b. The nurse contributes to individualized care planning with emphasis on:

        (1) Developmental stage and associated needs.

        (2) Emphasis on role modeling, family support, vocational and social skill training, peer-group issues, community support. (Kaminer & Bukstein, 1989).

The Adolescent Who Uses Drugs and Alcohol

B. The Nurse as Health Educator

1. Provides formal education programs in prevention approaches to alcohol and drug problems.

    a. These are most effective when the target student groups are composed of experimenters or occasional drug users.

    b. These include:

        (1) Building problem solving skills.

        (2) Reinforcing positive self-esteem.

        (3) Active recreational approaches to stress management.

        (4) Facilitating learning through positive outcomes of social experiences.

2. Participants in organizing student-based effects, such as student assistance programs.

3. Coordinates and assists community-based education efforts.

4. Participates with students and family in projects in grammar and secondary schools.

MODULE I.6
THE ADOLESCENT WHO USES DRUGS AND ALCOHOL

INSTRUCTOR'S GUIDE

Madeline A. Naegle, PhD, RN, FAAN

Madeline A. Naegle, PhD, RN, FAAN
Project Director
Janet S. D'Arcangelo, MA, RN, C
Project Coordinator

Project SAEN
SUBSTANCE ABUSE
EDUCATION IN NURSING

CONTENTS

MODULE DESCRIPTION

This module highlights adolescence as a life stage in which drug use begins or is reinforced in a developmental context. The module describes the prevalence and nature of patterns of use of alcohol, and illicit and prescription drugs and explores the motivations for, and risks of, use. Components of nursing assessment and intervention with implications for this age group are presented and implemented in the clinical setting. Relevant aspects of the nursing role are emphasized.

TIME FRAME

3 hours

PLACEMENT

Growth and Development, Fundamentals of Nursing, Nursing Care of the Adolescent, Adult Health, Psychiatric Mental-Health Nursing

LEARNER OBJECTIVES

Upon successful completion of this module, the learner will:

1. Describe commonly observed patterns of alcohol and other drug use/ abuse among adolescents.

2. List factors that appear to influence alcohol and other drug use among adolescents.

3. List factors that place adolescents at risk for the development of addiction and health problems related to drug abuse.

4. Identify components of nursing assessment of characteristics particular to drug-using adolescents.

5. Formulate nursing interventions implemented in prevention and care of drug-using adolescents.

6. Describe nursing roles implemented in prevention and in the care and rehabilitation of the drug-using adolescents.

Module I.6

RECOMMENDED READINGS

FACULTY READINGS

Fawzy, F. I., & Combs, R. H. (1983). Generational continuity in the use of substances: The impact of parental substance abuse on adolescent use. *Addictive Behavior, 8*(2), 109–114.

Groerer, J. (1987). Correlations between drug use by teenagers and drug use by older family members. *Drug and Alcohol Abuse, 13*(1–2), 95–108.

Henley, G., & Winters, K. (1988). Development of problem severity scales of the assessment of adolescent alcohol and drug abuse. *The International Journal of the Addictions, 23*(1), 65–85.

Khuri, E., Millman, R., & Hartman, N. (1984). Clinical issues concerning alcoholic and youthful narcotic abusers. *Advances in Alcohol and Substance Abuse, 3*(4), 69–86.

Levine, B. (1985). Adolescent substance abuse: Toward an integration of family systems and individual adaptation theories. *American Journal of Family Therapy, 13*(2), 3–16.

Meyer, D.C., & Phillips, W.M. (1990). No safe place: Parental alcoholism and adolescent suicide. *American Journal of Psychotherapy, 44*(4), 552–562.

Windle, M., & Barnes, G. M. (1988). Similarities and differences in correlates of alcohol and female adolescents. *International Journal of the Addictions, 23*(7), 707–728.

STUDENT READINGS

Deykin, E. Y., Levy, J. C., & Wells, V. (1987). Adolescent depression, alcohol and drug abuse. *American Journal of Public Health, 77*(2), 178–182.

Dishion, T.J., & Lieber, R. (1985). Adolescent marijuana and alcohol use: The role of parents and peers revisited. *American Journal of Drug and Alcohol Abuse, 11*(1–2), 11–25.

Martin, J.P., & Pritchard, M.E. (1991). Factors associated with alcohol use in late adolescents. *Journal of Alcohol Studies, 52*(1), 5–9.

Pallikkathayil, L., & Tweed, S. (1983). Substance Abuse: Alcohol and drugs during adolescence. *Nursing Clinics of North America, 18*(2), 313–321.

Schiff, M., & Caviola, A. (1988–1989). Adolescents at risk for chemical dependency: Identification and prevention issues. *Journal of Chemical Dependency Treatment, 2*(1), 25–47.

Singer, M., & Anglin, T. (1986). The identification of adolescent substance abuse by health care professionals. *International Journal of Addictions, 21*(2), 247–254.

Wodarski, J.S. (1990). Adolescent substance use: Practice implications. *Adolescence, 25*(99), 667–688.

RECOMMENDED AUDIOVISUAL AND OTHER RESOURCES

AUDIOVISUAL RESOURCES

1. Kids Talking to Kids About Drugs

Inner city kids discuss the experiences of living in a drug-infested city and the associated criminal, social and legal problems. Twenty-eight minutes. Video $250 purchase, $75 rental. Films for the Humanities & Sciences, P.O. Box 2053, Princeton, New Jersey, 08543-2053. Phone: 1-800-257-3126 or (609) 452-1128.

2. Kids Under the Influence

Examines legal, family, social, and health problems experienced as a result of alcohol consumption. Presents health and safety issues for children and adolescents and what can be done about alcohol abuse. Fifty-eight minutes. Video $159 purchase, $75 rental. Films for the Humanities & Sciences, P.O. Box 2053, Princeton, New Jersey, 08543-2053. Phone: 1-800-257-3126 or (609) 452-1128.

3. Portrait of a Teenager Drug Abuser

Documentary presenting young, recovering drug abusers. Self-disclosure and personal histories and common experiences. Presentations are honest and thought-provoking. Twenty-three minutes. Available from Barr Films. Barr Films, 3490 E. Foothill Blvd., P.O. Box 5667, Pasadena, CA 91107. (213) 681-2165.

4. Flip Tops

Saying "no" to alcohol. Looks at two young teenagers as they struggle to establish adult identities for themselves while learning that it is ok to say "no" to alcohol. Twenty-six minutes. Rental $50/100. 16mm Purchase $500. Video $195. Fanlight Productions, 47 Halifax Street, Boston, MA 02130. (617) 524-0950.

5. Body Building, Body Breaking

Prevent signs and risks of illegal steroid use for muscle building. Targets teen classroom audiences. (KC-5299M). Fourteen minutes. Video: $250. Coronet/ MTI Film and Video, 108 Wilmot Road, Deerfield, IL 60025-9925.

6. Athletes and Addiction: It's Not a Game

Interviews with recovering athlete addicts and alcoholics. Covers nature of addiction, components of 28-day treatment programs. Fifty-six minutes. Video $250. Produced by ABC Sports. An MTI Release. **Coronet/MTI Film, 108 Wilmot Road, Deerfield, IL 60015-9925.**

7. No Butts

Uses well-known personalities to discuss the pleasure and hazards of smoking. Techniques for quitting are included. Video purchase $80. Thirty minutes. **Coronet/ MTI Film & Video, 108 Wilmot Road, Deerfield, IL 60015-5196. Toll free: 1-800-621-2131.**

8. Steroids and Sports

Features interviews with athletes and individuals treated with growth hormone as well as comments and guidelines for use presented by an endocrinologist. 19 minutes. Video: $149. **Films for the Humanities & Sciences, P.O. Box 2053, Princeton, New Jersey, 08543-2053. Phone: 1-800-257-3126 or (609) 452-1128.**

OVERHEAD MASTERS

MODULE I.6 THE ADOLESCENT WHO USES DRUGS AND ALCOHOL

1. Lifetime Prevalence of Drug Use Among 12- to 13-year-olds

2. Any Lifetime Experience of Illicit Drug Use (1990)

3. Trends in Cocaine Use by Race/Ethnicity

4. Trends in Cocaine Use by 12- to 17-year-olds

5. Trends in Marijuana Use by 12- to 17-year olds

6. Trends in Perceived Harmfulness of Drugs by Age, 1985, 1988 and 1990

7. Trends in Perceived Harmfulness of Drugs Among 18- to 25-year-olds

8. Stages in Adolescent Involvement in Drugs and Alcohol Use

Module I.6—Overhead #1

LIFETIME PREVALENCE OF DRUG USE AMONG 12- TO 13-YEAR OLDS

1982, 1985, 1988, and 1990

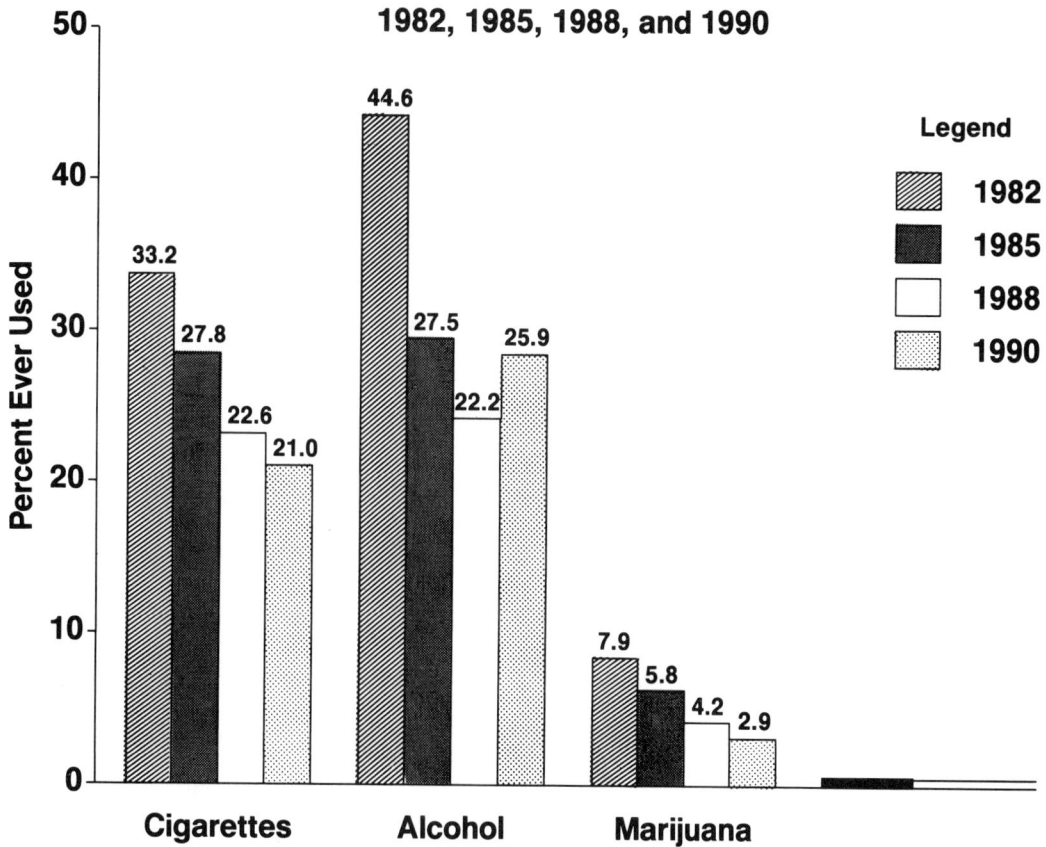

From: National Institute of Drug Abuse (NIDA). (1990). *National household survey on drug abuse.* Rockville, MD: NIDA.

Module I.6—Overhead #2

ANY LIFETIME EXPERIENCE
OF ILLICIT DRUG USE* 1990

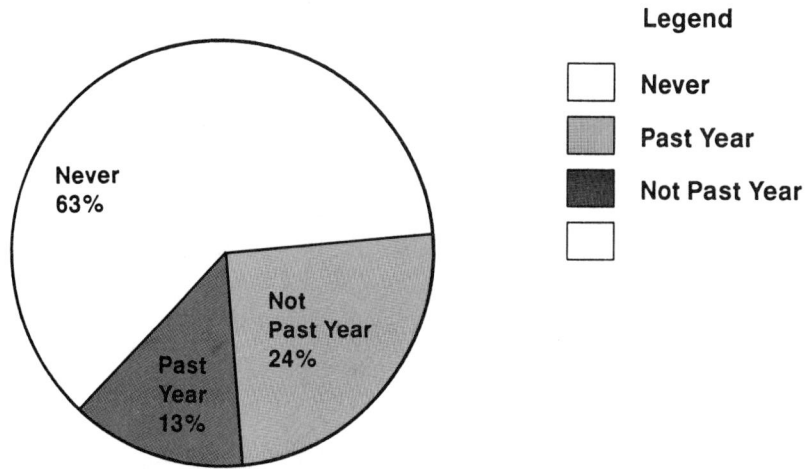

Legend

☐ Never

▨ Past Year

▬ Not Past Year

☐

Never
63%

Not
Past Year
24%

Past
Year
13%

	Youth 12–17	Young Adults 18–25	Adults 26–34	Adults 35 and Older
Never	77	44	37	74
Past Year	16	29	22	6
Not Past Year	7	27	41	20
	100	100	100	100

From: National Institute of Drug Abuse (NIDA). (1990). *National household survey on drug abuse.* Rockville, MD: NIDA.

*Includes marijuana, hallucinogens, inhalants, cocaine, heroin or prescription-type psychotherapeutic drugs (stimulants, sedatives, tranquilizers and analgesics) for nonmedical purposes.

TRENDS IN COCAINE
USE BY RACE/ETHNICITY

1985, 1988, and 1990

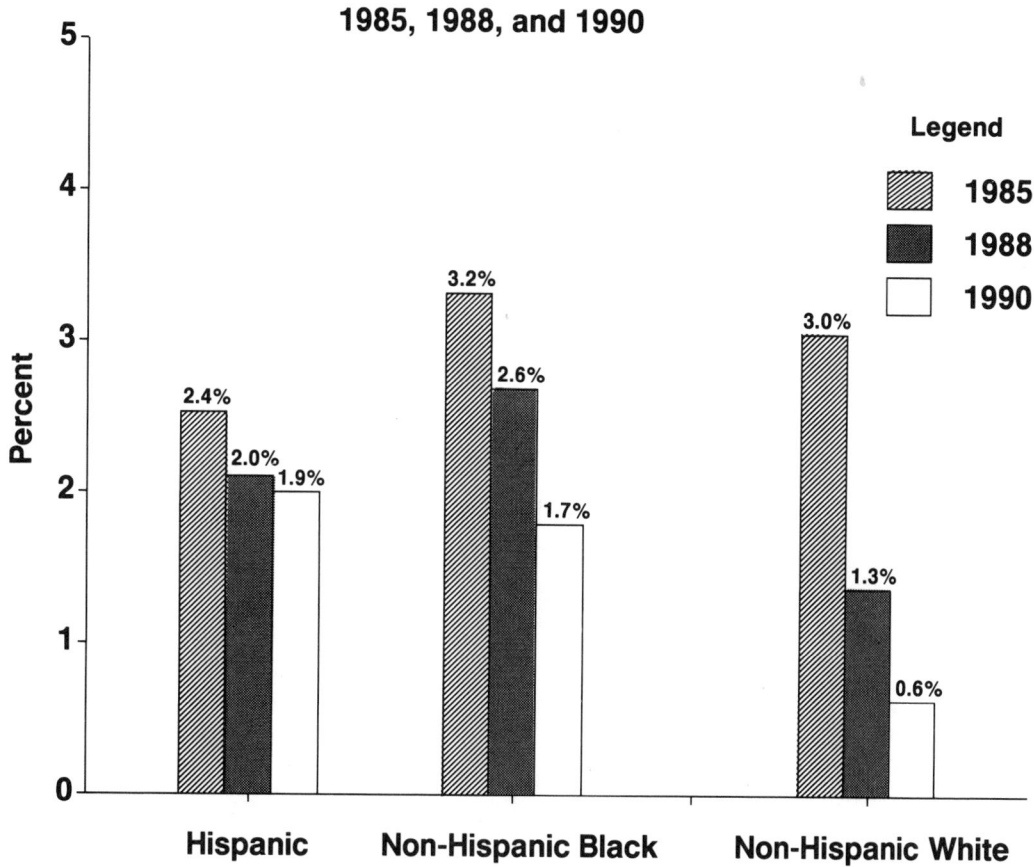

From: National Institute of Drug Abuse (NIDA). (1990). *National household survey on drug abuse.* Rockville, MD: NIDA.

TRENDS IN COCAINE USE
BY 12- TO 17-YEAR-OLDS

Use of Cocaine	1972	1974	1976	1977	1979	1982	1985	1988	1990
Lifetime	1.5	3.6	3.4	4.0	5.4	6.5	4.9	3.4	2.6
Past year	1.5	2.7	2.3	2.6	4.2	4.1	4.0	2.9	2.2
Past month	0.6	1.0	1.0	0.8	1.4	1.6	1.5	1.1	0.6

From: National Institute of Drug Abuse (NIDA). (1990). *National household survey on drug abuse.* Rockville, MD: NIDA.

*The difference between the 1988 and 1990 estimates is statistically significant at .05 level.

**Low precision

Module I.6—Overhead #5

TRENDS IN MARIJUANA USE
BY 12–17 YEAR OLDS

Use of Marijuana	1972	1974	1976	1977	1979	1982	1985	1988	1990
Lifetime	14.0	23.0	22.4	28.0	30.9	26.7	23.6	17.4	14.8
Past year	—	18.5	18.4	22.3	24.1	20.6	19.7	12.6	11.3
Past month	7.0	12.0	12.3	16.6	16.7	11.5	12.0	6.4	5.2

From: National Institute of Drug Abuse (NIDA). (1990). *National household survey on drug abuse.* Rockville, MD: NIDA.

*The difference between the 1988 and 1990 estimates is statistically significant at .05 level.

Module I.6—Overhead #6

TRENDS IN PERCEIVED HARMFULNESS OF DRUGS BY AGE, 1985, 1988 AND 1990

	Age Group	Percentage Perceiving "great risk"		
		1985	1988	1990*
Using cocaine occasionally	All ages	72.9	84.8	83.3
	ages 12–17	64.5	77.7	80.5
Using cocaine regularly	All ages	93.8	96.9	96.4
	ages 12–17	90.0	93.0	93.8
Using crack occasionally	All ages	NA	90.6	86.8
	ages 12–17	NA	78.9	75.7
Trying heroin	All ages	95.9	96.9	96.4
	ages 12–17	89.8	91.0	89.8
Smoking one or more packs of cigarettes per day	All ages	95.9	96.9	96.4
	ages 12–17	45.4	47.1	48.1
Having one or two alcoholic drinks per day	All ages	32.3	30.4	38.9+
	ages 12–17	26.7	25.5	35.1+
Having four to five alcoholic drinks per day	All ages	72.6	73.4	76.5+
	ages 12–17	66.0	63.3	67.9+
Having five or more alcoholic drinks once or twice a week	All ages	59.6	57.4	63.8+
	ages 12–17	56.1	51.6	59.2+
Taking anabolic steroids occasionally	All ages	NA	NA	63.8
	ages 12–17	NA	NA	53.1
Taking anabolic steroids regularly	All ages	NA	NA	87.0
	ages 12–17	NA	NA	80.2

From: National Institute of Drug Abuse (NIDA). (1990). *National household survey on drug abuse.* Rockville, MD: NIDA.

NA = data not available

*The difference between the 1988 and 1990 estimates is statistically significant at .05 level.

Module I.6—Overhead #7

TRENDS IN
PERCEIVED HARMFULNESS OF DRUGS
AMONG 18- TO 25-YEAR-OLDS

1985, 1988, and 1990

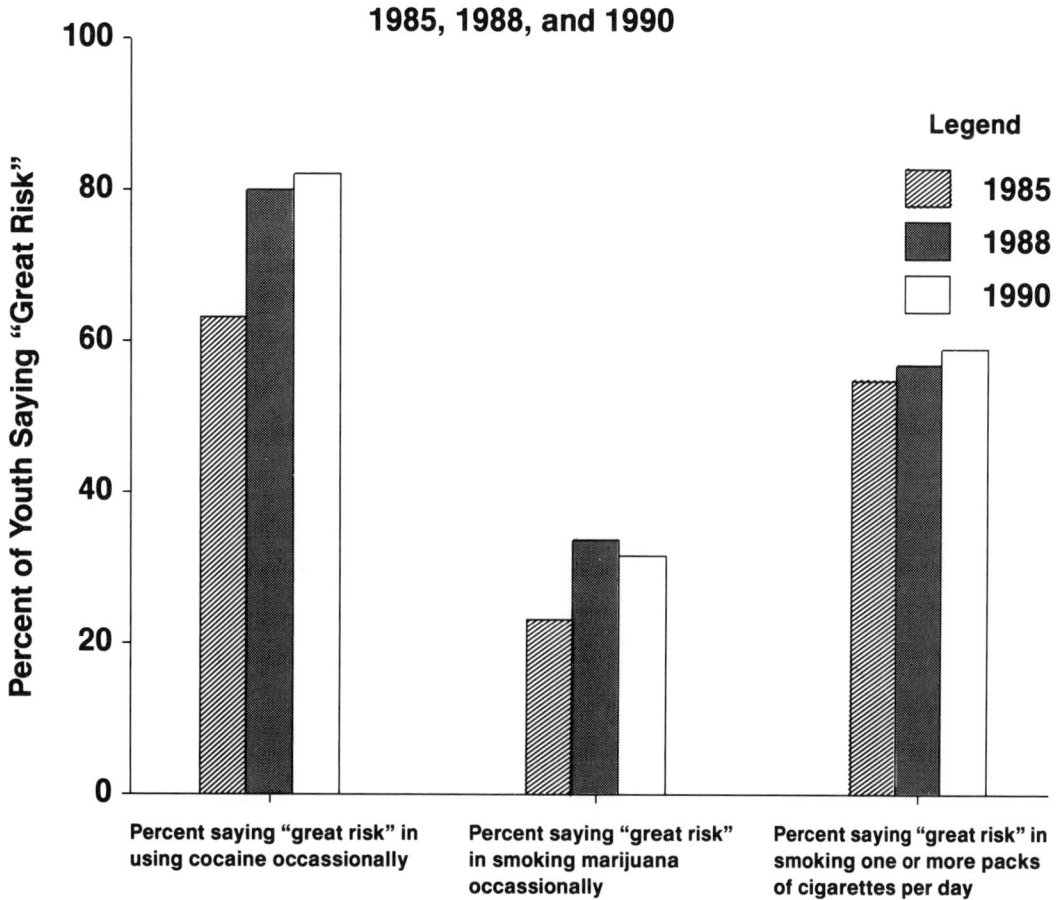

From: National Institute of Drug Abuse (NIDA). (1990). *National household survey on drug abuse.* Rockville, MD: NIDA.

Module I.6—Overhead #8

STAGES IN ADOLESCENT INVOLVEMENT WITH DRUGS AND ALCOHOL USE

Stage 1: Beer, wine

Stage 2: Hard liquor and/or cigarettes

Stage 3: Marijuana

Stage 4: Other illicit drugs

From: Kandel, D. (1975). Stages in adolescent involvement in drug use. *Science, 190.* 912–914.

HANDOUT MASTERS

MODULE I.6 THE ADOLESCENT WHO USES DRUGS AND ALCOHOL

1. Major Adverse Effects of Anabolic Steroids
2. Teen Developmental Needs Chart

MAJOR ADVERSE EFFECTS OF ANABOLIC STEROIDS

Females

1. Oily skin; acne
2. Decrease in breast size, ovulation, lactation, or menstruation
3. Hoarse and deep voice tone (usually irreversible)
4. Clitoral enlargement
5. Unusual hair growth and/or male type baldness (usually irreversible)

Males

Prepuberty

1. Increased size of penis, number of erections, and secondary male characteristics

Postpuberty

1. Priapism (continuous erection), difficult/increased urination
2. Increase in breast size (gynecomastia)
3. Testicular atrophy, oligospermia, erectile dysfunction

Both Sexes

1. Hypercalcemia
2. Edema of feet or legs
3. Jaundice, liver impairment
4. Liver carcinoma (rare)
5. Urinary calculi
6. Hypersensitivity
7. Insomnia
8. Iron deficiency anemia
9. Nausea, vomiting, anorexia, stomach pains

Module I.6—Handout #2

TEEN DEVELOPMENTAL NEEDS CHART

As an Individual

(To achieve a sense of self-esteem)

- Respect from parents/adults

- Respect from peers

- Appreciation and approval from adults and peers
- Opportunities to experience success
- Validation and reinforcement by others of teen's self-worth

(To establish an integrated personal identity)

- Recognition and choice of appropriate role models
- Development of socially acceptable and consistent levels of self-discipline and self-control
- Ability to assess personal strengths and weaknesses realistically
- Ability to establish and maintain friendships

As a Member of Society

(To acquire life-coping skills required for adult living)

- Ability to communicate thoughts and feelings effectively
- Opportunities to solve problems and perceive a range of options
- Chances to make appropriate decisions based on goals
- Opportunity to participate with others in activities involving shared investments and responsibility
- Capacity to negotiate and cooperate with others

(To explore career choices)

- Experience of paid employment

- Volunteer jobs to explore range of career choices
- Acceptance of personal accountability for behavior and choices

---

From: Youth Program staff, National Institute on Alcohol Abuse and Alcoholism's Clearinghouse for Alcohol Information (1981).

RECOMMENDED TEACHING STRATEGIES AND SAMPLE ASSIGNMENTS

RECOMMENDED TEACHING STRATEGIES

- Lecture
- Audiovisual materials
- Advancement at self-help meetings (such as Ala-Teen, Al-Anon)
- Small group discussion
- Role playing
- Clinical placement

SAMPLE ASSIGNMENT

Interview an adolescent in a clinical setting. Describe his or her physical, cognitive, social, psychological, and spiritual development according to a known growth and development theorist. Briefly describe the evident stressors.

Describe human and environmental patterns and factors that place this adolescent at risk for alcohol and substance abuse.

SAMPLE OF APPLICATION OF NURSING DIAGNOSIS

Nursing Diagnosis

Alteration in self-concept related to body image (7.1.2) Psychosocial

Defining Characteristics

- Verbal and/or nonverbal response to actual or perceived physical alteration.
- Altered social interactions due to a negative body image.
- Preoccupation with change.

Process Criteria: The Nurse

- Establishes with the individual a relationship characterized by trust.
- Provides individual and group experiences to review feelings regarding the self-concept.
- Assesses the risk of suicide.
- Assists in identification of co-dependency issues.

Outcome Criteria: The Individual

- Develops accurate, health body images.
- Increases self-esteem and confidence.
- Identifies her feelings within a group and in individual settings.

CASE VIGNETTE

The Adolescent Who Uses Drugs and Alcohol

Marci, a 16-year-old high-school sophomore, appears in the school health office at least three times a week. Her complaints are usually vague symptoms of gastric distress, headache, and nausea. The school nurse has noticed that she is frequently agitated and tremulous and appears to have been sleeping poorly. In addition to dark shadows under her eyes, Marci is about ten pounds underweight for her age and height, is poorly groomed and attired in clothes which are stylish in her peer group, but often wrinkled and in disrepair. During her latest visit to the school nurse, Marci complained of amenorrhea and expressed concerns about her gynecologic health.

Discussion Questions

1. What interventions are appropriate for the school nurse?
2. How should interventions be prioritized?
3. What additional sources of information would contribute to a comprehensive assessment of Marci's current situation?
4. What components of assessment should be included in the nursing intervention?
5. What ethical considerations are appropriate to the nursing intervention?

Nursing Diagnosis

Noncompliance (5.2.1.1) Cognitive

Defining Characteristics

- A personal behavior that deviates from health-related advice, or a person's informed decision not to adhere to a therapeutic recommendation by a health professional.

- Increased bio-psychosocial problems related to addictions.
- Inability to set goals or maintain goal-oriented behavior.

Process Criteria: The Nurse

- Identifies potential areas of high risk when individual does not comply with treatment.
- Confronts denial of effects of addiction by presenting assessment data from the individual's history.
- Teaches the family and significant others health coping skills.
- Encourages participation in a self-help group related to the addiction, such as Ala-Teen.

Outcome Criteria: The Individual

- Achieves and sustains compliance and abstinence related to the addictive process.
- Attends fellowship support groups.

Family Members

- Verbalize the difficulties in accepting the diagnosis of addiction and the issues related to relapse.

Nursing Diagnosis

Knowledge deficit related to learning (8.1.1) Cognitive

Defining Characteristics

- Lack of awareness or understanding of the disease concept of addiction.
- Verbalization of knowledge deficit.
- Inaccurate perception of health status.

Process Criteria: The Nurse

- Develops a teaching plan that includes the following concepts:
  - Disease states associated with addictions.
  - Developing positive communication skills.
  - Feelings associated with addictions.
  - Positive coping mechanisms.
- Reinforces learning with audiovisual aids and handouts.
- Fosters the individual's participation throughout the teaching and learning process.

Outcome Criteria: The Individual

- Defines the disease of addiction.
- Demonstrates positive communication skills in the classroom.

Nursing Diagnosis

Altered growth and development (6.6) Psychosocial

Defining Characteristics

- Children raised in families that are dysfunctional because of the disease process of substance abuse and addiction.
- Overdeveloped sense of responsibility.
- Delayed grief.

Process Criteria: The Nurse

- Identifies early symptoms of substance abuse and addiction and assists the family to recognize the symptoms and seek help.
- Provides appropriate counseling for children of alcohol and drug abusers.
- Educates the individual and family about issues related to adult children of alcoholics.
- Refers the family to individuals and agencies providing a variety of treatment modalities (such as nurse therapists and family counselors).

Outcome Criteria: The Individuals

- Demonstrate and verbalize an awareness of feelings and express them in an honest, health-promoting manner.
- Identify the need for help.

TEST QUESTIONS AND ANSWERS

TEST QUESTIONS

1. Identify the risk factor which is most likely to influence alcohol use by adolescents:
   a. traumatic losses in childhood.
   b. alcoholism in family members.
   c. sociopathic personality disorder.
   d. learning disabilities and poor school performance.
   e. ethnicity.

2. Characteristics of families of adolescent drug abusers often include:
   a. poor generational boundaries.
   b. flexible role structure.
   c. close parent-child relationships.
   d. an emphasis on individual autonomy.
   e. respect for different values.

3. Adolescent females vary from their male peers inasmuch as their drug use includes:
   a. heavier alcohol use.
   b. use of alcohol in combination with other drugs.
   c. more psychedelics.
   d. more nicotine and stimulants.
   e. the exchange of sex for drugs.

4. Trends in drug use by adolescents suggest:
   a. marked increase in alcohol use.
   b. overall declines in illicit drug use.
   c. increased reliance on cocaine.
   d. widespread use of inhalants.
   e. increased use of prescription drugs.

5. Assessment of the sero-positive adolescent requires:
   a. obtaining detailed data on sexual practices.
   b. patient teaching on safer sex practices.

    c. body fluid analysis for drug use.

    d. waiver of HIV testing.

    e. neurological evaluation.

6. Trends in drug use in economically disadvantaged youth include:

    a. widespread use of designer drugs.

    b. use of inhalants.

    c. abstinence by most females.

    d. cultural support for drug use.

    e. widespread psychedelic experimentation.

7. The primary intervention of the school nurse in relation to student drug using patterns is:

    a. assessment.

    b. counseling.

    c. identification.

    d. short-term treatment.

    e. screening.

8. Prevention programs appear most effective when they:

    a. build student self-esteem.

    b. teach coping strategies.

    c. provide education on the risks of drug use.

    d. are directed toward experimental users.

    e. are directed toward regular users.

9. Adolescent drinking is pathological when its pattern is one of:

    a. experimental use.

    b. regular use.

    c. use as a means of problem solving.

    d. use to increase sociability.

    e. use to avoid social rejection.

10. Identify the *most correct* statement about adolescent drug and alcohol use:

    a. depression predicts alcoholism in adolescent males.

    b. negative cultural norms deter adolescent drug experimentation.

    c. dysfunctional family patterns do not support adolescent drug use.

    d. adolescent alcohol use has accelerated since 1980.

    e. peer and family influence are significant predictors of adolescent drug use.

Module I.6

ANSWER KEY

1. b
2. a
3. d
4. b
6. b
7. c
8. d
9. c
10. e

BIBLIOGRAPHY

MODULE I.6 THE ADOLESCENT WHO USES DRUGS AND ALCOHOL

American Nurses' Association. (1988). *Standards of addictions nursing practice with selected diagnosis and criteria.* Kansas City, MO: Author.

Babow, I. (1990). A suicidal adolescent's Sleeping Beauty Syndrome: Cessation orientations toward dying, sleep and drugs. *Adolescence, 25*(100), 791–798.

Brook, R. C., & Whitehead, P. (1983). Values of adolescent drug abusers. *International Journal of Addiction, 18,* 1–8.

Brooks, J. S., Nomura, C., & Cohen, R. (1989). A network of influences on adolescent drug involvement: Neighborhood, school, peer, and family. *Genetic, Sociological and General Psychology Monographs, 115*(1), 123–145.

Deykin, E. Y., Levy, J. C., & Wells, V. (1987). Adolescent depression, alcohol and drug abuse. *American Journal of Public Health, 77*(2), 178–182.

Dishion, T. J., & Lieber, R. (1985). Adolescent marijuana and alcohol use: The role of parents and peers revisited. *American Journal of Drug and Alcohol Abuse, 11*(1–2), 11–25.

Fawzy, F. I., & Combs, R. H. (1983). Generational continuity in the use of substances: The impact of parental substance abuse on adolescent use. *Addictive Behavior, 8*(2), 109–114.

Frank, B., Marcel, R., & Schmeidler, J. (1988). The continuing problem of youthful solvent abuse in N.Y.S. *Research Monograph No. 85.* Rockville, MD: DHHS (ADM88-1577).

Groerer, J. (1987). Correlations between drug use by teenagers and drug use by older family members. *Drug and Alcohol Abuse, 13*(1–2), 95–108.

Haffner, D. W. (1988). AIDS and adolescents: School health education must begin now. *Journal of School Health, 58*(4), 154–155.

Harford, T. C., & Grant, B. F. (1987). *Alcohol consumption among youth: A national longitudinal survey.* Rockville, MD: Division of Biometry and Epidemiology, National Institute of Alcohol Abusing Adolescents.

Henderson, D. C., & Anderson, S. C. (1989). Adolescents and chemical dependency. *Social Work Health Care, 14*(1), 87–105.

Henley, G., & Winters, K. (1988). Development of a problem seventy scales for the assessment of adolescent alcohol and drug abuse. *The International Journal of the Addictions, 23*(1), 65–85.

Johnson, R. E., & Marcos, A. C. (1988). Correlates of adolescent use by gender and geographic location. *American Journal of Drug and Alcohol Abuse, 14*(1), 51–63.

Johnston, L. (1985). The etiology and prevention of substance abuse: What can we learn from recent historical changes? *Etiology of drug abuse, implications for prevention.* (NIDA Research Monograph 56). Rockville, MD: DHHS.

Johnston, L.D., O'Malley, P., & Bachman, J. (1988). *Illicit drug use, smoking, drinking in American high school students, college students, young adults.* Rockville, MD: DHHS (ADM8-1602).

Kaminer, Y., & Bukstein, O. (1989). Adolescent chemical use and dependence: Current issues in epidemiology, treatment and prevention. *Acta Psychiatric Scandinavia, 79,* 415–424.

Kandel, D. (1975). Stages in adolescent involvement in drug use. *Science, 190,* 912–914.

Kandel, D. (1989). State office of mental health researchers find teen drug use down. *Office of Mental Health News,* December 29, 1989.

Kandel, D. (1982). Epidemiologic and psychosocial perspectives on adolescent drug use. *Journal of the American Academy of Child Psychiatry, 21*(4), 328–347.

Kaufman, E., & Borders, L. (1984). Adolescent substance abuse in Anglo-America. *Journal of Drug Issues, 14*(2), 365–377.

Keyser-Smith, J. & Stoil, M. J. (1987). And I will stand the hazard of the die. *Alcohol Health and Research World, 11,* 48–53.

Khuri, E., Millman, R., & Hartman, N. (1984). Clinical issues concerning alcoholic and youthful narcotic abusers. *Advances in Alcohol and Substance Abuse, 3*(4), 69–86.

Levine, B. (1985). Adolescent substance abuse: Toward an integration of family systems and individual adaptation theories. *American Journal of Family Therapy, 13*(2), 3–16.

Maddahian, E., Newcomb, M., & Bentler, P. (1986). Adolescents' substance use: Impact of ethnicity, income and availability. *Advances in Alcohol and Substance Abuse, 5*(3), 63–78.

Martin, J. P., & Pritchard, M. E. (1991). Factors associated with alcohol use in late adolescents. *Journal of Alcohol Studies, 52*(1), 5–9.

McDermott, D. (1984). The relationship of parental drug use and parents' attitudes concerning adolescent drug use. *Adolescence, 19*(73), 89–99.

Meyer, D.C., & Phillips, L.M. (1990). No safe place: Parental alcoholism and adolescent suicide. *American Journal of Psychotherapy, 44*(4), 552–562.

Meyer, R. E. (1986). *Psychopathology and addictive disorders.* New York: Guilford Press.

National Institute of Drug Abuse (NIDA) (1990). *National household survey on drug abuse.* Rockville, MD: NIDA.

Newcomb, M. D., Bentler, P. M., & Fahy, B. (1987). Cocaine use and psychopathology: Association among young adults. *International Journal of Addictions, 22*(12), 1167–1188.

Oetting, E.R., Edwards, R.W., & Beauvais, F. (1988). *Social and psychological factors indulging inhalant abuse. Research Monograph 85.* Rockville, MD: DHHS (ADM88-8577).

Pallikkathayil, L. & Tweed, S. (1983). Substance abuse: Alcohol and drugs during adolescence. *Nursing Clinics of North America, 18*(2), 313–321.

Pandina, R.J., & Johnson, V. (1989). Familial drinking history as a predictor of alcohol and drug consumption in the adolescent children. *Journal of Studies on Alcohol, 50*(3), 245–250.

Perry, C. L. (1987). Results of prevention programs with adolescents. *Minnesota Drug and Alcohol Dependence, 20,* 13–19.

Pirie, P. L., Murray, D. M., & Luepker, R. V. (1988). Smoking prevalence in a cohort of adolescents, including absentees, drop-outs and transfers. *American Journal of Public Health, 78*(2), 176–178.

Potter-Efron, P., Potter-Efron, R. (1986). Treating the chemically dependent adolescent: The enabling inventory and other techniques for responsibility. *Alcoholism Treatment Oserfing, 3*(1), 59–72.

Radosevic, M.L., Lanza-Kaduce, R., Akens, & M. Krohn. (1980). The sociology of adolescent drug and drinking behavior: A review of the state of the field; part II. *Deviant Behavior: An Interdisciplinary Journal, 1,* 145–169.

Rohrbaugh, J., & Jessor, R. (1975). Religiosity in youth: A personal control against deviance. *Journal of Personality, 43,* 136–155.

Schiff, M., & Caviola, A. (1988–1989). Adolescents at risk for chemical dependency: Identification and prevention issues. *Journal of Chemical Dependency Treatment, 2*(1), 25–47.

Schiff, M., Caviola, A., & Harrison, L. (1989). Teaching prevention to professionals who work with abusive chemically dependent families. *Alcoholism Treatment Quarterly, 6*(2), 41–52.

Schubiner, H.H. (1989). Preventive health screening in adolescent patients. *Primary Care, 16*(1), 211–230.

Segal, J. (1983). Drugs and youth: A review of the problem. *The International Journal of Addictions, 18*(3), 429–433.

Singer, M., & Anglin, T. (1986). The identification of adolescent substance abuse by health care professionals. *International Journal of Addictions, 21*(2), 247–254.

Swadi, H., & Zeitlin, H. (1988). Peer influence and adolescent substance abuse: A promising side. *British Journal of Addiction, 83*(2), 153–157.

Todd, T.C., & Selekman, M. (1989). Principles of family therapy for adolescent substance abuse. *Journal of Psycho-Therapy and the Family, 6*(3–4), 49–70.

Wallack, L., & Corbett, K. (1987). Alcohol, tobacco & marijuana use among youth: An overview of epidemiological, program and policy trends. *Health Education Quarterly, 14*(29), 223–249.

White, H. R. (1988). Longitudinal patterns of cocaine use among adolescents. *American Journal of Drug and Alcohol Abuse, 14*(1), 1–15.

Windle, M., & Barnes, G. M. (1988). Similarities and differences in correlates of alcohol and female adolescents. *International Journal of the Addictions, 23*(7), 707–728.

Wodarski, J.S. (1990). Adolescent substance abuse: Practice implications. *Adolescence, 25*(99), 667–688.

APPENDIX

THE ADOLESCENT
ASSESSMENT/REFERRAL SYSTEM
MANUAL

National Institute on Drug Abuse
Editor
Elizabeth R. Rahdert, PhD

U.S. DEPARTMENT OF HEALTH
AND HUMAN SERVICES

Public Health Service
Alcohol, Drug Abuse, and Mental Health Administration

Publication #: ADM 91-1735

The Adolescent Assessment/Referral System was developed for the National Institute of Drug Abuse by West-over Consultants, Inc., 500 East Street, S.W., Suite 910, Washington, D.C. 20024, under contract number 271-87-8225, and by the Pacific Institute for Research and Evaluation, 7315 Wisconsin Avenue, Suite 900 East, Bethesda, MD 20814, under contract number 271-89-8252.

CHAPTER 3
PROBLEM ORIENTED SCREENING
INSTRUMENT FOR TEENAGERS

OVERVIEW OF THE POSIT

The Problem Oriented Screening Instrument for Teenagers (POSIT) is designed to identify problems in need of further assessment in the ten functional areas addressed by the
AARS. "Further assessment" refers to an in-depth assessment of identified functional
areas using the instruments recommended in the Comprehensive Assessment Battery
(Chapter 4). Adequate, in-depth assessments are not possible with the use of the **POSIT**
only. The **POSIT** simply points out areas where problems may exist.

Users of the **POSIT** and the **POSIT** scoring system presented in The Adolescent
Assessment/Referral System Manual must be aware of two important limitations:

The **POSIT** and the **POSIT** scoring system are based on expert clinical judgment.
Neither have been field-tested, and reliability and validity have not yet been established
through scientific studies. Any scores derived from administering this version of the
POSIT may be useful in clinical decision making, but must be viewed with caution.

The **POSIT** scoring system is very conservative. That is, a **POSIT** score might indicate
the need for further assessment even if there is a low probability that a severe problem
exists in that given functional area. Consequently, the fact that a particular score by itself
meets the **POSIT** criterion for "further assessment" cannot, by itself, be taken as an
indication that a problem will be shown to be severe enough after diagnostic assessment to
require further treatment.

Preliminary data on the **POSIT** which illustrate these points are presented at the end
of this chapter.

Materials

The version of the **POSIT** presented in the Manual consists of an eight-page questionnaire
containing 139 yes/no items. Adolescents record their responses directly on the **POSIT**
form. Both English and Spanish versions are provided.

The **POSIT** scoring kit consists of **POSIT** Scoring Sheets and a set of reusable scoring
templates. These templates indicate the functional area to which each item belongs, and
the interpretation that can be given to a "yes" or "no" response to that item. Because the
items for each of the ten functional areas addressed in the **POSIT** have been fully random-
ized, it is extremely difficult to score the **POSIT** without using the templates. Template 1
is used to score the first four pages of the **POSIT** and Template 2 is used to score the last
four pages. As the scores are counted for each page, they can be transferred to a **POSIT**
Scoring Sheet.

Module I.6

English and Spanish scoring templates for the **POSIT** are provided at the end of the Manual. To use them, they must be copied onto transparency stock. They may then be used to score as many **POSITS** as is required. Also, in the back of the Manual is a copy of the **POSIT** Scoring Sheet. This sheet should be copied onto plain paper. One scoring sheet is required for each **POSIT** scored.

The Logic of POSIT Scoring

In order to understand how the **POSIT** is scored, it is necessary to understand the types of items the **POSIT** contains. It will be helpful to have a copy of the **POSIT** and the clear plastic scoring templates in front of you as you read the following discussion.

The items in the **POSIT** are of three types:

General Purpose Items. Each item contributes one point to the total risk score for a functional area. The letter printed on the scoring template indicates which functional area is addressed and whether a "yes" or a "no" response is high risk and is therefore to be assigned the point. Some items contribute a point to more than one functional area. These items are identified by the presence of more than one letter on the scoring template.

General Purpose Age Related Items. Each age related item is similar to the general purpose items except that it will only be scored depending on whether the adolescent is over or under 16 years of age. The scoring templates indicate which items are age-related through a light grey screen, and indicate the age range (over or under 16 years) for which the item should be counted (e.g., "16+").

Red-Flag Items. These are items which alone indicate the need for further assessment. That is, if an adolescent gives the high risk response to any red-flag item for a given functional area, he or she should be assessed further in that functional area. The scoring templates indicate which items are red flags through a dark gray screen and the notation, "RF."

The Expert Clinician Researchers who designed the **POSIT** have assigned a cut-off score for each functional area. Each cut-off (e.g., 4 points for Mental Health Status) refers to the number of points assigned to an adolescent from responses to the general purpose and general purpose age related items that indicate a need for further assessment. If a high-risk response is given for any of the red flag items in a functional area, further assessment is indicated independent of the number of points assigned to that functional area. In two functional areas—Substance Use/Abuse and Peer Relations—all of the items are red flags. Thus, the cut-off score for each of these functional areas is one.

The assigned cut-off score for each functional area is given in Table 1.

Preliminary Data on the POSIT

In order to obtain a preliminary assessment of the adequacy of the current **POSIT** items to tap problem areas, and the assigned **POSIT** scoring system to discriminate, even to a modest degree, between a group of youth with some evidence of problems and a group of youth with as yet little or no evidence, NIDA administered the **POSIT** to 633 junior and senior high school students and 216 adolescents in substance abuse treatment. For each adolescent, **POSIT** scores in all 10 functional areas were computed using the assigned scoring system described above.

Table 1
Cut-off Scores For Posit

	Functional Area	Cut-off
A.	Substance Use/Abuse	1 point°
B.	Physical Health Status	3 points
C.	Mental Health Status	4 points
D.	Family Relationships	4 points
E.	Peer Relations	1 point°
F.	Educational Status	6 points
G.	Vocational Status	5 points
H.	Social Skills	3 points
I.	Leisure and Recreation	5 points
J.	Aggressive Behavior/Delinquency	6 points

°All items are red flag

Table 2 presents the percentage of school students and in-treatment adolescents who were identified as having a potential problem in one or more of the ten **POSIT** functional areas. "Identified as having a possible problem" means that the adolescent exceeded the cut-off and/or endorsed a red-flag item for that functional area, as defined by the aforementioned scoring system.

At least two conclusions can be drawn from the data in Table 2. First, the current items and the clinically derived scoring system successfully discriminate between adolescents in treatment and adolescents drawn from a school population. In every functional area, more in-treatment adolescents than students were identified as having a possible problem in the functional area. Moreover, all of these differences are statistically significant. Some of them are quite dramatic. This result suggests that the current items and scoring system have some validity.

Second, however, it is also clear that many of the school students were identified as having possible problems in each of the ten functional areas. For example, although almost 90% of the in-treatment adolescents were identified as having a possible problem in the Substance Use/Abuse functional area, almost 50% of the school students were identified as having possible problems in this functional area as well. In Mental Health Status, Peer Relations, and Educational Status, over 80% of the school students were identified as having possible problems in these functional areas. Of course, it is not clear what problems the school students may actually be having. However, on the face of it, these numbers seem too high.

As noted earlier, the **POSIT** cut-off scores were designed to be very sensitive to detecting problems when they are present. This sensitivity results in at least some "false alarms." Thus, the assigned **POSIT** scoring system may be too sensitive—that is, may result in too many false alarms. This fact must be kept in mind if the **POSIT** and assigned scoring system are to be used in actual clinical practice.

Module I.6

Table 2
Comprehensive Assessment
Battery Tools

Functional Area	Assessment Tool(s)
Substance Use/Abuse	Personal Experience Inventory (PEI) Adolescent Diagnostic Interview (ADI)
Physical Health Status	Physical examination and lab work Physician Report Form
Mental Health Status	Diagnostic Interview Schedule for Children (DISC-2.1C) Brief Symptom Inventory (BSI-53)
Family Relations	Family Assessment Measurement (FAM) Parent Adolescent Relationship Questionnaire (PARQ)
Peer Relations	Piers Harris Self-Concept Scale Behavior Problem Checklist
Educational Status	WAIS-R, WISC-R Woodcock-Johnson Psycho-educational Test Battery
Vocational Status	Career Maturity Inventory (CMI) Generalizable Skills Curriculum
Social Skills	
Leisure and Recreation	
Aggressive Behavior/ Delinquency	

Administering the POSIT

It is extremely important that adolescents feel free to answer all of the questions on the **POSIT** honestly. Instructions for the **POSIT** stress that the responses adolescents give will be used to help the adolescent. This point should be reiterated and stressed in verbal instructions. The **POSIT** administrator should stay with the adolescent to define words that the adolescent does not understand and may read the **POSIT** to youth who cannot read. However, an effort should be made to indicate that the administrator is not "watching over" the adolescent.

Before scoring a completed **POSIT**, look it over to make sure that all the questions have been answered. If items are missing, point this out to the adolescent, and give him/her an opportunity to respond to the missing items. If he/she refuses, leave the item blank.

Scoring the POSIT

Two sets of scoring templates are provided at the end of the Manual—one for scoring the English **POSIT** and one for scoring the Spanish **POSIT**. These templates are different. Make sure you use the correct template. Otherwise, scoring individual items on the English and Spanish **POSITS** are identical.

The first four pages of the **POSIT** are scored using Template 1. Place Template 1 over the first page of the **POSIT** such that the first column of the template covers the response

484

options (yes–no). Note that next to the response options for Item 1 of the **POSIT**, the template indicates that this question relates to Functional areas C (Mental Health) and F (Educational Status). Note also that there is a dark grey screen over the yes–no response options. This indicates that Item 1 is a red flag item. In this case, as indicated on the template (°RFF only), the item is a red flag for Functional area F only.

The high-risk response is indicated by a circle on the template. For Item 1, the high-risk response is "Yes." This means that if the adolescent has put an "X" through "Yes" for this question, further assessment is needed in Functional area F. (Question 1 is a red flag in this functional area.) A "Yes" response also means that one point should be counted for Functional area C.

Now look at Item 2. The template indicates that this question relates to Functional area J (Aggressive Behavior/Delinquency) and that the high-risk response is "Yes." This means that if the adolescent has put an "X" through "Yes" for Item 2, one point should be counted for Functional area J.

Scoring proceeds down the first column of Template 1 until all of the questions on the first page have been scored. Now, the second column of Template 1 is used to score the second page, the third column for the third page, and the fourth column for the fourth page. To score pages 5–8 of the **POSIT**, the four columns of Template 2 are used.

Points and red flags for each page of the **POSIT** are tallied using the **POSIT** Scoring Sheet. The eight columns of the Scoring Sheet correspond to the eight pages of the **POSIT**. The ten rows of the Scoring Sheet correspond to the 10 functional areas. For each page of the **POSIT**, indicate the number of points scored in each functional area. For example, if two points are scored for Functional area I (Leisure and Recreation) on Page 1, enter a "2" in the Functional area I row for page 1 on the **POSIT** Scoring Sheet. If the high-risk response is given for any red-flag item in a functional area on a given page, enter "RF" in the box for that functional area.

If a general-purpose item is age-related, count a point for a high-risk response only for the age group indicated on the template. If an item is blank (i.e., the adolescent has refused to respond), treat the item as though a high-risk response had been given. However, the fact that items are missing will lessen the utility of scores for that individual, and should be noted in the Scorer's Comments section on the Scoring Sheet.

If a given page has no items in a functional area, the appropriate box on the **POSIT** Scoring Sheet is blacked out. For example, there are no items related to Functional area B (Physical Health Status) on the fifth page. Thus, the box for Functional area B in the column for the fifth page is blacked out.

When all of the pages have been scored, total the points for each functional area in the Tally column of the **POSIT** Scoring Sheet. If any red flags have been recorded for a functional area, enter "RF" in the Tally column. The total points for each functional area may then be compared to the cut-off score noted above for each functional area.

If an adolescent exceeds the cut-off score or endorses one or more red-flag items in a given functional area, a problem may exist. However, the only way to determine if a problem does exist is to conduct a further assessment in the identified functional area using the appropriate assessment tool(s) from the Comprehensive Assessment Battery (CAB).

POSIT

Functional Areas

A. Substance Use/Abuse

B. Physical Health Status

C. Mental Health Status

D. Family Relationships

E. Peer Relations

F. Educational Status

G. Vocational Skills

H. Social Skills

I. Leisure and Recreation

J. Aggressive Behavior/Delinquency

CHAPTER 4
COMPREHENSIVE ASSESSMENT BATTERY

The Comprehensive Assessment Battery addresses the same 10 functional areas represented in the **POSIT**. The CAB instruments should only be used when the **POSIT** has indicated that a possible problem may exist in a given functional area. Uncritical application of the CAB instruments without reference to **POSIT** scores will unnecessarily burden adolescents and their families, and will result in a significant waste of time, energy, and money.

The instruments included in the Comprehensive Assessment Battery were selected based on the recommendations of national experts in adolescent assessment and treatment. In almost all cases, the instruments which comprise the CAB have been psychometrically validated on adolescents and have proven their utility in clinical settings. Where possible, instruments were selected that are readily available and that can be administered and scored with a minimum of training.

Table 2 presents the recommended assessment tools for each of the ten functional areas addressed by the AARS. The following sections provide descriptions of the instruments, along with information on how to obtain them, administration time, and cost. At the end of each description, key references are provided.

FUNCTIONAL AREA I: SUBSTANCE USE/ABUSE

Tools:

Part I of the Personal Experience Inventory (PEI)
Part II of the Personal Experience Inventory (PEI)
Adolescent Diagnostic Interview (ADI) available July 1991

Administration Time:

Part I of the PEI: 20–25 minutes
Part II of the PEI: 20–25 minutes
ADI: 40–50 minutes

Source for PEI and ADI:

Western Psychological Services
12031 Wilshire Blvd.
Los Angeles, CA 90025
(213) 478–2061 or (800) 222–2670

Cost:

PEI: $10–$17 per test depending on volume
ADI: $6–$9 per test depending on volume

Translations:

The PEI is available in French, and will be available in Spanish.

The Personal Experience Inventory (PEI) and Adolescent Diagnostic Interview (ADI), developed by a consortium of Minnesota Chemical Dependency service providers, comprise a comprehensive, clinically standardized set of assessments. These assessments are designed to measure adolescent substance involvement, psychosocial problems often associated with that involvement, and diagnostic signs and symptoms. The PEI and ADI are intended to provide professionals with a reliable and valid report for the identification, referral, and treatment of teenage alcohol and drug abuse.

The PEI is a self-report instrument for 12- to 18-year-olds written at a sixth-grade reading level. An effort has been made to construct short-sentence items and to avoid complicated double negatives. The PEI, which contains 33 scales, has been the norm on both chemical dependency treatment center adolescents and high-school student populations. Percentile and T-score norms based on nearly 2,000 adolescents are provided by age and sex. A user's manual and computerized scoring and interpretation reports are available.

The PEI is divided into two primary sections: chemical use problem severity, and psychosocial risk factors. The Problem Severity section (Part I) measures 10 scales associated with drug abusive and drug dependent-like characteristics such as personal consequences, social benefits, and loss of control. Also included is a detailed overview of drug use history and onset, and faking-good and faking-bad scales. The Psychosocial section (Part II) consists of eight scales that measure personal risk factors (e.g., negative self-image, deviant behavior) and four scales addressing environmental risk factors (e.g., peer chemical use). This section also includes six clinical problem screens, such as physical and sexual abuse, and another pair of faking-good and faking-bad response distortion scales.

Research on the PEI provides extensive evidence for the scales' reliability (internal consistency and test-retest) and construct validity (with respect to clinical diagnoses, treatment referral decisions, group status, Minnesota Multiphasic Personality Inventory [MMPI] scale scores, and other alternate measures of severity and psychosocial risk factors of problems).

The ADI primarily covers DSM-III-R symptoms of psychoactive substance disorders. The interview follows an easily administered structured format that reviews the adolescent's drug use history and signs of abuse or dependence for each of the major drug categories. Also included are measures of level of functioning and psychosocial stressors. Research on the ADI suggests high inter-rater agreement and temporal stability of diagnoses. In addition, ADI diagnoses are related to drug use frequency, self-report measures of problem severity, and independent clinical diagnostic decisions.

Information derived from the ADI can be used to supplement that obtained from the PEI, or may be used as the sole assessment in the Substance Use/Abuse Functional area if the adolescent is unable to take the PEI (e.g., is unable to read or comprehend it).

KEY REFERENCES

Henly, G. A., & Winters, K. C. (1988). Development of problem severity for the assessment of adolescent alcohol and drug abuse. *The International Journal of the Addictions, 23*:65–85.

Henly, G. A., & Winters, K. C. (1989). Development of psychosocial scales for the assessment of adolescent alcohol and drug involvement. *The International Journal of the Addictions, 24*:973–1001.

Winters, K. C., & Henly, G. A. (1989). *Personal experience inventory test and manual.* Los Angeles: Western Psychological Services.

Winters, K. C., & Henly, G. A. *Adolescent diagnostic interview schedule and manual.* Los Angeles: Western Psychological Services.

Module I.6

FUNCTIONAL AREA II: PHYSICAL HEALTH STATUS

Tools:

Physical Examination and Lab Work

Physician Report Form

Administration Time:

30 minutes

Source:

The Physician Report Form appears at the back of this Manual.

Cost:

Variable, depending on local health care costs and lab test ordered.

Although the use of illicit drugs and alcohol among adolescents does not usually lead to the organ system damage sometimes observed in adult abusers (e.g., liver cirrhosis, cardiomyopathy), such conditions are not unknown. Perhaps more important is the fact that the lifestyle of the chronic drug user increases the risk for accidental injury, infection (especially sexually transmittable diseases), unwanted pregnancy, malnutrition, and physical and sexual abuse. A variety of medical complications may also develop as the direct result of intravenous drug use, as well as drug inhalation and ingestion.

Because not all physicians feel competent to comprehensively evaluate an adolescent with possible substance abuse problems, a Physician Report Form has been prepared by adolescent medicine specialists at the Johns Hopkins University School of Medicine. This form can guide the physician in history taking, conducting the physical examination, and ordering lab work. The form can also be used as a vehicle for reporting findings to a case manager or treatment provider. The Physician Report Form appears at the end of this Manual, and may be copied without permission.

Health care professionals are strongly advised to be informed of their legal responsibilities with respect to obtaining, using, and disseminating the information obtained from a health status examination. This is especially relevant regarding HIV testing, pregnancy testing, and other aspects of the examination where patient confidentiality and public health considerations are factors influencing medical management.

KEY REFERENCES

Litt, I. F., & Cohen, M. I. (1970). The drug-abusing adolescent as a pediatric patient. *Journal of Pediatrics, 77*(2):195–202.

Litt, I. F., & Schonberg, S. K. (1975). Medical complications of drug abuse in adolescents. *Medical Clinics of North America, 56*(6).

A Guide for BCHS supported programs and projects: Adolescent health care, DHEW Publication No. (HSA) 79-5234, 1980. U.S. Government Printing Office, Stock No. 017-026-00083-6.

490

Appendix

Table 3

Diagnostic Categories Included in the DISC

Bipolar Affective Disorder   Anorexia Nervosa

Major Depression   Bulimia

Cyclothymic Disorder   Gender Identity

Anxiety Disorder-Avoidant   Tourette's Syndrome

Anxiety Disorder-Separation   Pervasive Dev. Disorder

Obsessive-Compulsive   Encopresis

Panic   Enuresis

Phobia   Schizophrenia

Attention Deficit   Alcohol Abuse

Conduct Disorder   Drug Abuse

Diagnostic Categories Not Included in the DISC

Adjustment Disorder   Schizoaffective

Generalized Anxiety   Schizoid Disorder

Sleep Disorder   Personality Disorder (Axis II)

Symptom Checklists

As an adjunct to the DISC2.1C, or where it is not possible to conduct the DISC2.1C, the self-report Symptom Checklist-90 (SCL-90) can be used to document psychopathology. While this type of evaluation is not a substitute for a comprehensive and objective structured interview, qualification of psychiatric symptoms using a self-report questionnaire can provide useful information about the presence and severity of mental and behavioral disturbances.

The adolescents' version of the SCL-90-R affords the opportunity to efficiently measure the severity of mental and behavioral disturbance across multiple dimensions. In addition to scores yielding a Global Severity Index, Symptom Distress Index, and total Positive Symptoms, this self-administered rating scale also contains scales measuring somatization, obsessive compulsive neurosis, interpersonal sensitivity, depression, anxiety, hostility, phobia, paranoid ideation, and psychoticism.

The Brief Symptom Inventory (BSI) is a modification of its longer parent instrument, the SCL-90-R. It reflects the same nine symptom dimensions and three global indices as the SCL-90-R. However, the BSI is comprised of 53 items instead of 90. Psychometric studies suggest that the BSI is an acceptable short alternative to the SCL-90. Both test-retest and internal consistency reliabilities are very good for the primary symptom dimensions of the BSI, and correlations between comparable dimensions of the BSI and SCL-90-R are quite high.

KEY REFERENCES

Costello, A., Edelbrock, C., Dulcan, M., Kalas, R., & Klaric, S. (1984). *Final report to NIMH on the diagnostic interview schedule for children* (Unpublished manuscript).

Costello, A. (1987). Structured interviewing for the assessment of child psychopathology In J. Noshpitz (Ed.), *Basic handbook of child psychiatry: Advances and new directions.* New York: Basic Books.

Derogatis, L., Rickels, K., & Rock, A. (1976). The SCL-90 and the MMPI: A step in the validation of a new self-report scale. *British Journal of Psychiatry, 128,* 280–289.

Derogatis, L., and Melisaratos, N. (1983). The brief symptom inventory: An introductory report. *Psychological Medicine, 1983, 13,* 595–605.

The organization of the family, patterns of communication, and cohesiveness are well known determinants of the psychosocial adjustment of children. Poor family management, including parental inconsistency, loose family structure, use of harsh physical punishment, lack of praise for doing well, family conflict, and poor family communication patterns have all been associated with increased risk of adolescent alcohol and other drug problems. In chaotic or disturbed families, parents cannot monitor children's behavior, nor can they be expected to do an adequate job of setting expectations and limits, communicating values, or serving as positive role models. Where the family system cannot effectively perform these tasks, the adolescent's potential for assuming socially normative adult roles is diminished.

It is also the case that substance use and abuse is not uncommon among youth from apparently normal, well-adjusted families. Here, the family comprises a major resource and a therapeutic ally for treating the substance abusing adolescent.

Either as a contributing factor or as a therapeutic resource, the family exerts a prime influence on the substance-abusing adolescent. The family is, therefore, an important component of the rehabilitative process—as an agent to assist in behavior change and/or as a system in need of change. It is also the case that substance use and abuse is not uncommon among youth from apparently normal, well-adjusted families. Here, the family comprises a major resource and a therapeutic ally for treating the substance abusing adolescent.

Either as a contributing factor or as a therapeutic resource, the family exerts a prime influence on the substance-abusing adolescent. The family is, therefore, an important component of the rehabilitative process—as an agent to assist in behavior change and/or as a system in need of change.

Where one or more members of the adolescent's family are alcohol or other drug abusers, special attention must be paid to the problems that living with such an individual may pose for the adolescent. If the Client Personal History Questionnaire indicates that a parent is involved in substance abuse, the assessment should also include a measure of family functioning specifically designed to assess the relationship between the adolescent and the abusing parent.

General Family Assessment

The Family Assessment Measure (FAM) consists of three interrelated instruments which, in combination, provide a comprehensive profile of the functioning of the family unit. Each of the three instruments addresses seven dimensions: a) Task Accomplishment, b) Role Performance, c) Communication, d) Affective Expression, e) Involvement, f) Control, and g) Values and Norms.

The 50-item General Scale measures the level of health in the family from a systems perspective. In addition to the seven dimensions listed above, the General State provides an overall index of family functioning. The 42-item Dyadic Relationship Scale documents the quality of relationship between specific family member pairs. Finally, the 42-item

Tool(s):

Family Assessment Measure (FAM)—General, Dyadic, and Self-Rating Scales

Parent-Adolescent Relationship Questionnaire (PARQ)

Administration Time:

FAM: 10–20 minutes for each of three scales

PARQ: 30 minutes

Source for FAM:

Lisa Johnson
FAM Coordinator
Addiction Research Foundation
33 Russell Street
Toronto, Ontario, Canada M5S-2S1
(416) 595-6000, ext. 7698

Source for PARQ:

Dwight J. McCall, PhD, LPC
Medical College of Virginia
The Forum
Executive Center
10124 W. Board Street, Suite N
Glen Allan, VA 23060
(804) 662-7172

Cost:

FAM: Test booklets (reusable) General, Dyadic, or Self-Rating Scale, 35 cents
each; Answer Sheets (not reusable) General, Dyadic, or Self-Rating Scale, 35
cents each; Profile Sheets (for Plotting FAM) General, Dyadic, or Self-Rating, 10
cents each; FAM Administration and Interpretation Guide, 25 pages, 1 free copy;
Brief FAM Administration and Interpretation Guide, 25 pages, 1 free copy; Brief
FAM, 25 cents

PARQ: Free of charge with permission of author

Translations:

FAM: French (Quebec), French (Parisian), Spanish, German, Japanese, Hebrew,
(Chinese in progress)

PARQ: English Only

Self-Rating Scale measures the individual's perception of his or her functioning in the family unit. The FAM, which is available in both paper-and-pencil and computer formats, can be completed without supervision.

Assessment for Families with a Substance-Abusing Parent

The Parent-Adolescent Relationships Questionnaire (PARQ) is based on the Acquaintance Description Form developed by Paul Wright for adult partners of chemically dependent people. The PARQ is a self-report instrument that assesses eight subscales: 1) worth dependency, 2) minimization of difficulties, 3) control, 4) unrealistic positive expectations, 5) exaggerated sense of responsibility, 6) rescue orientation, 7) change orientation, and 8) externalization of blame.

As yet, the psychometric properties of the PARQ have not been assessed, and no normative data are available. However, the PARQ represents one of the few assessments specifically designed to assess the problems that may be experienced by adolescents with a substance-involved parent.

KEY REFERENCES

Jacob, T., & Tennenbaum, D. (1987). Family Assessment Methods. In M. Rutter, H. Tuma and I. Lann (Eds.), *Assessment and diagnosis of child and adolescent psychopathology.* New York: Guilford Press.

Skinner, H. (1987). Self-report instrument for family assessment. In T. Jacob (Ed.), *Family intervention and psychopathology: Theories, methods, and findings.* New York: Plenum.

Skinner, H., Steinhauer, P., & Santa-Barbara, J. (1983). The family assessment measure. *Canadian Journal of Community Mental Health, 2,* 91–105.

Steinhauer, P. (1984). Clinical applications of the process model of family functioning. *Canadian Journal of Psychiatry, 29,* 98–111.

Wright, P., & Wright, K. Measuring co-dependents' close relationships: Progress and prospects. *Journal of Substance Abuse,* in press.

Wright, P. (1985). The acquaintance description form. In S. Duck and D. Perlman (Eds.), *Understanding personal relationships: An interdisciplinary approach.* London: Sage Publications.

Appendix

FUNCTIONAL AREA V: PEER RELATIONS

Tools:

Piers-Harris Children's Self-Concept Scale
Revised Problem Behavior Checklist

Administration Time:

Piers-Harris: 15–20 minutes
Revised Problem Behavior Checklist: 10–15 minutes

Source for Piers-Harris

Western Psychological Services
12031 Wilshire Blvd.
Los Angeles, CA 90025
(213) 478-2061 or (800) 222-2670

Source for Revised Problem Behavior Checklist:

Herbert C. Quay, PhD
Donald P. Peterson, PhD
P.O. Box 248074
Coral Gables, FL 33124
(305) 284-5208

Cost:

Piers-Harris: $55 per kit (25 test booklets, profiles, scoring forms, manual)
Revised Problem Behavior Checklist: $30 per kit (50 Checklists, scoring templates, and manual)

Translations:

Piers-Harris: English only
Revised Problem Behavior Checklist: Spanish

The peer group is a well documented and powerful influence on the behavior of adolescents. Although the specific mechanisms that underlie peer conformity are debated, there is likely to be a high level of consistency of behavior (risky or otherwise) within networks of close friends.

Much of the research into peer relations has focused on the *quality* of an adolescent's friendships. Here quality is defined in terms of the number of close friends an adolescent has, his or her perception of acceptance by these friends, the level of "closeness" or bonding the adolescent feels to friends, and so on.

Although issues of friendship quality are clearly of clinical importance—i.e., an adolescent who lacks close friendship relationships is generally considered to be at higher risk—they must be considered within the context of the general conventionality or deviance of the specific peers with whom the adolescent associates. An adolescent may have high-quality relationships with and be very attached to a deviant (e.g., drug abusing) peer group. In this case, the close attachment to the peer group may be a liability rather than a resource in the treatment and rehabilitation process. Accordingly, a comprehensive assessment in the functional area of peer relations must take into account both the quality of peer relations and the conventionality/deviance of the specific peers (if any) with whom the adolescent associates.

Quality of Peer Relations

The Piers-Harris Children's Self-Concept Scale ("The Way I Feel about Myself") is a well researched and commonly employed measure that provides self-evaluation along a number of dimensions. Among these is a "popularity" dimension that captures, in a simple 12-item subscale, a measure of the adolescent's perception of his or her peer relations. Other subscales address general behavior, intellectual and school status, physical appearance and attributes, anxiety, and happiness and satisfaction.

Over the years the Piers-Harris has been used in a wide variety of clinical and research applications with a number of different populations. Reliability and validity assessments of the scale generally suggest that reliability is good and validity is acceptable.

The Piers-Harris total score was the norm in the early 1960s in a population of 1,183 4th–12th graders in a single Pennsylvania school district. The manual that accompanies the Piers-Harris suggest that these norms, therefore, be viewed with some caution. The cluster (subscale) scores were norm on a sample of 485 public school children whose total scores differed somewhat from those of the original normative sample. These results again dictate caution in the interpretation of the Piers-Harris using the norms provided.

Deviance of the Peer Group

The Revised Problem Behavior Checklist provides, among other measures, an assessment of the deviance orientation of an adolescent's peer group. The Checklist is designed to be completed by a parent, teacher, child care worker, correctional officer, or other adult who knows the adolescent well. Eighty-five behaviors are rated as "not a problem," a "mild problem," or a "severe problem." From these ratings, six subscales are derived.

The 17-item Socialized Aggression subscale relates specifically to the deviance of the adolescent's peer group and/or the people the adolescent admires. The remaining five subscales of the Revised Problem Behavior Checklist include Conduct Disorder, Attention Problems-Immaturity, Anxiety-Withdrawal, Psychotic Behavior, and Motor Excess.

The reliability and validity of the Revised Problem Behavior Checklist have been well established. A 1987 *Manual for the Revised Problem Behavior Checklist* includes a description of the development of the scales, data on reliability and validity, and data on teacher, parent, and staff ratings for various normal and clinical samples. Also included are tables to convert raw scores to T scales by sex and grade or age for both normal and seriously emotionally disturbed youth.

KEY REFERENCES

Hagbord, W.J. (1990). The Revised problem behavior checklist and severely emotionally disturbed adolescents: Relationship to intelligence, academic achievement, and sociometric ratings. *Journal of Abnormal Child Psychology, 18,* 47–53.

Appendix

Morrison, D., Mantazicopoulos, P., & Carte, E. (1989). Pre-academic screening for learning and behavior problems. *Journal of the American Academy of Child and Adolescent Psychiatry, 28,* 101–106.

Piers, E.V. (1984). *Piers-Harris children's self-concept scale: Revised manual.* Los Angeles, CA: Western Psychological Services.

Rio, A.J., & Quay, H.C. (1989). Factor analytic study of a Spanish translation of the revised problem behavior checklist. *Journal of Clinical Child Psychology, 18,* 343–350.

FUNCTIONAL AREA VI: EDUCATIONAL STATUS

Tools:

Woodcock-Johnson Psycho-Educational Test Battery
Wechsler Intelligence Scale for Children-Revised (WISC-R)
Wechsler Adult Intelligence Scale-Revised (WAIS-R)

Administrative Time:

Woodcock-Johnson: approximately 2 hours
WISC-R: approximately 1 hour
WAIS-R: approximately 75 minutes

Source for Woodcock-Johnson:

DLM Teaching Resources
1 DLM Park, P.O. Box 4000
Allan, TX 78283-3954
(800) 228-0752

Cost:

Woodcock-Johnson: $445 ($525 with carrying case)

WAIS-R or WISC-R: $400 for the Complete Set. Includes all necessary equipment: Manual, 25 Record Forms, 25 Supplementary Record Forms, 25 Analysis Worksheets and Guides, and Mazes/Coding Booklet, with Attaché (Case).

Translations:

Woodcock-Johnson: English only

WAIS-R and WISC-R: Spanish (WISC-R adapted for use with hearing impaired.)

The coexistence of substance abuse and a pattern of learning disabilities is sufficiently common that a focus on assessing specific learning disabilities will be an important component of treatment planning for many adolescents. No single assessment of learning disabilities currently exists. Rather a diagnosis of learning disabilities is derived from a comparison between *ability* and *performance*.

The Woodcock-Johnson Psycho-Educational Test Battery and the Wechsler intelligence scales provide state-of-the-art measurement of ability and performance respectively. Comparison of an adolescent's scores on these two assessments will indicate the need for specialized educational services as part of the overall treatment plan. Deriving a diagnosis of learning disabilities from the Woodcock-Johnson and Wechsler tests generally requires assessment by a psychologist.

The Woodcock-Johnson Psycho-Educational Test Battery is designed to measure cognitive abilities, scholastic aptitude, academic achievement, and interest in a diversity of subjects such as reading, mathematics, writing, social studies, science, and physical activities. The Battery, which contains 27 subtests, can be used to identify weaknesses in different educational areas that might require remedial help. Whereas trained, experienced psychologists or educational diagnosticians usually administer, score, and interpret the results of the complete Battery, the Achievement and Interest tests can be administered by special education teachers or trained laypersons.

The Wechsler Intelligence Scales for Children—Revised (WISC-R) is appropriate for individuals age 6–16 years; the Wechsler Adult Intelligence Scales—Revised (WAIS-R) is suitable for youth 16 years and over. Both instruments sample similar verbal and nonverbal performance behaviors that comprise Wechsler's construct of "intelligence." The verbal sub-tests include: a) factual knowledge, b) comprehension of specific customs and mores, c) vocabulary and abstract conceptualizations, d) performance of computational tasks, and e) auditory recall. The performance sub-tests include: a) visual discrimination, b) visual memory, c) sequencing, d) visual comprehension, e) identification of relationships, f) non-verbal abstract concept formation, g) spatial relationships, and h) freedom from distractibility.

KEY REFERENCES

Salvia, J., & Yesseldyke, J. W. (1988). *Assessment in special education,* (4th ed.), Boston, MA: Houghton Mifflin Co.

FUNCTIONAL AREA VII: VOCATIONAL STATUS

Tools:

The Career Maturity Inventory (CMI) Attitude Scale, and Competence Test

The Generalizable Skills Assessments in Mathematics, Communications, Relations, and Reasoning (Performance Tests, Student Self-Ratings, Teacher Ratings)

Administration Time for CMI:

Attitude Scale: 30–40 minutes

Competence Test: Approximately 2 hours

Administration Time for Generalizable Skills Curriculum:

Performance Tests: 2½ hours

Student Self-Ratings: 10–20 minutes each

Teacher Ratings: 10–20 minutes each

Source for CMI:

MacMillan/McGraw-Hill Publishers Test Service
2500 Garden Road
Monterey, CA 93940
(800) 538-9547

Source for Generalizable Skills Curriculum:

Cirriculum Publications Clearinghouse
Western Illinois University
Horrabin Hall 46
Macomb, IL 61455
(800) 322-3905 (toll-free in Illiois)
(309) 298-1917 (outside Illinois)

Cost:

CMI: $14.60 for a Specimen Set including: Test Booklets, Administration and Users' Manual, Theory and Research Handbook, CompuScan Answer Sheet, Career Maturity Profile, and Test Reviewer's Guide. Individual test booklets. Attitude Scale: $46.90/35, Competence Test: $77.35/35. Answer Sheets, CompuScan: $11.50/50, Hand Scorable: $19.50/50.

Generalizable Interpersonal Relations Skills Assessment User Manual: $13.50; Generalizable Reasoning Skills Assessment User Manual: $13.50. Other User Manuals and Resource Directories available. Consult publisher.

Translations:

CMI: English only

Generalizable Skills Curriculum: English only

For many adolescents, entrance into the work force is the next step after high school. Moreover, for all adolescents, the motivation to seek work and earn money reflects an inclination to assume adult roles and strive for autonomy. The choice of and preparation for an occupation are major developmental milestones. Accordingly, adolescents lacking the skills to accomplish these milestones will require special considerations in treatment planning.

Two major approaches to the functional area of vocational status may be identified. The first stresses the skills required to successfully engage in the process of career choice. The second stresses the specific skills needed to successfully pursue a chosen occupation. The CAB offers two assessments, one focused on the process of career choice and the other focused on vocational skills.

The Process of Career Choice

The Career Maturity Inventory is designed to measure the maturity of attitudes and competencies necessary for realistic career decision making. The CMI consists of two parts: an Attitude Scale and a Competency Test.

The Attitude Scale measures five variables: 1) decisiveness in career decision making, 2) involvement in career decision making, 3) independence in career decision making, 4) orientation to career decision making, and 5) compromise in career decision making. Two versions of the Attitude Scale, a 50-item screening version and a 75-item counseling version, are available. The 100-item Competence Test measures 5 career choice competencies: 1) knowing yourself (self-appraisal), 2) knowing about jobs (occupational information), 3) choosing a job (goal selection), 4) looking ahead (planning), and 5) what should they do? (problem solving).

There exists almost two decades' research on the CMI. Reliability and validity have been extensively studied, and standard scores and percentile ranks have been established. The CMI has been used to study career development, screen for career immaturity, assess guidance needs, and evaluate career education.

Vocational Skills

The Generalizable Skills Curriculum protocol is a comprehensive method for evaluating adolescents employing self-ratings, teacher ratings, and direct performance measurement. The broad range of abilities measured include mathematics, communication, interpersonal relations, and reasoning. Over 70 types of vocational categories are identified to which the adolescent's abilities can best be matched.

The scales of the Generalized Skills curriculum assessments have been demonstrated to have high internal consistency and reliability. However, the self-ratings and teacher ratings demonstrate only a low-to-moderate correlation with the performance measures. It is probable that these low correlations reflect the fact that the self-ratings and teacher ratings are affected by psychological variables such as student self-esteem or self-concept.

KEY REFERENCES

Crites, J. O. (1974). The career maturity inventory. In D. E. Super (Ed.). *Measuring vocational maturity in counseling and evaluation.* Washington, D.C.: National Vocational Guidance Association.

Module I.6

Crites, J. O. (1978). *The career maturity inventory: Theory and research handbook,* (2nd ed.). Monterey, CA: McGraw-Hill.

Greenan, J. (1986). Curriculum and assessment in generalizable skills instruction. *The Journal for Special Needs Education, 9,* 3–10.

Greenan, J. (1983). Identification and validation of generalizable skills in vocational programs. *The Journal for Vocational Educational Research, 8,* 46–71.

Appendix

FUNCTIONAL AREA VIII: SOCIAL SKILLS

Tools:

Social Skills Rating System, Secondary Level (SSRS)

Student Form, Teacher Form, Parent Form.

Matson Evaluation of Social Skills with Youngsters (MESSY)

Administration Time:

SSRS: 10–25 minutes for Student, Parent and Teacher Forms

MESSY: 15 minutes

Source for SSRS:

American Guidance Service
Publishers' Building
P.O. Box 99
Circle Pines, MN 55014-1796
(800) 328-2560 (Outside Minnesota)
(800) 247-5053 (Inside Minnesota)

Source for MESSY:

International Diagnostic Systems
15127 South 73rd Avenue, Suite H-2
Orland Park, IL 60462
(800) 876-6360

Cost:

SSRS: $75.00 for a Secondary Level Starter Kit (includes 10 copies each of Teacher, Parent, and Student Questionnaires, 10 Assessment-Intervention Records, Manual, and storage folder).

MESSY: $80 for starter kit (Manual and 25 each of student forms, teacher forms, and hand score forms).

Translations:

SSRS: English only

MESSY: Spanish and German Available from the author.

John Matson, PhD
Department of Psychology
Louisiana State University
Baton Rouge, LA 70803

Adolescents who lack social skills are less able to form meaningful relationships with peers and significant adults. The resulting social isolation or rejection of such adolescents can lead to reduced probability of bonding to school, family, and other socializing institutions, increased susceptibility to negative influences, and increased anxiety, depression, and alienation. For these reasons, adolescents lacking social skills are believed to be at increased risk of alcohol and other drug problems and probably have poorer treatment prognoses. Social skills training and other remedial measures may, thus, form an important component of treatment planning.

The Social Skills Rating System (SSRS) is a paper-and-pencil checklist which provides student, parent, and teacher ratings of social skills in five areas: cooperation, assertion, responsibility, empathy, and self-control. In addition, a problem behavior scale derived from the Parent and Teacher Questionnaires provides assessments of externalizing problems, internalizing problems, and hyperactivity. Finally, an academic competence scale is available from the Teacher Questionnaire. Ratings of the perceived *importance* for successful functioning of each behavior addressed in the SSRS allow selection of specific behavioral targets for intervention and treatment planning.

The Secondary Level version of the SSRS is designed for grades 7–12; a preschool/ elementary version is also available.

The SSRS has been standardized on 4,000 children and youth aged 3–18 years. Separate norms are available for boys and girls on all versions of the SSRS, and for handicapped and non-handicapped students at the elementary level of the Teacher Form.

One problem that may arise with the SSRS concerns the fact that all items are worded in the positive format. This characteristic may introduce response biases, especially if data are derived only from adolescent self-reports (i.e., if parent and/or teacher ratings are not available). As an adjunct to the SSRS, clinicians may wish to gather additional information in the social skills functional area using the Matson Evaluation of Social Skills with Youngsters (MESSY). Although not as well researched as the SSRS, the MESSY includes items in both positive and negative formats, and may thus provide additional opportunities for adolescents to report negative social behaviors.

Factor analyses performed on MESSYs administered to children and to teachers revealed two factors common to both study populations: Appropriate Social Skills and Inappropriate Assertiveness. The analysis of the student data revealed three additional factors: Impulse/Recalcitrant, Overconfident, and Jealousy/Withdrawal.

KEY REFERENCES

Gresham, F. M. (1986). Conceptual and definitional issues in the assessment of children's social skills: Implications for classification and training. *Journal of Clinical Child Psychiatry, 15,* 16–25.

Elliot, S. N., & Gresham, F. M. (1987). Children's social skills: Assessment and classification practices. *Journal of Counseling and Development, 66,* 96–99.

Elliot, S. N., Gresham, F. M., Freeman, T., & McCloskey, G. (1988). Teachers and observers ratings of children's social skills. *Journal of Psycho-educational Assessment, 6,* 225–235.

Elliot, S. N., Sheridan, S. M., & Gresham, F. M. (1989). Assessing and treating social skills deficits: A case study for scientist-practitioners. *Journal of School Psychology, 27,* 197–222.

Matson, J. L., Rotatori, A. F., & Helsel, W. J. (1983). Development of a rating scale to measure social skills in children: The Matson evaluation of social skills with youngsters (MESSY). *Behavioral Research and Therapy, 21*(4), 335–340.

FUNCTIONAL AREA IX: LEISURE AND RECREATION

Tools:

Social Adjustment Inventory for Children and Adolescents (SAICA)

Leisure Diagnostic Battery, Physical Activity Assessment

Administration Time:

SAICA: 30 minutes

Leisure Diagnostic Battery:

Long form: 30–60 minutes

Short form: 15–45 minutes

Physical Activity Assessment: 15 minutes

Source for SAICA:

Venture Publishing, Inc.
1640 Oxford Circle
State College, PA 16803
(814) 234-4561

Source for Physical Activity Assessment:

The Physical Activity Assessment appears at the back of the Manual.

Cost:

SAICA: Free of charge with author's permission

Leisure Diagnostic Battery: Users Manual, $19.95; Long Form, $19.95 each; Short Form, 35 cents each

Physical Activity Assessment: May be copied from the Manual without permission.

Translation:

SAICA: English only

Leisure Diagnostic Battery: English only

Physical Activity Assessment: English only

The availability of leisure time and how it is used can greatly influence the adolescent's propensity to engage in drug taking as well as other non-normative and maladjusted behavior. The range of recreational activities available to adolescents is extensive and includes extracurricular activities at school, memberships in clubs, hobbies, and sports. It is also the case that engaging in strenuous physical activity can serve as a useful adjunct to alcohol and other drug treatment, and can assist in the maintenance of sobriety by providing a sense of accomplishment, mastery, and physical and mental well-being.

An assessment in the functional area of leisure and recreation should include two components: 1) an evaluation of use of leisure time, and 2) an assessment of participation in strenuous physical activity. If desired, a third component can be included to assess in more detail the nature of personal attitudes and experiences which have contributed to existing deficits in leisure and recreation.

Leisure Assessment

The Social Adjustment Inventory for Children and Adolescents (SAICA) assesses the types of activities engaged in and the intensity of involvement. The SAICA is a semi-structured interview that provides assessments of the use of leisure time in four areas: 1) Spare time activity, 2) Spare time TV watching, 3) Spare time alone/with others, and 4) Overall spare time functioning. The SAICA can be administered to either adolescents or their parents. It may be used to assess current functioning (defined as no more than one school year), and can be re-administered to cover previous school year. To shorten the assessment, summary items only may be used to assess adjustment in earlier grades. The SAICA also provides assessments of school functioning, peer relationships, and functioning at home.

A study of 124 children, ages 6–18, of parents with and without a history of major depression support the construct, convergent, and divergent validity of the SAICA. Normative data are not currently available on the SAICA.

Assessment of Participation in Strenuous Physical Activity

Most adolescents are capable of participating in strenuous physical activity without medical risk. Thus, unless otherwise indicated by medical history, cardiopulmonary testing or other assessments of physical fitness are generally not necessary in developing an exercise regimen for adolescents. However, an assessment of current level of physical activity provides a useful starting point for determining the overall level of conditioning, and for determining those areas of physical activity in which the adolescent shows (or has shown) interest.

A simple assessment of current physical activity may be derived from the Physical Activity Assessment provided at the end of the Manual. The assessment includes: 1) self-reports of level of involvement in a number of active physical pursuits, 2) an assessment of participation in organized team sports, 3) a general assessment of cardiovascular conditioning, and 4) an assessment of physical problem that may limit participation in physical activities.

Attitudes Towards Leisure

The Leisure Diagnostic Battery examines attitudes and attributions associated with leisure activities as a way of determining if these attitudes and attributions may contribute to deficits in the use of leisure time. The Leisure Diagnostic Battery is a self-administered paper-and-pencil test for use with children 9–18 years of age consisting of five scales: Perceived Leisure Competence, Perceived Leisure Control, Leisure Needs, Depth of Involvement in Leisure, and Playfulness. The combined scores from these scales yield a measure of Perceived Freedom in Leisure. There are 95 items in these scales. A short form is available to measure Perceived Freedom in Leisure consisting of 25 items. If deficits are identified in these five scales, an additional three scales may be administered: Barriers to Leisure Involvement, Leisure Preferences Inventory, and Knowledge of Leisure Opportunities.

The battery has been administered to a variety of handicapped and non-handicapped populations, and to substance abusing and non-substance abusing populations from junior high school students to college students. This testing supported the reliability, and convergent, predictive, and discriminant validity of the battery. Normative data from the various groups tested are available.

KEY REFERENCES

Ellis, G. & Witt, P. (1982). *The leisure diagnostic battery: Theoretical and empirical structure*. Denton, Texas: University of North Texas, Leisure Diagnostic Battery Project.

John, K., Gammon, G. D., Prushoff, B. A., & Warner, V. (1989). The social adjustment inventory for children and adolescents (SAICA): Testing of a new semi-structured interview. *Journal of the American Academy of Child and Adolescent Psychiatry, 26*(6), 89–1253.

National Center for Health Statistics (1989). Assessing physical fitness and physical activity in population-based surveys. *DHHS Publication Number (PHS)*, 89–125.

Module I.6

FUNCTIONAL AREA X: AGGRESSIVE BEHAVIOR/DELINQUENCY

Tools:

Youth Self-Report (YSR) of the Child Behavior Checklist (CBCL)
National Youth Survey (NYS) Delinquency Scale

Administration Time:

YSR: 15–20 minutes
NYS Delinquency Scale: 15–20

Source for YSR:

Thomas M. Achenbach
University Associates in Psychiatry
University of Vermont
1 So. Prospect Street
Burlington, VT
(802) 656-4563

Source for NYS Delinquency Scale:

The NYS Delinquency Scale appears at the end of the *Manual* and may
be copied without permission.

Cost:

YSR: Sample Packet–$15.00

Translations:

YSR: Afrikaans, Arabic, Cambodian, Chinese, Dutch, Finnish, French,
German, Greek, Hebrew, Hindi, Hungarian, Icelandic, Italian,
Japanese, Korean, Norwegian, Portuguese, Russian, Spanish, Swedish,
Thai, Turkish, and Vietnamese

NYS Delinquency Scale: English only

Aggressive, acting-out behavior has been observed to be both a precursor to and consequence of alcohol and other drug involvement in some youth. Moreover, substance use/abuse appears to be prevalent among adolescents who contact the juvenile justice system, suggesting a strong correlation between alcohol and drug involvement and delinquency. Finally, the economic demands of an addict lifestyle may involve some substance-abusing adolescents in serious crime. Treatment programs who admit youth of aggressive or delinquent tendencies may need to make special arrangements for their supervision and care.

The Child Behavior Checklist (CBCL) quantifies behavioral disturbance across a variety of behavioral dimensions. The version of the CBCL applicable to the widest age range of adolescents is the Youth Self-Report (YSR), a paper-and-pencil instrument designed for adolescents 11–18 years of age. The YSR measures aggressive behaviors, delinquent activities, and self-destructive behavior. In addition, it measures social competency (social and

508

job-related/recreational activities), depression, social unpopularity, somatic complaints, and disordered thoughts.

Other CBCL forms have been developed and standardized for use by parents and by teachers. The use of the parent and teacher forms allows comparisons of the adolescent's viewpoint with the views of significant adults, thereby adding to the comprehensiveness of the assessment. Moreover, the use of essentially equivalent forms for teachers and parents enables detection of problem behaviors that may be situationally specific to school or home.

The CBCL does not provide a direct assessment of all the specific delinquent acts that an adolescent may have committed. Such an assessment is available from the National Youth Survey Delinquency Scale.

Conducted in 1977, the National Youth Survey (NYS) interviewed 1,726 adolescents who were representative of the U.S. population aged 11–17. The NYS Delinquency Scale as modified by researchers at the University of South Florida Department of Criminology asks the frequency of 23 delinquent acts and the age at which these acts were first committed. Five summated indices may be calculated for the scale: 1) General Theft, 2) Crimes Against Persons, 3) Index Offenses, 4) Drug Sales, and 5) Total Delinquency.

KEY REFERENCES

Achenbach, T. M., & Edelbrock, C. (1978). The classification of child psychopathology: A review and analyses of empirical efforts. *Psychological Bulletin, 85,* 1275–1301.

Achenbach, T. M., & Edelbrock, C. (1978). *Manual for the youth self-report and profile.* Burlington, VT.

Edelbrock, C., & Achenbach, T.M. (1980). A typology of child behavior profile patterns: Distribution and correlates for disturbed correlates for disturbed children age 6 to 16. *Journal of Abnormal Child Psychology, 8,* 441–470.

PROBLEM ORIENTED SCREENING INSTRUMENT FOR TEENAGERS (POSIT)

INSTRUCTIONS

The purpose of these questions is to help us choose the best ways to help you. So, please try to answer the questions honestly.

Please answer *all* of the questions. If a question does not fit you exactly, pick the answer that is *mostly* true.

You may see the same or similar questions more than once. Please just answer each question as it comes up.

Please put an "X" through your answer.

If you do not understand a word, please ask for help.

You may begin.

QUESTIONS

1.	Do you have so much energy you don't know what to do with it?	Yes	No
2.	Do you brag?	Yes	No
3.	Do you get into trouble because you use drugs or alcohol at school?	Yes	No
4.	Do your friends get bored at parties when there is no alcohol served?	Yes	No
5.	Is it hard for you to ask for help from others?	Yes	No
6.	Has there been adult supervision at the parties you have gone to recently?	Yes	No
7.	Do your parents or guardians argue a lot?	Yes	No
8.	Do you usually think about how your actions will affect others?	Yes	No
9.	Have you recently either lost or gained more than 10 pounds?	Yes	No
10.	Have you ever had sex with someone who shot up drugs?	Yes	No
11.	Do you often feel tired?	Yes	No
12.	Have you had trouble with stomach pain or nausea?	Yes	No
13.	Do you get easily frightened?	Yes	No
14.	Have any of your best friends dated regularly during the past year?	Yes	No
15.	Have you dated regularly in the past year?	Yes	No

16. Do you have a skill, craft, trade or work experience?   Yes   No

17. Are most of your friends older than you are?   Yes   No

18. Do you have less energy than you think you should?   Yes   No

19. Do you get frustrated easily?   Yes   No

20. Do you threaten to hurt people?   Yes   No

21. Do you feel alone most of the time?   Yes   No

22. Do you sleep either too much or too little?   Yes   No

23. Do you swear or use dirty language?   Yes   No

24. Are you a good listener?   Yes   No

25. Do your parents or guardians approve of your friends?   Yes   No

26. Have you lied to anyone in the past week?   Yes   No

27. Do your parents or guardians refuse to talk with you when they are mad at you?   Yes   No

28. Do you rush into things without thinking about what could happen?   Yes   No

29. Did you have a paying job last summer?   Yes   No

30. Is your free time spent just hanging out with friends?   Yes   No

31. Have you accidentally hurt yourself or someone else while high on alcohol or drugs?   Yes   No

32. Have you had any accidents or injuries that still bother you?   Yes   No

33. Are you a good speller?   Yes   No

34. Do you have friends who damage or destroy things on purpose?   Yes   No

35. Have the whites of your eyes ever turned yellow?   Yes   No

36. Do your parents or guardians usually know where you are and what you are doing?   Yes   No

37. Do you miss out on activities because you spend too much money on drugs or alcohol?   Yes   No

38. Do people pick on you because of the way you look?   Yes   No

39. Do you know how to get a job if you want one?   Yes   No

40. Do your parents or guardians and you do lots of things together?   Yes   No

41. Do you get A's and B's in some classes and fail others?   Yes   No

42. Do you feel nervous most of the time?   Yes   No

43. Have you stolen things?   Yes   No

44. Have you ever been told you are hyperactive?   Yes   No

45. Do you ever feel you are addicted to alcohol or drugs?   Yes   No

46. Are you a good reader?   Yes   No

47. Do you have a hobby you are really interested in?	Yes	No
48. Do you plan to get a diploma (or already have one)?	Yes	No
49. Have you been frequently absent or late for work?	Yes	No
50. Do you feel people are against you?	Yes	No
51. Do you participate in team sports which have regular practices?	Yes	No
52. Have you ever read a book cover to cover for your own enjoyment?	Yes	No
53. Do you have chores that you must regularly do at home?	Yes	No
54. Do your friends bring drugs to parties?	Yes	No
55. Do you get into fights a lot?	Yes	No
56. Do you have a hot temper?	Yes	No
57. Do your parents or guardians pay attention when you talk with them?	Yes	No
58. Have you started using more and more drugs or alcohol to get the effect you want?	Yes	No
59. Do your parents or guardians have rules about what you can and cannot do?	Yes	No
60. Do people tell you that you are careless?	Yes	No
61. Are you stubborn?	Yes	No
62. Do any of your best friends go out on school nights without permission from their parents or guardians?	Yes	No
63. Have you ever had or do you now have a job?	Yes	No
64. Do you have trouble getting your mind off things?	Yes	No
65. Have you ever threatened anyone with a weapon?	Yes	No
66. Do you have a way to get to a job?	Yes	No
67. Do you ever leave a party because there is no alcohol or drugs?	Yes	No
68. Do your parents or guardians know what you really think or feel?	Yes	No
69. Do you often act on the spur of the moment?	Yes	No
70. Do you usually exercise for a half hour or more at least once a week?	Yes	No
71. Do you have a constant desire for alcohol or drugs?	Yes	No
72. Is it easy to learn new things?	Yes	No
73. Do you have trouble with your breathing or with coughing?	Yes	No
74. Do people your own age like and respect you?	Yes	No
75. Does your mind wander a lot?	Yes	No
76. Do you hear things no one else around you hears?	Yes	No
77. Do you have trouble concentrating?	Yes	No

78. Do you have a valid driver's license? — Yes No
79. Have you ever had a paying job that lasted at least one month? — Yes No
80. Do you and your parents or guardians have frequent arguments which involve yelling and screaming? — Yes No
81. Have you had a car accident while high on alcohol or drugs? — Yes No
82. Do you forget things you did while drinking or using drugs? — Yes No
83. During the past month have you driven a car while you were drunk or high? — Yes No
84. Are you louder than other kids? — Yes No
85. Are most of your friends younger than you are? — Yes No
86. Have you ever intentionally damaged someone else's property? — Yes No
87. Have you ever stopped working at a job because you just didn't care? — Yes No
88. Do your parents or guardians like talking with you and being with you? — Yes No
89. Have you ever spent the night away from home when your parents didn't know where you were? — Yes No
90. Have any of your best friends participated in team sports which require regular practices? — Yes No
91. Are you suspicious of other people? — Yes No
92. Are you already too busy with school and other adult supervised activities to be interested in a job? — Yes No
93. Have you cut school at least 5 days in the past year? — Yes No
94. Are you usually pleased with how well you do in activities with your friends? — Yes No
95. Does alcohol or drug use cause your moods to change quickly—like from happy to sad or vice versa? — Yes No
96. Do you feel sad most of the time? — Yes No
97. Do you miss school or arrive late for school because of your alcohol or drug use? — Yes No
98. Is it important to you now to get or keep a satisfactory job? — Yes No
99. Do your family or friends ever tell you that you should cut down on your drinking or drug use? — Yes No
100. Do you have serious arguments with friends or family members because of your drinking or drug use? — Yes No
101. Do you tease others a lot? — Yes No
102. Do you have trouble sleeping? — Yes No
103. Do you have trouble with written work? — Yes No

104. Does your alcohol or drug use ever make you do something you would not normally do—like breaking rules, missing curfew, breaking the law or having sex with someone?   Yes   No

105. Do you feel you loose control and get into fights?   Yes   No

106. Have you ever been fired from a job?   Yes   No

107. During the past month, have you skipped school?   Yes   No

108. Do you have trouble getting along with any of your friends because of your alcohol or drug use?   Yes   No

109. Do you have a hard time following directions?   Yes   No

110. Are you good at talking your way out of trouble?   Yes   No

111. Do you have friends who have hit or threatened to hit someone without any real reason?   Yes   No

112. Do you ever feel you can't control your alcohol or drug use?   Yes   No

113. Do you have a good memory?   Yes   No

114. Do your parents or guardians have a pretty good idea of your interests?   Yes   No

115. Do your parents or guardians usually agree about how to handle you?   Yes   No

116. Do you have a hard time planning and organizing?   Yes   No

117. Do you have trouble with math?   Yes   No

118. Do your friends cut school a lot?   Yes   No

119. Do you worry a lot?   Yes   No

120. Do you find it difficult to complete class projects or work tasks?   Yes   No

121. Does school sometimes make you feel stupid?   Yes   No

122. Are you able to make friends easily in a new group?   Yes   No

123. Do you often feel like you want to cry?   Yes   No

124. Are you afraid to be around people?   Yes   No

125. Do you have friends who have stolen things?   Yes   No

126. Do you want to be a member of any organized group, team, or club?   Yes   No

127. Does one of your parents or guardians have a steady job?   Yes   No

128. Do you think it's a bad idea to trust other people?   Yes   No

129. Do you enjoy doing things with people your own age?   Yes   No

130. Do you feel you study longer than your classmates and still get poorer grades?   Yes   No

131. Have you ever failed a grade in school?   Yes   No

132. Do you go out for fun on school nights without your parents' or guardians' permission?   Yes   No

133. Is school hard for you? Yes No

134. Do you have an idea about the type of job or career that you want to have? Yes No

135. On a typical day, do you watch more than two hours of TV? Yes No

136. Are you restless and can't sit still? Yes No

137. Do you have trouble finding the right words to express what you are thinking? Yes No

138. Do you scream a lot? Yes No

139. Have you ever had sexual intercourse without using a condom? Yes No

POSIT SCORING SHEET—ENGLISH

Client Name _____ Age _____ Sex _____

Date of Posit Administration _____ Posit Scored by _____

Domain	1	2	3	4	5	6	7	8	Tally
A-Substance use/abuse (All items are red flags)									
B-Physical Health Status (Cut-off = 3 points)									
C-Mental Health Status (Cut-off = 4 points)									
D-Family Relationships (Cut-off = 4 points)									
E-Peer Relations (All items are red flags)									
F-Educational Status (Cut-off = 6 points)									
A-Substance use/abuse (All items are red flags)									
B-Physical Health Status (Cut-off = 3 points)									
G-Vocational Status (Cut-off = 5 points)									
H-Social Skills (Cut-off = 3 points)									
I-Leisure and Recreation (Cut-off = 5 points)									
J-Aggressive Behavior/Delinquency (Cut-off = 6 points)									
Scorer's Comments:									

CLIENT PERSONAL HISTORY QUESTIONNAIRE

ENGLISH VERSION

Client Personal History Questionnaire

Name: _____
          Last   First   Middle

Your Zip Code: _____

Age: _____   Birth Date: _____

Sex: _____ Male   Marital Status: Single   _____

_____ Female   Married   _____

                                           Divorced   _____

                                           Separated _____

Which of the following best describes you?

_____ Black

_____ White

_____ Hispanic/Chicano/Latino

_____ American Indian

_____ Asian

_____ Other

What language are you most comfortable reading? _____

What language are you most comfortable writing? _____

What language are your parents most comfortable speaking? _____

In which religion were you raised?

_____ Protestant

_____ Catholic

_____ Jewish

_____ None

_____ Other   Which? _____

Module I.6

How often do you attend religious services?

_____ Every week

_____ A few times a month

_____ About once a month

_____ A few times a year

_____ Rarely

_____ Never

With whom are you currently living?

_____ Both parents

_____ Mother only

_____ Father only

_____ Mother and stepfather

_____ Father and stepmother

_____ Other relatives

_____ Foster parents

_____ Friends

_____ Spouse

_____ Boyfriend/Girlfriend

_____ Other

_____ No one

In what type of place do you live?

_____ No regular place

_____ Rooming or boarding house

_____ Hotel

_____ Apartment

_____ Single family house

_____ Jail

_____ Institution or hospital

_____ Therapeutic community, halfway house, or similar place

_____ Shelter

How many times in the past year have you changed the people with whom you live?

_____ Once   _____ Twice   _____ Three times or more

Do you have any children?

1. No   2. Yes

Appendix

If Yes: Do they live with you?

1. No   2. Yes

Are you currently in school?

1. No   2. Yes

If Yes: What grade are you in? _____

What type of program (Check one)?

_____ Academic

_____ Vocational

_____ Commercial/Business

_____ Alternative

_____ Other   Which? _____

What is your grade average (Circle one)?

A   B   C   D   Fail

Do you currently have a job?

1. No   2. Yes

If Yes: Is it full or part time?

_____ Full

_____ Part

What kind of job? _____

Are you a member of a street gang?

1. No   2. Yes

How many times have you been to a doctor in the last twelve months?

_____ Never

_____ Once

_____ Twice

_____ 3–5 Times

_____ More Often

Have you been kept overnight in a hospital in the last 6 months?

1. No   2. Yes

If Yes: Why? _____

Are you currently taking any medications prescribed by your doctor?

1. No   2. Yes

If Yes: What medication(s) are you taking? _____

Module I.6

What does your father or male head of household do for a living? (Please do not list *where* he works but *what job* he does.)

_____

What does you mother or female head of household do for a living?

_____

Is your family receiving public assistance?

1. No   2. Yes

Have you been arrested or had any other trouble with the law in the past twelve months?

1. No   2. Yes

If Yes, what? _____

Has any member of your family or household family besides yourself ever had problems with alcohol abuse?

1. No   2. Yes

If Yes, has this person been in a treatment program? _____

Has any member of your family or household family besides yourself ever had problems with other drug use?

1. No   2. Yes

If Yes, has this person been in a treatment program? _____

Has any member of your family or household family besides yourself ever had involvement with the police or courts?

1. No   2. Yes

If Yes, have any of them been (Check all that apply):

_____ Arrested.

_____ Held in jail or detention.

_____ Convicted of a crime.

_____ Put on probation.

_____ Sent to a training school or prison.

Are you currently seeing a psychiatrist, psychologist, counselor, or social worker because you needed help with an emotional or behavioral problem?

1. No   2. Yes

Have you ever been in special education classes?

Below is a list of experiences or events. Put an "X" next to the items that have happened to you *within the past 12 months.*

1. _____ An important friend moved away.

2. _____ You changed schools.

3. _____ Your parents argued or fought with each other.

4. _____ One or both of your parents got married.

5. _____ Your parents got divorced or separated.

6. _____ There were serious money problems at home.

7. _____ A family member had a serious accident or illness that worried you.

8. _____ Someone in your family had a drinking or drug problem.

9. _____ You started earning your own money.

10. _____ You feared that someone might physically hurt you.

11. _____ You feared that someone might make sexual advances towards you.

12. _____ A brother or sister was born or adopted by your family.

13. _____ You found a new group of friends.

14. _____ You broke up with someone you were dating on a regular basis.

15. _____ (for girls) You became pregnant or gave birth to a child or did not complete pregnancy.

16. _____ (for boys) Your girlfriend became pregnant.

17. _____ You moved to a new home or neighborhood.

18. _____ You got poor grades in school.

19. _____ You had problems at work or school.

20. _____ You had a serious accident or illness.

21. _____ You started dating regularly.

22. _____ You had sex for the first time.

23. _____ You got in trouble with the law.

24. _____ You were expelled or suspended from school.

25. _____ You gained a lot of weight.

26. _____ You had a sexual experience with someone of your own sex.

27. _____ A close friend died.

28. _____ You thought about hurting or killing yourself.

29. _____ You had trouble with a brother or sister.

30. _____ Your mother or father lost a job.

31. _____ A brother or sister moved out.

32. _____ You had trouble with a school teacher.

33. _____ Someone in your family died.

34. _____ You were bothered by a lack of affection and kindness toward you by one or both of your parents.

Module I.6

35. _____ You were placed in a new living situation, for example, in a foster home, residential setting, or institution.

36. _____ A close friend became seriously ill or had serious medical problems.

37. _____ You stole something valuable.

38. _____ One or both of your parents changed jobs.

39. _____ You ran away from home.

40. _____ You have been a victim of a crime.

INSTRUMENTO PARA LA EVALUACION DE PROBLEMAS PROPIOS DE LA ADOLESCENCIA

INSTRUCCIONES

El propósito de estas preguntas es ayudarnos a nosotros a escoger la forma en que mejor podemos ayudarte a ti. Por consiguiente, trata de contestar las preguntas con franqueza.

Contesta *todas* las preguntas. Si alguna de ellas no se aplica exactamente a ti, escoge la contestación que *más* se acerque a la verdad en tu caso.

Es posible que encuentres la misma pregunta, o preguntas semejantes, más de una vez. Contéstalas cada vez que aparezcan en el cuestionario.

Por favor, ponga una "X" sobre su repuesta.

Si no comprendes alguna palabra, pide ayuda.

Puedes comenzar.

QUESTIONS

1. ¿Tienes tanta energia que no sabes qué hacer con ella?   Sí No

2. ¿Eres jactancioso(a)?   Sí No

3. ¿Te encuentras a veces en dificultades porque consumes drogas o bebidas alcohólicas en la escuela?   Sí No

4. ¿Se aburren tus amigos en las fiestas donde no se sirven bebidas alcohólicas?   Sí No

5. ¿Se te hace dificil pedir ayuda a otra persona?   Sí No

6. ¿Han estado supervisadas por adultos las fiestas a que has asistido recientemente?   Sí No

7. ¿Argumentan demasiado tus padres o guardianes?   Sí No

8. ¿Reflexionas a menudo sobre las consecuencias que tienen tus actos para los demás?   Sí No

9. ¿Has adelgazado o engordado más de 5 kilos recientemente?   Sí No

10. ¿Has tenido alguna vez relaciones sexuales con alguien que se inyecta drogas?   Sí No

11. ¿Te cansas con frecuencia?   Sí No

12. ¿Has tenido trastornos de salud que te ocasionen dolores de estómago o náuseas?   Sí No

Module I.6

13. ¿Te asustas con facilidad? Sí No
14. ¿Hay entre tus amigos intimos parejas que salían juntas regularmente el año pasado? Sí No
15. ¿Saliste tu regularmente con un muchacho o una muchacha del sexo opuesto el año pasado? Sí No
16. ¿Tienes alguna destreza, artesania, oficio o experiencia de trabajo? Sí No
17. ¿Son la mayoría de tus amigos mayores que tu? Sí No
18. ¿Tienes menos energia que la que crees que deberias tener? Sí No
19. ¿Te sientes frustrado(a) con facilidad? Sí No
20. ¿Amenazas a otros con hacerles daño? Sí No
21. ¿Te sientes solo(a) la mayor parte del tiempo? Sí No
22. ¿Duermes demasiado, o muy poco? Sí No
23. ¿Dices groserías o vulgaridades? Sí No
24. ¿Escuchas cuidadosamente cuando alguien te habla? Sí No
25. ¿Son tus amigos del agrado de tus padres o guardianes? Sí No
26. ¿Le mentiste a alguien la semaña pasada? Sí No
27. ¿Si niegan tus padres o guardianes a hablarte cuando se enfadan contigo? Sí No
28. ¿Actúas impulsivamente y sin pensar en las consecuencias que tendrán tus actos? Sí No
29. ¿Tuviste un empleo con sueldo el verano pasado? Sí No
30. ¿Pasas tus horas libres holgazaneando con tus amigos? Sí No
31. ¿Te has hecho daño o le has hecho daño a otra persona accidentalmente estando bajo el efecto del alcohol o de drogás? Sí No
32. ¿Has tenido algún accidente o sufrido alguna lesión cuyos efectos que te molestan todavía? Sí No
33. ¿Sabes escribir o de letrear bien? Sí No
34. ¿Tienes amigos que causan daño o destrucción intencionalmente? Sí No
35. ¿Si te ha puesto amarilla alguna vez la parte blanca de los ojos? Sí No
36. Generalmente, ¿Saben tus padres o guardianes dónde estás y lo que estás haciendo? Sí No
37. ¿Sueles perderte de actividades o acontecimientos porque has gastado demasiado dinero en drogas o bebidas alcohólicas? Sí No
38. ¿Te molesta cuando se ríen de ti la gente por tu apariencia personal? Sí No
39. Sabes cómo encontrar un empleo si lo deseas? Sí No
40. ¿Participas en muchas actividades en compañia de tus padres o guardianes? Sí No
41. ¿Obtienes buenas notas en algunas clases y fracasas en otras? Sí No

42. ¿Te sientes nervioso(a) la mayor parte del tiempo?   Sí No

43. ¿Has robado alguna vez?   Sí No

44. ¿Te han dicho alguna vez que eres hiperactivo(a)?   Sí No

45. ¿Sientes a veces que eres adicto(a) al alcohol o a las drogas?

46. ¿Sabes leer bien?   Sí No

47. ¿Tienes algún pasatiempo a afición que realmente te interesa?   Sí No

48. ¿Has estado ausente o has llegado tarde a tu trabajo? (o tienes ya uno)   Sí No

49. ¿Has estado ausente o llegado tarde a tu trabajo con frecuencia?   Sí No

50. ¿Sientes que la gente está en contra tuya?   Sí No

51. ¿Eres miembro de un equipo deportivo que practica regularmente?   Sí No

52. ¿Has leído alguna vez un libro de principio a fín por tu propío gusto que no debería leer por tareas escolares?   Sí No

53. ¿Tienes ciertas tareas que debes hacer regularmente en tu casa?   Sí No

54. ¿Llevan tus amigos drogas a las fiestas?   Sí No

55. ¿Peleas a o muchas veces?   Sí No

56. ¿Tienes mal genio?   Sí No

57. ¿Te prestan atención tus padres o guardianes cuando les hablas?   Sí No

58. ¿Has comenzado a consumir mayores cantidades de drogas o alcohol para obtener el efecto que deseas?   Sí No

59. ¿Han fijado tus padres o guardianes ciertas reglas en cuanto a lo que te está permitido o no te está permitido hacer?   Sí No

60. ¿Te dice la gente que eres descuidado(a)?   Sí No

61. ¿Eres testarudo(a)?   Sí No

62. ¿Tienes amigos intimos que salen en noches de semana sin el permiso de sus padres o guardianes?   Sí No

63. ¿Has tenido alguna vez o tienes actualmente un empleo?   Sí No

64. ¿Se te hace dificil quitarte ciertas cosas de la mente?   Sí No

65. ¿Has amenazado alguna vez a alguien con un arma?   Sí No

66. ¿Tienes algún medio de obtener empleo?   Sí No

67. ¿Te vas a veces de las fiestas porque no hay en ellas bebidas alcohólicas o drogas?   Sí No

68. ¿Saben tus padres o guardianes cómo realmente piensas o te sientes?   Sí No

69. ¿Actuas impulsivamente con frecuencia?   Sí No

70. Generalmente, ¿Haces ejercicio media hora o más por lo menos una vez por semaña?   Sí No

71. ¿Sientes un deseo constante de consumir bebidas alcohólicas o drogas?   Sí No

72. ¿Es fácil aprender cosas nuevas?　　　　　　　　　　　　　　Sí　No

73. ¿Síentes dificultad al respirar? ¿Toses?　　　　　　　　　　　Sí　No

74. ¿Te quieren y te respetan las personas de tu edad?　　　　　Sí　No

75. ¿Pierdes el hil o del pensamiento con mucha frecuencia?　　Sí　No

76. ¿Oyés cosas que nadie más oyé a tu alrededor?　　　　　　Sí　No

77. ¿Tienes dificultad en concentrar te en tus pensamientos?　　Sí　No

78. ¿Tienes una licencia de manejar válida?　　　　　　　　　　Sí　No

79. ¿Has tenido alguna vez un empleo con sueldo que hayas durado por lo menos un mes?　　　　　　　　　　　　　　　　　　　　Sí　No

80. ¿Discutes frecuentemente con tus padres o guardianes, levantando la voz y gritando?　　　　　　　　　　　　　　　　　　　　Sí　No

81. ¿Has tenido un accidente automovilístico estando bajo el efecto del alcohol o de edrogas?　　　　　　　　　　　　　　　　　　Sí　No

82. ¿Olvidas lo que haces cuando bebes o te endrogas?　　　　Sí　No

83. El mes pasado, ¿Manejaste un automóvil estando borracho(a) o endrogado(a)?　　　　　　　　　　　　　　　　　　　　Sí　No

84. ¿Levantas la voz más que los demás muchachos de tu edad?　Sí　No

85. ¿Son la mayoria de tus amigos más jóvenes que tu?　　　　Sí　No

86. ¿Has ocasionado daños a la propiedad ajena intencionalmente alguna vez?　Sí　No

87. ¿Has dejado un empleo sencillamente porque no te importaban las consecuencias de dejarlo?　　　　　　　　　　　　　　　　Sí　No

88. ¿Le gusta a tus padres o guardianes hablar y estar contigo?　Sí　No

89. ¿Has pasado alguna noche fuera de tu casa sin que tus padres o guardianes supieran dónde estabas?　　　　　　　　　　　　　　　Sí　No

90. ¿Tienes amigos intimos que han sido miembros de equipos deportivos que requieren prácticas regulares?　　　　　　　　　　　　　　Sí　No

91. ¿Desconfías de la gente?　　　　　　　　　　　　　　　　Sí　No

92. ¿Te consideras demasiado ocupado(a) con las actividades escolares y demás actividades supervisadas por adultos para interesarte en un empleo?　Sí　No

93. ¿Tuviste más de cinco ausencias no autorizadas de la escuela el año pasado?　Sí　No

94. ¿Te sientes generalmente satisfecho(a) de tu conducta cuando participas en actividades con tus amigos?　　　　　　　　　　　　　Sí　No

95. ¿Te ócasiona el uso del alcohol o de las drogas cambios repentinos de humor, como pasar de estar contento(a) a estar triste, o viceversa?　Sí　No

96. ¿Te sientes triste la mayor parte del tiempo?　　　　　　Sí　No

97. ¿Pierdes días de clase o llegas tarde a la escuela por haber consumido bebidas alcohólicas o drogas?　　　　　　　　　　　　　Sí　No

98. Actualmente, ¿Es importante para ti conseguir o conservar un empleo satisfactorio?   Sí   No

99. ¿Te han dicho alguna vez tus familiares o amigos que debes reducir el uso de bebidas alcohólicas o drogas?   Sí   No

100. ¿Discutes seriamente con tus amigos o familiares por el uso que haces de bebidas alcohólicas o drogas?   Sí   No

101. ¿Embromas mucho a tus amigos?   Sí   No

102. ¿Tienes dificultad en dormir?   Sí   No

103. ¿Tienes dificultad con trabajos escritos?   Sí   No

104. ¿Te inducen a veces las bebidas alcohólicas o las drogas a hacer algo que normalmente no harias, como a desobedecer alguna regla o ley, o la hora de llegar a casa, o a tener relaciones sexuales con alguien?   Sí   No

105. ¿Síentes que a veces pierdes control de ti mismo(a) y terminas peleando?   Sí   No

106. ¿Te han despedido alguna vez de un empleo?   Sí   No

107. ¿Faltaste a la escuela sin autorización el mes pasado?   Sí   No

108. ¿Tienes dificultad en tus relaciones con alguno de tus amigos debido a las bebidas alcohólicas o drogas que consumes?

109. ¿Tienes dificultad en seguir instrucciones?   Sí   No

110. ¿Sabes "hacer cuentos" para salir de apuros con facilidad?   Sí   No

111. ¿Tienes amigos que han golpeado o amenazado a alguien sin razon?   Sí   No

112. ¿Síentes a veces que no puedes controlar el deseo de consumir bebidas alcohólicas o drogas?   Sí   No

113. ¿Tienes buena memoria?   Sí   No

114. ¿Tienen tus padres o guardianes una idea relativamente buena de lo que te interesa?   Sí   No

115. Generalmente, ¿Estan tus padres o guardianes de acuerdo en cuanto a la forma en que te deben manejar a tí?   Sí   No

116. ¿Se te hace dificil hacer planes o organizar tus actividades?   Sí   No

117. ¿Tienes dificultad con las matemáticas?   Sí   No

118. ¿Faltan tus amigos a la escuela sin autorización con mucha frecuencia?   Sí   No

119. ¿Te preocupas mucho?   Sí   No

120. ¿Se te hace dificil terminar tus proyectors o tareas escolares?   Sí   No

121. ¿Te hace la escuela a veces sentirte estúpido(a)?   Sí   No

122. ¿Haces amistades con facilidad cuando te encuentras entre un groupo de gente nueva?   Sí   No

123. ¿Síentes deseos de llorar frecuentemente?   Sí   No

124. ¿Te da miedo estar con la gente?   Sí   No

Module I.6

125. ¿Tienes amigos que han robado?   Sí No

126. ¿Deseas ser miembro de un grupo, equipo o club organizado?   Sí No

127. ¿Tiene uno de tus padres o guardianes un empleo permanente?   Sí No

128. ¿Te parece mala idea confiar en otros?   Sí No

129. ¿Te gusta participar en actividades con personas de tu edad?

130. ¿Tienes la impresión de que a pesar de que estudias más que tus compañeros siempre sacas peores notas que ellos?   Sí No

131. ¿Has frascasado algun año en la escuela?   Sí No

132. ¿Sales a divertirte en noches de semana sin el permiso de tus padres o guardianes?   Sí No

133. ¿Es dificil la escuela para ti?   Sí No

134. ¿Tienes alguna idea del trabajo o la carrera que deseas?   Sí No

135. ¿En un dia tipicio, ves televisión más de dos horas?   Sí No

136. ¿Eres una persona nerviosa, de las que no pueden estar sentadas mucho tiempo?   Sí No

137. ¿Tienes dificultad en encontrar palabras apropriadas para expresar tus pensamientos?   Sí No

138. ¿Gritas mucho?   Sí No

139. ¿Has tenido relaciones sexuales sin usar un condon?   Sí No

CLIENT PERSONAL HISTORY QUESTIONNAIRE

SPANISH VERSION

Cuestionario De Información Personal

_____   _____   _____
Apellido Paterno   Primer Nombre   Segundo Nombre

Código Postal (Zip Code): _____ Edad: _____

Fecha de Nacimiento: _____/_____/_____
                      mes   dia   año

Sexo: _____ Masculino   Estado Civil o matrimonial: _____ Soltero

_____ Fememino   _____ Casado

                                                           _____ Divorciado

                                                           _____ Separado

¿Cúal de las siguientes razas es la que mejor te describe?

_____ Negro

_____ Blanco

_____ Hispano/Chicano/Latino

_____ Indio Americano

_____ Asiático

_____ Otra

¿Cúal lengua está ud. más confortable para leer? _____

¿Cúal lengua está ud. más confortable para escribir? _____

¿Cúal lengua usan sus padres más confortable de hablar? _____

¿En que religíon crecío ud?

_____ Protestante

_____ Católico

_____ Judío

Module I.6

_____ Ninguna

_____ Otra   ¿Cúal? _____

¿Cúantas veces va ud. a servicios religiosos?

_____ Cada semana

_____ Unos pocos veces cada mes

_____ Una vez cada mes

_____ Unos pocos veces cada año

_____ Rara vez

_____ Nunca

¿Con quién vive ud. actualmente?

_____ Con los dos padres

_____ Solo con la madre

_____ Solo con el padre

_____ Madre y padrasto

_____ Padre y madrasta

_____ Otros patientes/deudos

_____ Padres adoptivos

_____ Amigos

_____ Esposo (a)

_____ Novio/Novia

_____ Otro

_____ Ninguna

¿En qué clase de lugar vive vd?

_____ Sín dirreción fija

_____ Casa de huéspedes

_____ Hotél

_____ Apartamento

_____ Casa unifamiliar

_____ Cárcel

_____ Hospital o Institutión

_____ Comunidad terpéutica o lugar similar

_____ Refugio

¿Cúantas veces en el año pasado ha cambiado ud. las personas con quien vive?

_____ Una vez

_____ Dos veces

_____ Tres veces o más

¿Tiene ud. hijos?

No   Sí

(Sí la respuesta es sí:)

¿Viven con ud.?

No   Sí

¿Asiste ud. a las escuela actualmente?

No   Sí

(Sí la respuesta es sí) ¿En que grado ustás? _____

¿En que tipo de programa (escoge uno)?

_____ Académico

_____ Vocational

_____ Comercial/Negocios

_____ Alternativa

_____ Otra   ¿Cúal? _____

¿Cúal es su promedio de calificaciónes?

   A   B   C   D   Desaprobado

¿Tiene ud. trabajo actualmente?

No   Sí

(Sí la respuesta es sí:)

¿Su trabajo es a tiempo completo o parcial?

_____ Tiempo completo

_____ Tiempo parcial/Medio tiempo

¿Qué tipo de trabajo? _____

¿Es ud. miembro de una pandilla o (ganga)?

No   Sí

¿Cúantas veces ha visitado ud. al doctor en los últimos 12 meses?

_____ Nunca

_____ Una vez

_____ Dos veces

_____ 3–5 veces

_____ Más de 5 veces

¿Ha tenido que permanecer en el hospital toda la noche en los últimos 6 meses?

No   Sí

(Sí la respuesta es sí:)

¿Porque? _____

¿Está ud. tomando algún medicamento recetado por algún médico actualmente?

No   Sí

(Sí la respuesta es sí:)

¿Qué medicamentos has tomado, o está tomando?

_____

¿En que trabaja su padre?

(Por favor, no enscriba *en dónde*, sino *que trabajo realiza*)

_____

¿En que trabaja su madre?

(Por favor, no enscriba *en dónde*, sino *que trabajo realiza*)

_____

¿Está su familia viviendo con las asistencia pública?

No   Sí

¿Ha sído arrestado, o ha tenido problemas con la ley en los últimos 12 meses?

No   Sí

(Sí la repuesta es sí:) ¿Porque? _____

Además de ud, ¿Ha tenido un miembro de su familia problemas con el abuso de alcohol?

No   Sí

(Sí la repuesta es sí:)

¿Ha estado esta persona en una programa de tratemiento?

_____

Además de ud., ¿Ha tenido un miembro de su familia problema con el abuso de otras drogas?

No   Sí

(Sí la repuesta es sí:)

¿Ha estado esta persona en una programa de tratemiento?

_____

No   Sí

Además de ud., ¿Ha tenido un miembro de su familia problemas con la policia o tribunales?

No   Sí

(Sí la repuesta es sí:)

¿Ha estado un miembro de su familia:

(Ponga un "X")

_____ Arrestado

_____ Detenido en el cárcel o detención

_____ Declarado convicto de un crimen

_____ Puesto en un periodo de prueba

_____ Puesto en el cárcel

¿Está ud. actualmente viendo algún psiquiatra, psicólogo, consejero o trabajador social; porque necesita ayuda en un problema emocional o de comportamiento?

No   Sí

¿Ha estado en una clase de educación especial?

No   Sí

Aqui está una lista de experiencias o eventos. Ponga una "X" al lado de las experiencias que le han pasado a ud. *durante el año pasado.*

1. _____ Un amigo importante se ha mudado.

2. _____ Te cambiaste de escuela.

3. _____ Tus padres discuten o pelean uno con el otro.

4. _____ Uno o tus dos padres se han casado nuevamente.

5. _____ Tus padres se han separado o divorciado.

6. _____ Hay problemas serios de dinero en tu hogar.

7. _____ Un miembro de tu familia ha sufrido un accidente serio o una enfermedad que te procupa.

8. _____ Alguíen en tu familia tiene problemas con alcohol o drogas.

9. _____ Has comenzado a ganar tu propio dinero.

10. _____ Has sentido miedo porque alguíen pudiera hacerte algun daño fisico.

11. _____ Has sentido miedo porque alguíen posiblemente quiere tomar ventaja sexual sobre ti.

12. _____ Un hermano o hermana ha nacido o adoptado en tu familia.

13. _____ Has emcontrado un nuevo grupo de amigos.

14. _____ Has terminado con alguíen con quien venías saliendo en forma seria.

15. _____ (Para chicas) Has salido embarazada o has dado a luz a un bebe o no has completado tu embarazo.

16. _____ (Para chicos) Tu enamorada o novia ha salido embarazada.

17. _____ Te has mudado a un nuevo vecindario.

18. _____ Has obtenido bajas calificaciones en la escuela.

19. _____ Tienes problemas en el trabajo o en la escuela.

20. _____ Has tenido un accidente o enfermedad seria.

21. _____ Has comenzado a salir regularmente, con alguíen del sexo opuesto.

22. _____ Has tenido relaciones sexuales por primara vez.

23. _____ Has tenido problemas con la ley.

24. _____ Has sido suspendido o expulsado de la escuela.

25. _____ Has aumentado mucho de peso.

26. _____ Has tenido alguna experiencia sexual con alguíen de tu mismo sexo.

27. _____ Un(a) amigo(a) muy cercano (a) ha muerto.

28. _____ Has pensado en hacerte daño a ti mismo o suicidarte.

29. _____ Tienes problemas con un hermano(a).

30. _____ Tu madre o padre han perdido el trabejo.

31. _____ Un hermano o hermana se ha mudado de tu casa.

32. _____ Has tenido problemas con un(a) maestro de la escuela.

33. _____ Algún miembro de tu familia ha muerto.

34. _____ Te has sentido mal o molestado por falta de afecto y cariño de parte de uno o tus dos padres.

35. _____ Te has cambiado de lugar de vivienda últimamente, por ejemplo, a un asilo de niños, una nueva casa o una institucion benéfica.

36. _____ Un amigo muy cercano se ha enfermado seriamente o tenido problemas médicos serio.

37. _____ Has robado algo de valor.

38. _____ Uno o tus dos Padres han cambiado de trabajo.

39. _____ Te has ido de tu casa.

40. _____ Has sido una victima de un crimen.

MODULE I.7
PREVENTION OF DRUG AND
ALCOHOL PROBLEMS IN THE
SCHOOL-AGE CHILD

Jeremy Leeds, PhD
Janet S. D'Arcangelo, MA, RN, C

Madeline A. Naegle, PhD, RN, FAAN
Project Director
Janet S. D'Arcangelo, MA, RN, C
Project Coordinator

Project SAEN
SUBSTANCE ABUSE
EDUCATION IN NURSING

CONTENT OUTLINE

I. Introduction to Prevention
   A. Definitions of Prevention
   B. Perspectives
   C. Prevention Intervention
   D. Integration of Concepts of Prevention, Addiction, and Nursing

II. Patterns of Drug Use in School-Age Children
   A. Issues Affecting Data about Drug Use in This Population
   B. Patterns of Use
   C. Prevention Intervention
   D. Integration of Concepts of Prevention, Addiction, and Nursing

III. Familial and Social Contexts Which Influence Drug Use in School-Age Children
   A. Prevention in Social Context
   B. Etiology of Youth Drug Abuse

IV. Nursing Assessment of the School-Age Child
   A. Prevention Issues and Values
   B. Developmental Issues

V. Prevention Activities Utilized with School-Age Children
   A. Goals
   B. Kinds of Prevention Programs
   C. Family Interventions

VI. Identifying Substance Abuse Problems in the Child
   A. Spectrum of Risk Factors
   B. Signs and Symptoms in Context
   C. Referrals

CONTENTS

I. INTRODUCTION TO PREVENTION

A. Definitions of Prevention

1. Primary: Activities to prevent the occurrence of a disease.

2. Secondary: Early detection of and intervention in a problem.

3. Tertiary: Attempts to minimize the long-term effects of the disease.

4. Definition of prevention as a concept.

    a. Prevention is a proactive process utilizing an interdisciplinary approach designed to empower people with their resources to constructively confront stressful life situations (National Institute on Drug Abuse, 1980).

    This module will focus mainly on primary and secondary prevention.

B. Perspectives

1. Prevention is a *proactive* stance.

2. "The prevention of drug problems is nothing less than the promotion of healthy, competent and informed children with positive attitudes and well-developed life skills. The challenge is to *empower* children (Schwebel, 1989).

C. Prevention Intervention

1. Prevention interventions for alcohol and other drug abuse are those actions which simultaneously alter and probabilistically direct human and environmental patterns toward constructive outcomes.

2. Rather than a discrete act, prevention intervention should be perceived as a process. Forestalling negative consequences and promoting positive consequences result in altered patterns.

3. Simultaneity is necessary in choosing prevention interventions. Both immediate and advanced moves are appropriate.

D. Integration of Concepts of Prevention, Addiction and Nursing

1. Prevention is a proactive process utilizing an interdisciplinary approach designed to empower people with their resources to constructively confront stressful life conditions.

2. Key words.

    a. *Proactive:* Commitment to awareness of the problem; commitment to nursing principles, actual and potential health problems; countermove to the denial inherent in the addictive process.

    b. *Process:* A dynamic mechanism characterized by interrelated goals, prevention of current and future problems simultaneously, and ongoing outcomes.

    c. *Interdisciplinary:* Refers to diverse practice settings, multidimensional components of addictions.

    d. *Empowerment:* Informed choices made about actions which can effect change in behaviors, thinking and feelings.

    e. *Resources:* A database comprised of human components, environmental components, applicable knowledge and skills, diverse theory-based frameworks, extant and evolving.

    f. *Constructive confrontation:* A process initiating positive advance moves while simultaneously forestalling negative consequences.

    g. *Stressful life conditions:* Actual and potential health problems; addictions, specifically alcoholism and other drug abuse.

II. PATTERNS OF DRUG USE IN SCHOOL-AGE CHILDREN

A. Issues Affecting Data about Drug Use in This Population

1. This is well-studied, compared to available information on adolescent drinking and drug behavior. In any case, most information is skewed toward the middle class and dependent on self-report (*New York Times*, 1991).

2. When analyzing data on these issues, the researcher should consider.

    a. Age range.

    b. Limitations of self-report data.

    c. Difference between use and abuse.

    d. Possible skewing of data to one segment of the population.

3. Whatever the validity of the data, there are two important issues:

    a. Use of some substances does begin in school-age children.

        (1) A NIDA (1990) self-report survey of households on drug use shows 41% of 12- to 17-year-olds have used alcohol in the past month; 22.2% have smoked cigarettes; 11.3% have used marijuana.

        (2) National Council on Alcoholism figures show 50% of seventh graders have tried alcohol. The average age for first drink is 13 (Felsted, 1986).

        (3) In a study of two New England towns, initiation to alcohol use occurred prior to the middle school years. "By the time students reach sixth, seventh and eighth grades, a relatively high percentage of them have begun experimenting with alcohol and refusal rates are relatively low" (Grady et al., 1986).

        (4) In a study of Midwest suburban communities, the critical period for tobacco use occurred prior to sixth grade (Reid, Martinson & Weaver, 1987).

        (5) Use of "gateway" drugs (alcohol, cigarettes, marijuana, inhalants)— i.e., those drugs that *might* lead to more serious drug use—can begin

at early ages. Trend analyses of four surveys of high school use from 1977 to 1986 show that the largest increases in use since 1983 are in "gateway" drugs (Pascale & Sylvester, 1988).

b. As a result of these studies, there is ample evidence of specific prevention needs for school-age children.

(1) "Therefore the sixth grade may be an appropriate time to initiate a preventive intervention regarding smoking but may be already somewhat late regarding alcohol use" (Gersick, Grady & Snow, 1988, p. 66).

(2) Results from an urban Pennsylvania school district questionnaire showed that ". . . sixth-grade students were significantly more advanced than the fourth- or fifth-grade students, in terms of conformity to peer pressure and positive attitudes toward the use of drugs and alcohol" (Pisano & Rooney, 1988, p. 1).

c. Along with information on actual use, there are information and controversy about behavioral and other predispositions in school-age children to later problem drug use (see section III.B, below).

B. Patterns of Use

1. Definition of "patterns."

   a. Differentiation between use and abuse.

   b. There is controversy over whether all youthful drug use is abuse.

2. Beschner and Friedman (in Archambault, 1989) speak of two kinds of users:

   a. Experimental, situational or recreational.

   b. The user with serious personal problems.

3. Beschner and Friedman (in Archambault, 1989) found that 5% of 14- to 18-year-olds are in this second group.

4. "Many researchers in the field believe that occasional intoxication, if conducted in a protective environment, may be harmless" (Finn, 1986, p. 39).

5. "From an educational point of view, it is also important to recognize that trying a drug does not mean that the user automatically becomes dependent—a large minority, if not the majority, of those who try cannabis or tobacco discontinue use of these drugs" (Goodstadt, 1989, p. 199) (see Section III.B, below).

III. FAMILIAL AND SOCIAL CONTEXTS WHICH INFLUENCE DRUG USE IN SCHOOL-AGE CHILDREN

A. Prevention in Social Context

1. Drug use is actually a spectrum of problems, itself imbedded in a larger spectrum of problems.

   a. "Broader variables, such as socioeconomic status (SES), race, school environments and community resources, have rarely been considered of central interest by researchers involved in the field of drug abuse. These variables, however, can provide important information concerning the adolescent's risk for substance abuse" (Rhodes & Jason, 1988, p. 19).

2. The relationship between drugs and other problems may not be a one-way causal one; there may be interaction.

   a. The stressors that lead to substance abuse, perhaps more than the specific effects of a substance (e.g., marijuana), are the same that may lead to problems in school, among the peer group, or other contexts.

3. Thorough knowledge of the population for prevention is critical.

   a. There are many different drug problems and causes of drug problems in different settings. As one example, Grady et al. (1986) found different patterns of drug use in sixth to eighth graders for two different but comparable New England towns.

   b. There has not been enough attention paid to specific needs of specific populations, especially minority populations (Howard et al., 1988; Shaw, 1989).

4. Use has *adaptive* consequences; in other words, there are *reasons* why people use drugs. These adaptive consequences may be different for different groups and individuals (Lawson, 1989). It is important for prevention experts to assess the adaptive consequences in their target population.

B. Etiology of Youth Drug Abuse

1. There are numerous models of the predispositions and developmental processes by which drug use becomes a problem for a young individual.

2. One group speaks of *psychological and behavioral predispositions to drug use.*

   a. Jessor and Jessor (1980) posit a range of "problem behaviors" of which drug use is only a part: "drug use; drinking and problem drinking; sexual experience; activist protest; and general deviance, including lying, stealing and aggression" (p. 102). Whatever the validity of parts of this view, the conservative value orientation is clear.

   b. Brook, Gordon, Whiteman, and Cohen (1989) did an extensive study of white males.

      (1) Based on their findings, they posit that childhood personality factors are associated with adolescent personality factors, which in turn are associated with drug use.

      (2) This is a "mediational model," which encourages the parent and the professional to look at childhood behavior as a possible precursor to the adolescent behavior that leads to drug abuse.

      (3) "Unconventionality, such as deviant behavior, rebelliousness, lack of social conformity, and low law abidance, are associated with drug use" (p. 709).

3. One of the most important models of progression to problem drug use was developed by Kandel (1980). There are several key concepts in Kandel's model:

a. Lower (i.e., less "serious") drug use almost always precedes higher drug use, but progression is not automatic from one level to the next. Marijuana smokers do not automatically become heroin addicts, as the old "scare" movies depicted.

b. There are various combinations of predictor variables—parental influence, peer influence, adolescent involvement in various behaviors, and beliefs and values. These have different valances at each stage of drug behavior (Kandel, 1980).

c. "Participation in various deviant behaviors is most relevant in starting to use alcohol, least for illicit drugs. . . . By contrast, initiation into illicit drugs other than marijuana appears to be a conscious response to intrapsychic pressures of some sort or other" (Kandel, 1980, p. 126).

d. There are four progressive stages of drug use in Kandel's model:

   (1) Beer or wine.

   (2) Cigarettes or hard liquor.

   (3) Marijuana.

   (4) Other illicit drugs.

4. Rhodes and Jason (1988) have developed a "Social Coping Model" which, while it does not invalidate Kandel's or other individual predisposition models, puts drug use in a larger perspective.

   a. "The social stress model suggests that in addition to focusing on individual, family and peer variables, we need to examine the large-scale social, political and economic issues that may impact on substance use" (Rhodes & Jason, 1988, p. 18).

   b. "Children who (1) have not identified with parent figures and consequently have failed to incorporate their values and standards, (2) have failed to acquire the necessary skills to offset the pressures to use drugs and (3) have not had adequate educational and employment opportunities may be less certain of their own abilities and less equipped to cope with a variety of social stressors during adolescence" (Rhodes & Jason, 1988, p. 12).

5. In an important longitudinal study published recently, Shedler and Block (1990) followed, from age three on, a cohort of 101 eighteen-year-olds in the San Francisco Bay area.

   a. They found the children to be divided into three groups: non-users, abusers and experimenters. Shedler and Block (1990) reported that "it is difficult to escape the inference that experimenters are the psychologically healthiest subjects" (p. 625).

   b. They characterized the *frequent user* as "a troubled adolescent, an adolescent who is interpersonally alienated, emotionally withdrawn and manifestly unhappy, and who expresses his or her maladjustment through undercontrolled, overtly antisocial behavior" (Shedler & Block, 1990, p. 617).

(1) They found that such adolescents were also maladjusted as children. "As early as age 7, the frequent users show signs of the alienation, undercontrol and emotional distress that will characterize them at age 18" (Shedler & Block, 1990, p. 626).

c. The *abstainer* is "a relatively tense, overcontrolled, emotionally constricted individual who is somewhat socially isolated and lacking in interpersonal skills" (Shedler & Block, 1990, p. 618).

d. They found that mothers of both frequent users and abstainers "are perceived as relatively cold and unresponsive" (Shedler & Block, 1990, p. 621).

IV. NURSING ASSESSMENT OF THE SCHOOL-AGE CHILD

A. Prevention Issues and Values

1. One of the most important problems in substance abuse prevention efforts is: Prevention of what? The first task of the nurse is to clarify the policy of setting and his/her own values as to what is being prevented.

2. The overall goal is the prevention of diagnosable problems and family dysfunction. The prevention goals may be defined by:

   a. The treatment setting: Some settings by their nature are specifically designed for primary, secondary or tertiary prevention. The nurse must be informed of the policy of the setting, and must develop a perspective on the available supports and resources for intended goals. A reasonable amount of congruity must exist in order for the goals to be achievable.

   b. The nurse's own attitudes and values: The nurse's own knowledge base and experience are the foundation of attitudes and values. Skills and experience in self-awareness, self-reflection and evaluation of feedback are taught as basic affective education in generalist programs.

3. Professionals may disagree about prevention objectives (Moskowitz, 1983). This may be a function of the model of addiction which they espouse. For example, the "disease concept" recognizes abstinence as a goal.

4. The consensus among nursing professionals is expressed in the American Nurses' Association's *Standards of addiction nursing practice with selected diagnoses and criteria* (1988).

B. Developmental Issues

1. Young children need to hear the message that drugs are not for them, because adults know what is best. In addition, however, they need:
   a. Role models.
   b. To feel good about themselves.
   c. To know how to have fun.
   d. To know how to cope with stress without drugs (Schwebel, 1989).

2. In elementary school, children need a safe place to ask questions about drugs and alcohol. In junior high school, when the peer group takes on more

importance, children need information about effects of alcohol (and other drugs) and need to know peers will support non-use (cf. Milgram, 1990).

3. Growth and development norms for the school-age child.

    a. The ages of 6–12 are considered to define "school-age." The school-age child is in a period of highly active psychosocial, physical and emotional growth.

    b. Psychosocial issues.

        (1) 6 years—Egocentric; generally displays positive attitudes.

        (2) 7 years—Begins to internalize experiences; becomes more sensitive to criticism; more anxious to please and cooperate with peers.

        (3) 8 years—Becomes more curious and gregarious; same-sex peers predominate.

        (4) 9 years—Begins to refine behavior and develop self-confidence, responsibility.

        (5) 10 years—Peer-oriented; responsive to group norms; increased powers of reasoning.

        (6) 11–12 years—Becomes critical of authority, especially parents; displays moodiness, need for independence (Jones, Lepley, & Baker, 1984).

    c. Developmental tasks.

        (1) Activities reveal drive for exploration.

        (2) Characteristic behavior may be loud and energetic.

        (3) Slower physical growth than during pre-school.

        (4) Gross motor skills being refined; still ahead of fine motor skills.

        (5) A period of mastery over tasks, with the school setting predominating.

        (6) Erickson's period of industry vs. inferiority.

        (7) Piaget's period of concrete operational thought.

        (8) Freud's period of latency, development of superego.

        (9) Development of sense of moralism.

    d. Health needs.

        (1) Maintenance of adequate patterns of nutrition, sleep/rest to support the developmental needs of the age group.

        (2) Monitoring of developmental milestones in order to identify and intervene in a timely way.

        (3) Health promotion.

e. Risk factors.

   (1) Environmental factors.

      (a) Lead paints.

      (b) Asbestos.

      (c) Accidents, including accidental ingestion of substances.

      (d) Passive inhalation of pollutants, including cigarette smoke.

   (2) Economic factors.

      (a) Inappropriate responsibilities.

      (b) Inadequate financial resources for material needs.

      (c) Lack of transportation.

      (d) Lack of supervisory care.

      (e) Inadequate access to health care.

   (3) Social factors.

      (a) Divorce, single parent adoptions, and other alternative family configurations demand attention and innovative ways in relation to meeting the developmental, psychosocial, and health needs of the school-age child.

4. Growth and development norms for the pre-adolescent.

   a. The ages of 10–13 are considered to be the preadolescent period. Many developmental frameworks do not consider this a discrete stage.

   b. The psychosocial issues, developmental tasks and physical growth during the pre-adolescent years have very broad ranges that display components of both school-age and adolescent norms. These ranges are also characterized by frequent, unpredictable shifts within the same individual.

   c. There is an unevenness between males and females that is accentuated in the pre-adolescent period.

   d. The breadth and overlap which define this age group also present difficulty in establishing norms.

   e. Choosing a target for the focus of a prevention program for pre-adolescents is problematic under these circumstances.

      (1) A chronological framework may not be the most efficient method for pre-adolescents.

      (2) The school organization of community (for example, K–6/ 6–8/ 9–12) may be a helpful organizer of norms for a presentation.

      (3) Other frameworks may be drawn from cultural characteristics, geographic features, or social features of a given population and specific prevention content goals, such as smoking prevention.

V. PREVENTION ACTIVITIES UTILIZED WITH SCHOOL-AGE CHILDREN

A. Goals

1. Scope of the prevention program.

   a. *Is there a different goal for different substances?*

   b. *Is there a difference between use, misuse and abuse (see below)?*

   c. *What is the role of legality in decisions about use?*

   d. *Is the prevention goal a specific behavior, e.g., not driving drunk, or more broadly conceived?*

2. Values clarification.

   a. Goals will need to be geared first to the age of the target population. However, even when working with young children, where the message will be that drug use is always a problem, the role of values is crucial in presenting the rationale.

   b. What kind of person is the optimal "graduate" of the prevention program?

3. Interrelatedness of goals.

   a. With youth, consider two interrelated goals: prevention of current and future problems.

   b. Beauchamp (1980) advocates that teenage drinking and drug problems be considered in their own right, rather than as precursors to adult problems. These need not be mutually exclusive choices.

4. Advocacy.

   a. According to the Rand Corporation (Polich, Ellickson, Reuter & Kahan, 1984) and other sources, prevention is not given enough attention in federal substance abuse efforts. More attention and funding are directed toward enforcement and treatment.

   b. Is this the best use of funds? Why does prevention not have a greater place in policy and implementation?

B. Kinds of Prevention Programs

1. There are three general categories of prevention programs:

   a. Knowledge/attitudes.

   b. Values/decision-making.

   c. Social competency (Moskowitz, 1983).

2. There are problems with each and all of these program approaches. Increases in knowledge do not necessarily lead to changes in attitudes. In fact, there is some evidence that factual presentations sometimes increase propensity to substance use.

3. No substance abuse prevention program for school-age children has shown much efficacy: ". . . effective prevention has proven to be as elusive as effective treatment (and effective law enforcement)" (Abadinsky, 1989, p. 170).

4. Examples of well-known programs.

   a. "Here's Looking at You": In an evaluation of this program, it was found that information level was increased but there was little attitude change (Green & Kelley, 1989).

   b. "I'm Special": In a follow-up of this program for fourth graders, it was found that program recipients used less drugs in grades 5–7 than controls; by high school, the pattern was almost random (Kim, McLeod & Palmgren, 1989). (Note that use in this evaluation was defined as one use per month or more.)

5. The Rand Corporation (Polich et al., 1984) found that informational, or affective educational programs are not successful.

   a. Based on a smoking program for seventh and eighth graders, they found that what works best is inoculation against pro-smoking influences taught by peers.

   b. Other studies as well report this finding, that peer education is preferable.

   c. The Rand Corporation recommends programs targeted to specific drugs, not to substance abuse in general.

6. Kim, McLeod and Shantzis (1989) advocate early education, comprehensive programs, and "booster" components.

7. Goodstadt (1986) puts forward five principles for prevention programs:

   a. Programs should be targeted to specific subpopulations.

   b. Programs should have a sound theoretical basis.

   c. Programs should be explicit and realistic in their objectives.

   d. Programs which involve hypothesized intervention variables or processes should be evaluated with caution and skepticism.

   e. Programs should incorporate or be associated with as much evaluation research as is feasible.

C. Family Interventions

1. Opportunities for health professionals for primary and secondary prevention exist in various settings.

   a. Child health maintenance.

   b. Well-child care settings.

   c. School health.

   d. Community settings.

2. Parental guidance in connection with other parental interventions for primary care of children and families.

3. Referral to appropriate care providers may be an outcome of child and family assessment.

4. Family counseling.

VI. IDENTIFYING SUBSTANCE ABUSE PROBLEMS IN THE CHILD

A. Spectrum of Risk Factors

1. Given the perspective on substance abuse as a part of a spectrum of problems, the "risk factors" include any stress under which a child does not perceive adequate social support. "The list could be endless" (Archambault, 1989, p. 233).

B. Signs and Symptoms in Context

1. Schwebel (1989) gives a list of signs and symptoms that *could* indicate drug use or other problems:

   a. School.

      (1) Increased absenteeism and tardiness to classes.

      (2) Drop in grades.

      (3) Behavior problems in school.

      (4) Negative attitudes about school.

   b. Social life/friends.

      (1) Dropping out of old activities.

      (2) Dropping old friends and making new friends who are drug users.

      (3) Strange-sounding phone calls, with covert communication about drugs.

   c. Emotional life.

      (1) Basic mood changes: was outgoing, now withdrawn; was withdrawn, now outgoing; was relaxed, now fidgety.

      (2) Incidence of inexplicable mood changes: euphoria followed by tenseness and edginess.

      (3) Caring less about everything: school, sports, other activities.

   d. Family.

      (1) Very secretive (not to be confused with need for privacy).

      (2) Estrangement from family.

      (3) Less responsible at home.

      (4) More conflict at home.

   e. Physical effects.

      (1) Red eyes.

      (2) Deterioration in personal hygiene.

     (3) Weight loss.

     (4) Sleep disturbances.

     (5) Fatigue or hyperactivity.

C. Referrals

1. Most school districts will have in-house programs or referral networks for potential or actual substance abuse problems. Some of these operate as "Student Assistance Programs," based on an Employee Assistance Program model (Milgram, 1989).

2. Family involvement should be evaluated and sought, in most cases, when facing substance abuse problems in school-age children. Nurses must be aware of laws, professional ethics, and school procedures in deciding on the possible and optimal involvement of parents in such situations, and the possibility of problems within the family of greater scope.

3. The prevalence of depression and suicide in the school-age population suggests that signs of these problems, whether associated with substance use or not, should be comprehensively evaluated through psychiatric referral.

MODULE I.7
PREVENTION OF DRUG AND ALCOHOL PROBLEMS IN THE SCHOOL-AGE CHILD

INSTRUCTOR'S GUIDE

Jeremy Leeds, PhD
Janet S. D'Arcangelo, MA, RN, C

Madeline A. Naegle, PhD, RN, FAAN
Project Director
Janet S. D'Arcangelo, MA, RN, C
Project Coordinator

Project SAEN
SUBSTANCE ABUSE
EDUCATION IN NURSING

CONTENTS

Module I.7

MODULE DESCRIPTION

This module assists the student in understanding factors which influence drug and alcohol use by children. Identification of family and social contexts, peer influences which relate to the initiation of drug use, and recognition of "at risk" children are emphasized. Prevention activities with children and families are explored in relation to the nursing role. The use of community resources for referral and education are discussed.

TIME FRAME

2 hours

PLACEMENT

Nursing Care in Childhood, Pediatric Nursing, Family Development

LEARNER OBJECTIVES

Upon successful completion of this module, the learner will:

1. List street names and classes of drugs used by the school-age and pre-adolescent child.

2. Describe behaviors commonly associated with drug use by the school-age child.

3. List parental and peer influences associated with the initiation and continuation of drug use by the school-age child.

4. Identify components of the nursing health assessment which relate to the identification of drug use by the school-age child.

5. Identify factors which place the child at risk for substance abuse.

6. Describe nursing interventions which utilize parental guidance, community and school programs and resources in prevention and treatment activities.

7. Identify referrals to social and community agencies in the provision of health teaching to children and their families.

RECOMMENDED READINGS

FACULTY READINGS

Baumrind, D. (1987). Familial antecedents of adolescent drug use: A developmental perspective. In C. L. Jones & R. L. Battjes (Eds.), *Etiology of drug abuse: Implications for prevention* (pp. 13–44). Rockville, MD: National Institute on Drug Abuse.

Bonagura, J. A., Rhonehouse, M., & Bonagura, E. W. (1988). Effectiveness of four school health education projects upon substance use, self-esteem and adolescent stress. *Health Education Quarterly, 15*(1), 81–92.

Goodwin, D. W. (1977). Genetic and experiential antecedents of alcoholism: A prospective study. *Alcoholism: Clinical and Experimental Research, 1*(3), 259–265.

Hawkins, J. D., Lishner, D. M., & Catalano, R. F. (1987). Childhood predictors and the prevention of adolescent substance abuse. In C. L. Jones & R. L. Battjes (Eds.), *Etiology of drug abuse: Implications for prevention* (pp. 75–126). Rockville, MD: National Institute on Drug Abuse.

Lewis, C. E., & Lewis, M. (1984). Peer pressure and risk-taking behaviors in children. *American Journal of Public Health, 74*, 580–584.

STUDENT READINGS

Globetti, G. (1988). Alcohol education and minority youth. *Journal of Drug Issues, 18*, 115–129.

Hanson, D. J. (1980). Drug education: Does it work? In F. S. Scarpitti & S. K. Datesman (Eds.), *Drugs and youth culture* (pp. 251–282). Beverly Hills, CA: Sage.

Reid, L. D., Martinson, O. B., & Weaver, L. C. (1987). Factors associated with the drug use of fifth through eighth grade students. *Journal of Drug Education, 17*(2), 149–161.

Stuart, R. B. (1974, April). Teaching facts about drugs: Pushing or preventing? *Journal of Educational Psychology, 66*, 189–201.

Vejnoska, J. (1981). Parent action groups: A prevention resource. *Alcohol Health and Research World, 6*(4), 13–17.

RECOMMENDED AUDIOVISUAL
AND
OTHER RESOURCES

AUDIOVISUAL RESOURCES

1. A Story about Feelings

This is an effective and eye-catching film about alcoholism and other drug dependencies narrated by five- to eight-year-old children. Presented in cartoon form, the film helps children recognize the role that feelings play in their lives. They also learn that some people drink, smoke and use drugs in order to change their feelings. 10 minutes. Available from Johnson Institute and New York State Council on Alcoholism, Film Library, 155 Washington Avenue, Albany, New York 12210. Phone: (518) 432-8281 or 1-800-252-2557.

2. Alcohol . . . Drugs . . . And Kids

The earlier kids start drinking or using drugs, the greater the risk of addiction. Why do kids start? In this program four teenagers who started drinking or using drugs at an early age share their experiences. The film dramatizes their stories in flashback while the teens talk about why they started. They each reveal how alcohol or a drug came to control their lives. A counselor in a drug and alcohol rehabilitation unit of a hospital discusses peer pressure, self-esteem and the problems these kids have because of their addictions. She points out that they all had one thing in common—the belief that they'd never get into trouble drinking alcohol or taking drugs. The recovering teens stress that help is always available for problems young people may be facing—they need never turn to alcohol or drugs. 18 minutes. Available from AIMS Media, 6901 Woodley Avenue, Van Nuys, California 91406-4878. Phone: 1-800-267-2467 or (818) 785-4111. #8036, rental ($50) or purchase ($345).

3. Cincinnati Bones and the Treasure of Health

Explorer Cincinnati Bones discovers the ruins of a giant body machine and uncovers the devastating effects of drugs in this exciting journey through the human body, presented in live action with special effects. Long ago, an ancient tribe called the Hitecs lived in a beautiful city deep in the jungle. They were a strong, healthy people and they built many wonderful things. But when the Hitecs began taking drugs, their minds became clouded and their bodies were destroyed. As the tribe was dying, they built the body machine to warn future generations about the dangers of drugs. Cincinnati Bones faces great perils as he explores the damage done by different types of drugs to the heart, brain, lungs, stomach and eyes. He also views the harm done to muscles and bones. Barely surviving his exploration of the ruins, Cincinnati Bones carries the message of the Hitecs back to civilization: Staying away from drugs leads to the greatest treasure of all—a healthy body. 15 minutes. **Available from AIMS Media, 6901 Woodley Avenue, Van Nuys, California 91406-4878. Phone: 1-800-267-2467 or (818) 785-4111. #9987, rental ($30) or purchase ($295).**

4. **Dugout**

In this film designed for children ages 6–12, former major league pitcher Bo Belinsky befriends a group of Little Leaguers who have turned to beer and marijuana to lift their spirits after a sound defeat. Especially helpful for young boys involved in Little League or other team sports, the film makes young athletes aware of the temptations and the consequences of alcohol and drug use. It effectively shows how even though alcohol and drugs may help ease the disappointment of defeat, a real winner is one who can say no. 16 minutes. **Available from Hazelden Educational Materials, Pleasant Valley Road, P.O. Box 176, Center City, Minnesota 55012-1076. #8796H, purchase ($150).**

5. **Families and Chemical Dependency**

A slide show starring Mr. Learn About, the charming cartoon character who has led countless readers through the entertaining and educational titles in Hazelden's *Learn About* series. In this full-color slide presentation, Mr. Learn About visits the Smith family and learns about the effects of chemical dependency on families. Designed as a community awareness tool, the show contains information that may be used by businesses, schools, churches, and other community groups to prevent or deal with alcohol and other drug use problems. 15 minutes. **Available from Hazelden Educational Materials, Pleasant Valley Road, P.O. Box 176, Center City, Minnesota 55012-0176. #5800, purchase ($70).**

6. **How to Raise a Drug-Free Child**

Mary Tyler Moore narrates this serious documentary that presents information on the fact that all kinds of kids from all social, economic and ethnic backgrounds use drugs, most commonly under the pressure of peers. Many kinds of drugs such as cocaine, LSD, crack, tranquilizers and barbiturates are shown as well as the paraphernalia a child might use in imbibing them such as pipes, spoons and rolled up dollar bills. **Available from HBO TV, 1100 Avenue of the Americas, New York, New York 10036.**

7. **McGruff's Drug Alert**

McGruff the Crime Dog warns children about legal and illegal drugs. He explains that even medicines can be dangerous if they're prescribed for someone else. Since children understand that poison is dangerous, McGruff compares drugs to poison. But he cautions that, unlike poison, drugs have no warning labels. McGruff teaches children how to stand up to peer pressure and protect themselves from people who try to persuade them to take drugs. 13 minutes. Available from AIMS Media, 6901 Woodley Avenue, Van Nuys, California 91406-4878. Phone: 1-800-267-2467 or (818) 785-4111. #9913, rental ($50) or purchase ($260).

8. Say No to Drugs—It's Your Decision

Combining testimony from former drug users, professional counselors and leaders of drug abuse organizations, this film is a persuasive program sure to make viewers evaluate their attitudes towards drug use. Narrated by the New York Yankees outfielder Dave Winfield, this program covers a wide spectrum of issues dealing with drug use, but won't bury viewers in a mountain of laboratory statistics. Students will see drugs and their abuses from different angles— medically, sociologically and legally—thus better preparing them to say "no" and *know* that it's the right decision. The program doesn't focus on any one drug nor does it draw conclusions, making it well-suited for audiences in businesses, schools and industry. 17 minutes. Available from National Audiovisual Center, 8700 Edgeworth Drive, Capitol Heights, Maryland 20743.

OVERHEAD MASTERS

MODULE I.7 PREVENTION OF DRUG AND ALCOHOL PROBLEMS IN THE SCHOOL-AGE CHILD

1. Gateway Drugs

2. Marijuana as a Predictor of Cocaine Use

3. Etiology of Youth Drug Abuse—Models of Psychological and Behavioral Predispositions

4. Key Concepts of Rhodes and Jason's Social Coping Model

5. Key Concepts of Kandel's Model of Progression to Problem Drug Use

6. Issues for Nurses in Setting Goals for Prevention

7. Developmental Issues to be Considered in Prevention Planning

8. Growth and Development Norms for the School-Age Child: Age-Specific Psychosocial Issues and Developmental Tasks (8A, 8B)

9. Kinds of Prevention Programs/Principles of Prevention Programming

10. Signs and Symptoms in Context (10A, 10B)

Module I.7—Overhead #1

GATEWAY DRUGS

Definition

Those drugs that might lead to more serious drug use.

Common Gateway Drugs

Alcohol

Cigarettes

Marijuana

Inhalants

Prevalence of Gateway Drug Use among Adolescents

Ever Used, Ages 12–17

Alcohol	48.2%
Cigarettes	40.2%
Marijuana	14.8%
Inhalants	7.8%

From: National Institute on Drug Abuse. (1990). *National Household Survey on Drug Abuse: Population estimates, 1990* (DHHS Publication No. (ADM) 91-1732). Rockville, MD: National Institute on Drug Abuse.

Module I.7—Overhead #2

MARIJUANA AS A PREDICTOR OF COCAINE USE

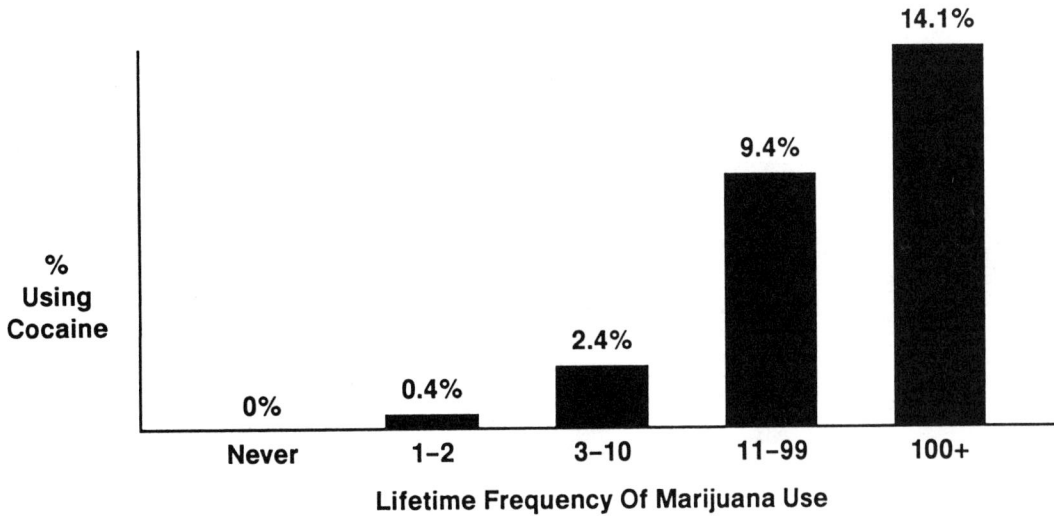

From: National Institute on Drug Abuse. (1990). *National Household Survey on Drug Abuse: Population estimates, 1990* (DHHS Publication No. (ADM) 91-1732). Rockville, MD: National Institute on Drug Abuse.

ETIOLOGY OF YOUTH DRUG ABUSE MODELS OF PSYCHOLOGICAL AND BEHAVIORAL PREDISPOSITIONS

1. *Problem Behavior:*

   An individual manifests a range of "problem behaviors," including "drug use, drinking and problem drinking, sexual experience, activist protest and general deviance, including lying, stealing and aggression" (Jessor & Jessor, 1980).

2. *Mediational Model:*

   Childhood behavior is a precursor to the adolescent behavior which leads to drug use; "unconventionality, such as deviant behavior, rebelliousness, lack of social conformity and low law abidance, are associated with drug use" (Brook, Gordon, Whiteman & Cohen, 1989).

3. *Social Coping Model:*

   In addition to focusing on individual, family and peer variables, large scale social, political and economic issues impact on substance use and need to be examined (Rhodes & Jason, 1988).

4. *Use Intensity:*

   Children may be divided into three groups: non-users, abusers and experimenters. It is inferred that "experimenters" are healthiest. Frequent users and abstainers manifest various indicators of maladjustment (Shedler & Block, 1990).

KEY CONCEPTS OF RHODES' AND JASON'S SOCIAL COPING MODEL (1988)

I. $$\frac{\text{Stress}}{\text{Attachments + Coping Skills + Resources}} = \text{Risk for Substance Abuse}$$

In a demonstration of this fractional equation, hypothetically quantify the components (1 = lowest risk):

Example A:

High Stress (Low = 0, High = 30) = 30

Few Attachments, Coping Skills and Resources
(Low = 0, High = 30) = 3

30/3 = 10 = Risk for Substance Abuse

Example B:

High Stress = 30

Adequate Attachments, Coping skills and Resources = 15

30/15 = 2 = Risk for Substance Abuse

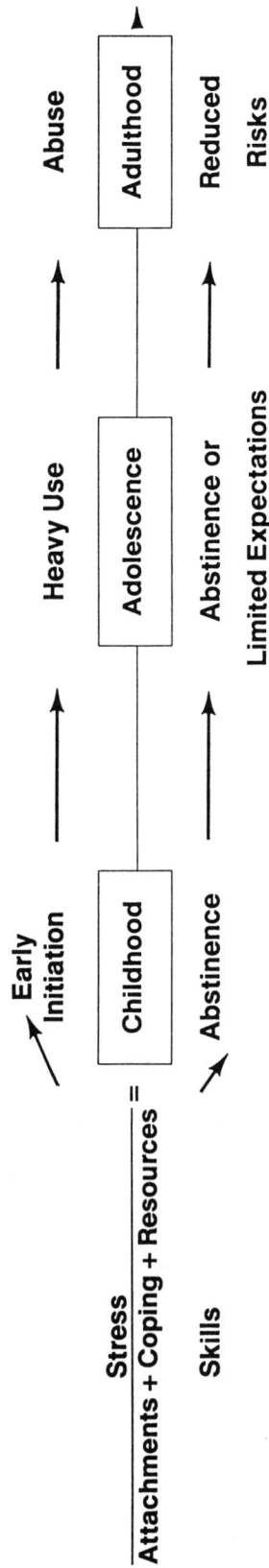

$$\frac{\text{Stress}}{\text{Attachments + Coping + Resources}} =$$
Skills

Childhood → Adolescence → Adulthood

Abstinence → Early Initiation → Heavy Use → Abuse

Abstinence or → Reduced
Limited Expectations → Risks

KEY CONCEPTS OF KANDEL'S MODEL OF PROGRESSION TO PROBLEM DRUG USE (1980)

1. Lower (i.e., less "serious" drug use) almost always precedes higher; but progression is not automatic from one to the next. Marijuana smokers do not automatically become heroin addicts, as the old "scare" movies would depict.

2. There are various combinations of predictor variables—parental influence, peer influence, adolescent involvement in various behaviors, and beliefs and values. These have different predictive valence at each stage of drug behavior.

3. "Participation in various deviant behaviors is most relevant in starting to use alcohol, least for illicit drugs. . . . By contrast, initiation into illicit drugs other than marijuana appears to be a conscious response to intrapsychic pressures of some sort or other" (Kandel, 1980, p. 126).

4. There are four stages: beer or wine; cigarettes or hard liquor; marijuana; other illicit drugs.

ISSUES FOR NURSES IN SETTING GOALS FOR PREVENTION

Professional Issues

- Identification of *what* is being prevented; policy of the treatment setting guides this identification.

- Awareness of nurse's own attitudes and values.

- Awareness of own or prevailing model of addiction; for example, disease concept, etc.

- Consensus among nursing professionals is expressed in standards of practice of addictions nursing.

DEVELOPMENTAL ISSUES TO BE CONSIDERED IN PREVENTION PLANNING

Needs of Young Children:

- Communication of message that drugs are harmful.
- Role models.
- Self-esteem.
- Ability to have fun.
- Ability to cope with stress without street drugs.
- A safe place to ask questions about drugs and alcohol.
- Information about consequences of substance abuse.
- Peer support for non-use.

Consideration of Age-Specific Developmental Norms:

- Psychosocial needs.
- Developmental tasks.
- Health needs.

Knowledge of Risk Factors:

- Environmental.
- Economic.
- Social factors.

Module I.7—Overhead #8A

GROWTH AND DEVELOPMENT NORMS FOR THE SCHOOL-AGE CHILD AGE-SPECIFIC PSYCHOSOCIAL ISSUES

The ages of 6 through 12 are considered to define "school-age." The school-age child is in a period of highly active psychosocial, physical and emotional growth (Jones, Lepley, & Baker, 1984).

(1) 6 years—Egocentric; generally displays positive attitudes.

(2) 7 years—Begins to internalize experiences; becomes more sensitive to criticism; more anxious to please and cooperate with peers.

(3) 8 years—Becomes more curious and gregarious; same-sex peers predominate.

(4) 9 years—Begins to refine behavior and develop self-confidence, responsibility.

(5) 10 years—Peer-oriented; responsive to group norms; increased powers of reasoning.

(6) 11–12 years—Becomes critical of authority, especially parents; displays moodiness, need for independence.

GROWTH AND DEVELOPMENT NORMS FOR THE SCHOOL-AGE CHILD

Developmental Tasks

(1) Activities reveal drive for exploration.

(2) Characteristic behavior may be loud and energetic.

(3) Slower physical growth than during pre-school.

(4) Gross motor skills being refined; still ahead of fine motor skills.

(5) A period of mastery over tasks, with the school setting predominating.

(6) Erickson's period of industry vs. inferiority.

(7) Piaget's period of concrete operational thought.

(8) Freud's period of latency, development of superego.

(9) Development of sense of moralism.

KINDS OF PREVENTION PROGRAMS

Knowledge/Attitudes

Values/Decision Making

Social Competency

PRINCIPLES OF PREVENTION PROGRAMMING (GOODSTADT, 1986)

- Should be targeted to specific subpopulations.
- Should have a sound theoretical basis.
- Should be explicit and realistic in their objectives.
- Should be critically evaluated if involving hypothesized variables or processes.
- Should incorporate or be associated with as much evaluation research as possible.

SIGNS AND SYMPTOMS IN CONTEXT (SCHWEBEL, 1989)

Signs and symptoms that *could* indicate drug use or other problems:

1. *School:*

    a. Increased absenteeism and tardiness to classes.

    b. Drop in grades.

    c. Behavior problems in school.

    d. Negative attitudes about school.

2. *Social Life/Friends:*

    a. Dropping out of old activities.

    b. Dropping old friends and making new friends who are drug users.

    c. Strange-sounding phone calls, with covert communication about drugs.

3. *Emotional Life:*

    a. Basic mood changes: was outgoing, now withdrawn; was withdrawn, now outgoing; was relaxed, now fidgety.

    b. Incidence of inexplicable mood changes: euphoria followed by tenseness and edginess.

    c. Caring less about everything: school, sports, other activities.

SIGNS AND SYMPTOMS IN CONTEXT (SCHWEBEL, 1989)

Signs and symptoms that *could* indicate drug use or other problems (continued):

4. *Family:*

   a. Very secretive (not to be confused with need for privacy).

   b. Estrangement from family.

   c. Less responsible at home.

   d. More conflict at home.

5. *Physical Effects:*

   a. Red eyes.

   b. Deterioration in personal hygiene.

   c. Weight loss.

   d. Sleep disturbances.

   e. Fatigue or hyperactivity.

HANDOUT MASTERS

MODULE I.7 PREVENTION OF DRUG AND ALCOHOL PROBLEMS IN THE SCHOOL-AGE CHILD

1. Etiology of Youth Drug Abuse—Models of Psychological and Behavioral Predispositions

2. Key Concepts of Kandel's Model of Progression to Problem Drug Use

3. Growth and Development Norms for the School-Age Child: Age-Specific Psychosocial Issues and Developmental Tasks (3A, 3B)

4. Signs and Symptoms in Context

Module I.7—Handout #1

ETIOLOGY OF YOUTH DRUG ABUSE
MODELS OF PSYCHOLOGICAL AND BEHAVIORAL PREDISPOSITIONS

1. *Problem Behavior:*

An individual manifests a range of "problem behaviors," including "drug use, drinking and problem drinking, sexual experience, activist protest and general deviance, including lying, stealing and aggression" (Jessor & Jessor, 1980).

2. *Mediational Model:*

Childhood behavior is a precursor to the adolescent behavior which leads to drug use; "unconventionality, such as deviant behavior, rebelliousness, lack of social conformity and low law abidance, are associated with drug use" (Brook, Gordon, Whiteman & Cohen, 1989).

3. *Social Coping Model:*

In addition to focusing on individual, family and peer variables, large scale social, political and economic issues impact on substance use and need to be examined (Rhodes & Jason, 1988).

4. *Use Intensity:*

Children may be divided into three groups: non-users, abusers and experimenters. It is inferred that "experimenters" are healthiest. Frequent users and abstainers manifest various indicators of maladjustment (Shedler & Block, 1990).

KEY CONCEPTS OF KANDEL'S MODEL OF
PROGRESSION TO PROBLEM DRUG USE (1980)

1. Lower (i.e., less "serious" drug use) almost always precedes higher; but progression is not automatic from one to the next. Marijuana smokers do not automatically become heroin addicts, as the old "scare" movies would depict.

2. There are various combinations of predictor variables—parental influence, peer influence, adolescent involvement in various behaviors, and beliefs and values. These have different predictive valence at each stage of drug behavior.

3. "Participation in various deviant behaviors is most relevant in starting to use alcohol, least for illicit drugs. . . . By contrast, initiation into illicit drugs other than marijuana appears to be a conscious response to intrapsychic pressures of some sort or other" (Kandel, 1980, p. 126).

4. There are four stages: beer or wine; cigarettes or hard liquor; marijuana; other illicit drugs.

Module I.7—Handout #3A

GROWTH AND DEVELOPMENT NORMS FOR THE SCHOOL-AGE CHILD AGE-SPECIFIC PSYCHOSOCIAL ISSUES

The ages of 6–12 are considered to define "school-age." The school-age child is in a period of highly active psychosocial, physical and emotional growth (Jones, Lepley & Baker, 1984).

1. 6 years—Egocentric; generally displays positive attitudes.

2. 7 years—Begins to internalize experiences; becomes more sensitive to criticism; more anxious to please and cooperate with peers.

3. 8 years—Becomes more curious and gregarious; same-sex peers predominate.

4. 9 years—Begins to refine behavior and develop self-confidence, responsibility.

5. 10 years—Peer-oriented; responsive to group norms; increased powers of reasoning.

6. 11–12 years—Becomes critical of authority, especially parents; displays moodiness, need for independence.

GROWTH AND DEVELOPMENT NORMS FOR THE SCHOOL-AGE CHILD
DEVELOPMENTAL TASKS

1. Activities reveal drive for exploration.
2. Characteristic behavior may be loud and energetic.
3. Slower physical growth than during pre-school.
4. Gross motor skills being refined; still ahead of fine motor skills.
5. A period of mastery over tasks, with the school setting predominating.
6. Erickson's period of industry vs. inferiority.
7. Piaget's period of concrete operational thought.
8. Freud's period of latency, development of superego.
9. Development of sense of moralism.

Module I.7—Handout #4

SIGNS AND SYMPTOMS IN CONTEXT (SCHWEBEL, 1989)

Signs and symptoms that *could* indicate drug use or other problems:

1. *School:*
   a. Increased absenteeism and tardiness to classes.
   b. Drop in grades.
   c. Behavior problems in school.
   d. Negative attitudes about school.

2. *Social Life/Friends:*
   a. Dropping out of old activities.
   b. Dropping old friends and making new friends who are drug users.
   c. Strange-sounding phone calls, with covert communication about drugs.

3. *Emotional Life:*
   a. Basic mood changes: was outgoing, now withdrawn; was withdrawn, now outgoing; was relaxed, now fidgety.
   b. Incidence of inexplicable mood changes: euphoria followed by tenseness and edginess.
   c. Caring less about everything: school, sports, other activities.

4. *Family:*
   a. Very secretive (not to be confused with need for privacy).
   b. Estrangement from family.
   c. Less responsible at home.
   d. More conflict at home.

5. *Physical Effects:*
   a. Red eyes.
   b. Deterioration in personal hygiene.
   c. Weight loss.
   d. Sleep disturbances.
   e. Fatigue or hyperactivity.

RECOMMENDED TEACHING STRATEGIES AND SAMPLE ASSIGNMENTS

RECOMMENDED TEACHING STRATEGIES

- Lecture
- Discussion
- Attendance at Ala-Teen and Al-Anon meetings
- Utilize games such as the "Don't Start" game as a teaching strategy
- Micro-teaching techniques

SAMPLE ASSIGNMENT

Essay Questions

1. Plan a health teaching session to address the child's needs in relation to drugs and alcohol.
2. Develop a nursing intervention using age appropriate teaching materials.
3. Review and critique media offerings designed for the school-age child.
4. Utilize role-playing to maximize understanding of communication approaches to the school-age child.
5. List (discuss, describe) some barriers to successful prevention programming in schools.
6. What are the conceptual differences between elementary school and junior high school prevention and knowledge goals?
7. List three of the principles of effective prevention programming you have learned.
8. Describe the concept of "adaptive consequences" for drug use.
9. Explain your evaluation of the "JUST SAY NO" slogan as a tool for drug abuse prevention in school-age children.
10. Pick a particular school-age population with whom you are or will be working. What are three goals that you would hope to accomplish with a successful prevention program? How would you evaluate whether or not you have met these goals?

CASE VIGNETTE

The Bentley School for Boys

Mr. Chrisholm wants to incorporate some drug prevention content in his lesson plans for his third grade class at the Bentley School for Boys. He was surprised to learn that the school administration does not allow this kind of material to be presented during valuable class time, when students are expected to pay serious attention to classwork designed for academically superior, college-bound students. The administration further maintains that alcohol and drug addiction have never been a problem among either the Bentley Boys or their families. Mr. Chrisholm consults with the local Council on Alcoholism for advice. They encourage him to persist in educating the school administrators, especially since he has observed evidence that the boys have been curious about drugs and several have shared information about their fear and shame regarding some of their family experiences.

Role-Play—School Nurse's Script

You are the School Nurse with whom Mr. Chrisholm consults. Your task in this role-play is to:

1. Identify parental and peer influences associated with the initiation and continuation of drug use by school-age children.

2. Identify components of the nursing health assessment which relate to the identification of drug use by these children and for which Mr. Chrisholm can observe among the students.

3. Describe community resources which can be utilized in this school-based prevention effort.

4. Encourage the development of a teaching plan that includes:

    a. Feelings associated with drug use or abuse.

    b. Facts about the disease of addiction.

    c. Positive coping mechanisms.

TEST QUESTIONS AND ANSWERS

TEST QUESTIONS

1. Jane is a 7-year-old girl who was referred for mental health evaluation and services by the school system. She does not enter into any activities with other children but instead seeks to be at the teacher's side at all times. She cannot concentrate on doing any schoolwork independently but can do her work if an adult sits with her. She is the fourth child in a family of five children. When assessing Jane, the nurse should gather information from:

   a. as many family members as possible, Jane and teachers.

   b. the mother and Jane.

   c. the siblings only.

   d. the parents only.

2. What does the nurse need to know about Jane before any plans for treatment can be made?

   a. The chance of parental alcoholism or drug abuse.

   b. Jane's scores on intelligence tests.

   c. Jane's behavior pattern in other situations.

   d. All of the above.

3. Which of the following questions gives the nurse the best chance of getting information about parents' values and attitudes?

   a. How would you like your child to be today?

   b. Do you believe all children should try to go to college?

   c. Did you plan to have this child?

   d. Is there any alcoholism in the family?

4. Effective primary prevention programs for children at risk for alcoholism focus on all of the following except:

   a. disturbed and chaotic environments for children.

   b. maturational crises involving children.

   c. situational crises involving children.

   d. identified clients younger than 20 years.

5. Why is play an especially effective form of involvement with children?

   a. They don't know the meaning of words describing feelings.

   b. It is more cost-effective than other forms of psychotherapy.

   c. It is easy to understand children's conflicts when they show them directly in play.

   d. It is a child's natural medium for self-expression.

6. What does a nurse look for in family therapy with dysfunctional families in order to successfully intervene?

   a. Family patterns that exclude a child.

   b. Family patterns that are ambiguous.

   c. Family patterns that support the child's symptoms.

   d. Role strain among the family members.

7. Which of the following is *not* within the child advocacy role of addictions nurses?

   a. Teaching mental health concepts to children in elementary schools.

   b. Talking about children's rights in parenting classes.

   c. Working to overcome budget restrictions for services for children.

   d. Testifying in a court case on a child's behalf.

8. A "gateway" drug is most closely defined as:

   a. one which is used to enter into certain peer groups.

   b. one available without a prescription.

   c. one that might lead to more serious drug use.

   d. one's first experiment with drug use.

9. Kandel's model of problem drug use includes all the following concepts except:

   a. large scale social, political, and economic issues.

   b. predictor variables/behaviors.

   c. progression from less serious to more serious drugs, though not necessarily automatic.

   d. four stages: beer or wine, cigarettes or hard liquor, marijuana, other illicit drugs.

10. The Social Coping model of Rhodes and Jason is significant in that:

    a. it invalidates the "individual predisposition" model.

    b. it provides the most popular scale for school-age child drug assessment.

    c. it puts the etiology of drug use in a larger perspective.

    d. it focuses only on alcohol use.

11. A study by Shedler and Block which studied 101 eighteen year olds from age three on suggested that the "psychologically healthiest subjects" were:

    a. abstainers.

    b. frequent users.

    c. those who attended Ala-Teen.

    d. experimenters.

12. Prevention programs usually fall in the following category:

    a. Knowledge/Attitudes.

    b. Values/Decision Making.

    c. Social Competency.

    d. All of the above.

13. The efficacy of prevention programs is:

    a. proven with the Social Competency model.

    b. difficult to measure with accuracy.

    c. the most highly funded by government agencies.

    d. demonstrated by a recent 60% decrease in alcohol use by 13-year-olds.

ANSWER KEY

1. a
2. d
3. a
4. d
5. d
6. c
7. a
8. c
9. a
10. c
11. d
12. d
13. b

BIBLIOGRAPHY

MODULE I.7 PREVENTION OF ALCOHOL AND OTHER DRUG PROBLEMS IN THE SCHOOL-AGE CHILD

Abadinsky, H. (1989). *Drug abuse: An introduction.* Chicago: Nelson-Hall.

American Nurses' Association, & National Nurses Society on Addictions. (1988). *Standards of addictions nursing practice with selected diagnoses and criteria.* Kansas City, MO: American Nurses' Association.

American Social Health Association. (1972). *Guidelines: A comprehensive community program to reduce drug abuse. I: Overview.* New York: American Social Health Association.

Archambault, D. (1989). Adolescence: A physiological, cultural and psychological no-man's-land. In G. Lawson & A. Lawson (Eds.), *Alcoholism and substance abuse in special populations* (pp. 223–246). Baltimore, MD: Aspen Publishers, Inc.

Baumrind, D. (1987). Familial antecedents of adolescent drug use: A developmental perspective. In C. L. Jones & R. L. Battjes (Eds.), *Etiology of drug abuse: Implications for prevention* (pp. 13–44). Rockville, MD: National Institute on Drug Abuse.

Beauchamp, D. E. (1980). *Beyond alcoholism: Alcohol and public health policy.* Philadelphia: Temple University Press.

Beauvais, F., & Oetting, E. R. (1988). Inhalant abuse by young children. *Research Monograph No. 85* (DHHS Publication No. (ADM) 88–1577). Washington, DC: National Institute on Drug Abuse.

Bingham, A., & Barger, J. (1985). Children of alcoholic families: A group treatment approach for latency age children. *Journal of Psychosocial Nursing and Mental Health Services, 23*(12), 13–15.

Blakeslee, S. (1988, July 21). Eight-year study finds two sides to teenage drug use. *New York Times,* 1, 13.

Bonagura, J. A., Rhonehouse, M., & Bonagura, E. W. (1988). Effectiveness of four school health education projects upon substance use, self-esteem and adolescent stress. *Health Education Quarterly, 15*(1), 81–92.

Brook, J. S., Gordon, A. S., Whiteman, M., & Cohen, P. (1989). Changes in drug involvement: A longitudinal study of childhood and adolescent determinants. *Psychological Reports, 65,* 707–726.

Brotman, R., & Suffet, F. (1975). The concept of prevention and its limitations. *Annals, 417,* 53–65.

Bush, P. J., & Iannotti, R. (1987). The development of children's health orientations and behaviors: Lessons for substance abuse prevention. In C. L. Jones & R. L. Battjes (Eds.), *Etiology of drug abuse: Implications for prevention* (pp. 45–74). Rockville, MD: National Institute on Drug Abuse.

Chein, I., Gerard, D. L., Lee, R. S., & Rosenfeld, E. (1964). *The road to H: Narcotics, delinquency and social policy.* New York: Basic Books.

Duster, T. (1970). *The legislation of morality: Law, drugs and moral judgment.* New York: Free Press.

Felsted, C. M. (Ed.) (1986). *Youth and alcohol abuse: Readings and resources.* Phoenix, AZ: Oryx Press.

Finn, P. (1986). Teenage drunkenness: Warning signal, transient boisterousness, or symptom of social change? In C. M. Felsted (Ed.), *Youth and alcohol abuse: Readings and resources* (pp. 36–51). Phoenix, AZ: Oryx Press.

U.S. General Accounting Office. (1987). *Drug abuse prevention: Further efforts needed to identify programs that work.* Washington, DC: U.S. Government Printing Office.

Gersick, K. E., Grady, K., & Snow, D. L. (1988). Social-cognitive skill development with sixth graders and its initial impact on substance use. *Journal of Drug Education, 18*(1), 55–70.

Globetti, G. (1988). Alcohol education and minority youth. *Journal of Drug Issues, 18,* 115–129.

Goodstadt, M. S. (1986). Alcohol education research and practice: A logical analysis of the two realities. *Journal of Drug Education, 16*(4), 349–365.

Goodstadt, M. S. (1987). *Drug education.* Rockville, MD: National Institute on Drug Abuse.

Goodstadt, M. S. (1989). Drug education: The prevention issues. *Journal of Drug Education, 19*(3), 197–208.

Goodwin, D. W. (1977). Genetic and experiential antecedents of alcoholism: A prospective study. *Alcoholism: Clinical and Experimental Research, 1*(3), 259–265.

Grady, K., Gersick, K. E., Snow, D. L., & Kessen, M. (1986). The emergence of adolescent substance use. *Journal of Drug Education, 16*(3), 203–219.

Green, J. J., & Kelley, J. M. (1989). Evaluating the effectiveness of a school drug and alcohol prevention curriculum: A new look at "Here's Looking At You, Two." *Journal of Drug Education, 19,* 9–13.

Greenspan, S. I. (1985). Research strategies to identify developmental vulnerabilities for drug abuse. *Research Monograph No. 56* (pp. 136–154). Washington, DC: National Institute on Drug Abuse.

Hanson, D. J. (1980). Drug education: Does it work? In F. S. Scarpitti & S. K. Datesman (Eds.), *Drugs and youth culture* (pp. 251–282). Beverly Hills, CA.: Sage.

Hawkins, J. D., Lishner, D. M., & Catalano, R. F. (1987). Childhood predictors and the prevention of adolescent substance abuse. In C.L. Jones & R. Battjes (Eds.), *Etiology of drug abuse: Implications for prevention* (pp. 75–126). Rockville, MD: National Institute on Drug Abuse.

Hendler, H. I., & Stephens, R. C. (1977). The addict odyssey: From experimentation to addiction. *International Journal of the Addictions, 12,* 25–42.

Howard, J., Taylor, J. A., Ganikos, M. L., Holder, H. D., Godwin, D. F., & Taylor, E. D. (1988). An overview of prevention research: Issues, answers and new agendas. *Public Health Reports, 103*(6), 674–683.

Jessor, R., & Jessor, S. (1980). A social-psychological framework for studying drug use. In D. Lettieri, M. Sayers, & H. W. Pearson (Eds.), *Theories on drug abuse* (NIDA Research Monograph No. 30, pp. 102–109). Rockville, MD: National Institute on Drug Abuse.

Jones, D., Lepley, M., & Baker, B. (1984). *Health assessment across the lifespan.* New York: McGraw-Hill.

Kandel, D. (1980). Developmental stages in adolescent drug involvement. In D. Lettieri, M. Sayers, & H. W. Pearson (Eds.), *Theories on drug abuse* (NIDA Research Monograph No. 30, pp. 120–127). Rockville, MD: National Institute on Drug Abuse.

Kim, S., McLeod, J., & Palmgren, C. L. (1989). The impact of the "I'm Special" program on student substance abuse and other related student problem behavior. *Journal of Drug Education, 19*(1), 83–95.

Kim, S., McLeod, J. H., Shantzis, E. (1989). An outcome evaluation of refusal skills program as a drug abuse prevention strategy. *Journal of Drug Education, 19*(4), 363–371.

Lawson, G. (1989). A rationale for planning treatment and prevention of alcoholism and substance abuse for specific populations. In G. Lawson & A. Lawson (Eds.), *Alcoholism and substance abuse in special populations* (pp. 1–10). Rockville, MD: Aspen Publishers, Inc.

Lewis, C. E., & Lewis, M. (1984). Peer pressure and risk-taking behaviors in children. *American Journal of Public Health, 74,* 580–584.

May, C. D. (1988, June 6). Drug enforcement: Once-lonely voice finds an audience. *New York Times,* A-12.

Milgram, G. (1989). Impact of a student assistance program. *Journal of Drug Education, 19*(4), 327–335.

Milgram, G. (1990). Alcohol/Drug education: School and community factors. In R. Engs (Ed.), *Controversies in the addictions field: Volume One.* Baltimore, MD: American Council on Alcoholism.

Moskowitz, J. (1983). Preventing adolescent substance abuse through drug education. In T. J. Glynn, C. G. Leukefeld, & J. P. Ludford (Eds.), *Preventing adolescent drug abuse* (NIDA Research Monograph No. 47, pp. 233–249). Rockville, MD: National Institute on Drug Abuse.

National Council on Alcoholism, Inc. (1986). Facts on teenage drinking. In C. M. Felsted (Ed.), *Youth and alcohol abuse: Readings and resources.* Phoenix, AZ: Oryx Press.

National Institute on Drug Abuse. (1980). The developmental approach to preventing problem dependencies. In H. S. Glenn & J. W. Warner (Eds.), *Community-based prevention specialist: Participant manual* (pp. 133–153). Rockville, MD: National Institute on Drug Abuse.

National Institute on Drug Abuse. (1987). *Drug abuse and drug abuse research.* Rockville, MD: National Institute on Drug Abuse.

National Institute on Drug Abuse. (1990). *National household survey on drug abuse: Population estimates, 1990* (DHHS Publication No. (ADM) 91–1732). Rockville, MD: National Institute on Drug Abuse.

Oetting, E. R., & Beauvais, F. (1987). Common elements in youth drug abuse: Peer clusters and other psychosocial factors. *Journal of Drug Issues, 17,* 133–151.

Pascale, P. J., & Sylvester, J. (1988). Trend analyses of four large-scale surveys of high school drug use. *Journal of Drug Education, 18*(1), 221–233.

Pisano, S., & Rooney, J. F. (1988). Children's changing attitudes regarding alcohol: A cross-sectional study. *Journal of Drug Education, 18*(1), 1.

Polich, J. M., Ellickson, P. L., Reuter, P., & Kahan, J. (Eds.). (1984). *Strategies for controlling adolescent drug use.* California: Rand Corporation.

Reid, L. D., Martinson, O. B., & Weaver, L. C. (1987). Factors associated with the drug use of fifth through eighth grade students. *Journal of Drug Education, 17*(2), 149–161.

Rhodes, J., & Jason, L. (1988). *Preventing substance abuse among children and adolescents.* New York: Pergamon Press.

Schwebel, R. (1989). *Saying no is not enough.* New York: Newmarket Press.

Scipien, G., Chard, M., & Jones, D. (1984). *Health assessment across the life span.* New York: McGraw-Hill.

Shaw, S. W. (1989). The impact of culture on prevention programming for high risk youth in inner cities. *Prevention Pipeline, 2*(6), 15–16.

Shedler, J., & Block, J. (1990). Adolescent drug use and psychological health. *American Psychologist, 45*(5), 612–630.

Stuart, R. B. (1974, April). Teaching facts about drugs: Pushing or preventing? *Journal of Educational Psychology, 66,* 189–201.

Swadi, H., & Zeitlin, H. (1987). Drug education to children: Does it really work? *British Journal of Addictions, 82,* 741–746.

Treaster, J. B. (1991, February 24). From the front lines of the war on drugs, few small victories. *The New York Times,* Section E, p. 5.

Vejnoska, J. (1981). Parent action groups: A prevention resource. *Alcohol Health and Research World, 6*(4), 13–17.

Wald, P. M., & Abrams, A. (1972). Drug education. In P. M. Wald, P. B. Hutt, & J. V. DeLong (Eds.), *Dealing with drug abuse: A report to the Ford Foundation* (pp. 123–172). New York: Praeger.

Wald, P. M., Hutt, P. B., & DeLong, J. V. (Eds.) (1972). *Dealing with drug abuse: A report to the Ford Foundation.* New York: Praeger.

Waldorf, D. (1983, Spring). Natural recovery from opiate addiction. *Journal of Drug Issues, 13,* 237–280.

Zinberg, N. E. (1984). *Drug, set and setting: The basis for controlled intoxicant use.* New Haven, CT: Yale University Press.